Neuroimaging of Treatment-Related Conditions in the Brain

Marialuisa Zedde • Rosario Pascarella
Editors

Neuroimaging of Treatment-Related Conditions in the Brain

Springer

Editors
Marialuisa Zedde
Neurology Unit, Stroke Unit
Azienda Unità Sanitaria Locale-IRCCS
di Reggio Emilia
Reggio Emilia, Italy

Rosario Pascarella
Neuroradiology Unit
Ospedale Santa Maria della Misericordia
AULSS 5 Polesana
Rovigo, Italy

ISBN 978-3-032-23617-3 ISBN 978-3-032-23618-0 (eBook)
https://doi.org/10.1007/978-3-032-23618-0

This Springer imprint is published by the registered company Springer Nature Switzerland AG
The registered company address is: Gewerbestrasse 11, 6330 Cham, Switzerland

Contents

Encephalopathy: Definition and Diagnostic Criteria

1

Maria Sessa

1.1 Nomenclature and Classification

Encephalopathy is generally defined as a pathobiological brain process characterized by a global disturbance in cognition, which can occur hyperacutely (over the course of seconds to minutes), acutely (over hours to days), subacutely (over weeks to months), or chronically (over years).

In the acute setting, until recently, several terms have been used to define the clinical syndrome including delirium, acute confusional state, acute brain dysfunction, acute brain failure, and altered mental status, underscoring the lack of a uniform definition. This represents an obstacle to epidemiological studies, identification of triggering factors, correct clinical management, prognostic evaluation, as well as scientific progress in the field. Recently, consensus recommendations on nomenclature have been reached by a panel of experts in the field and endorsed by ten professional societies. According to these recommendations:

– the term acute encephalopathy refers to a rapidly developing (≤ 4 weeks) pathobiological brain process;
– it can lead to a subsyndromal delirium, delirium, or coma, all representing a change from baseline cognitive status.

The term delirium refers to a clinical state defined according to the criteria of the DSM-5 [1] (see Table 1.1). Additionally, according to Liptzin and Levkoff criteria, three subtypes of delirium are recognized (see Table 1.2) [2]. The term subsyndromal delirium refers to acute cognitive changes that are compatible with delirium, but do not fulfill all DSM-5 delirium criteria. The term coma refers to a state of severely depressed responsiveness, defined by diagnostic systems such as the Glasgow Coma Scale (GCS) [3] or the Full Outline of UnResponsiveness (FOUR) score [4].

The panel discourages the use of acute confusional state, acute brain dysfunction, acute brain failure, and altered mental status in addition or as synonymous.

M. Sessa (✉)
Neurology, ASST Grande Ospedale Metropolitano Niguarda, Milan, Italy
e-mail: maria.sessa@ospedaleniguarda.it

M. Zedde, R. Pascarella (eds.), *Neuroimaging of Treatment-Related Conditions in the Brain*,
https://doi.org/10.1007/978-3-032-23618-0_1

Table 1.1 Criteria for delirium of the DSM-5

A. A disturbance in attention (i.e., reduced ability to direct, focus, sustain, and shift attention) and awareness (reduced orientation to the environment).
B. The disturbance develops over a short period of time (usually hours to a few days), represents a change from baseline attention and awareness, and tends to fluctuate in severity during the course of a day.
C. An additional disturbance in cognition (e.g., memory deficit, disorientation, language, visuospatial ability, or perception).
D. The disturbances in criteria A and C are not explained by another pre-existing, established, or evolving neurocognitive disorder and do not occur in the context of a severely reduced level of arousal, such as coma.
E. There is evidence from the history, physical examination, or laboratory findings that the disturbance is a direct physiological consequence of another medical condition, substance intoxication or withdrawal (i.e., due to a drug of abuse or to a medication), or exposure to a toxin, or is due to multiple etiologies.

From: Ref. [1]

Table 1.2 Liptzin and Levkoff criteria

Hyperactive type	
Three or more of the following	Hypervigilance, restlessness, fast or loud speech, anger or irritability, combativeness, impatience, uncooperativeness, swearing, singing, laughing, euphoria, wandering, easy startling, distractibility, nightmares, persistent thoughts
Hypoactive type	
Four or more of the following	Unawareness, decreased alertness, sparse or slow speech, lethargy, decreased motor activity, staring, apathy
Mixed type	
Met the criteria for both (a) and (b) above	

From: Ref. [2]

In nonsedated patients, mental status is assessed by the Confusion Assessment Method (CAM) for patients outside the ICU and Confusion Assessment Method for the Intensive Care Unit (CAM-ICU) for patients admitted to the ICU. The CAM has been validated for use in diagnosis of delirium in this setting and shows excellent sensitivity (94–100%) and positive predictive value (91–94%) [5, 6]. However, it has to be acknowledged that the majority of the studies have been carried out in research settings, and that CAM-ICU has only about 41–47% sensitivity when used by regular ICU nurses, although the specificity remains excellent (98%) [7, 8]. CAM is most likely to miss patients with hypoactive delirium. The Assessment to Intensive Care Environment (ATICE) score, which enables assessment of awakening, comprehension, and calmness, may indicate delirium when the score is less than 10 (maximum value being 20) [9]. Unstructured delirium assessments or the Intensive Care Delirium Screening Checklist (ICDSC) also seems to have greater sensitivity for detecting delirium in the ICU than does the CAM-ICU [10, 11]. Thus, in spite of a number of screening tools, the most appropriate delirium screening tool for ICU is still a controversy.

Encephalopathy is a syndrome, which recognizes many underlying causes, including both primary neurologic and systemic conditions. Revision of the literature offers different classification schemes [12, 13].

A practical scheme for clinicians, which can serve as a guide to navigate the difficult differential diagnosis, can group encephalopathies according to time course and to the underlying cause, either primary neurologic or systemic (see Table 1.3).

Table 1.3 Acquired encephalopathies

	Hyperacute	Acute	Subacute	Chronic
Primary neurologic				
	Vascular	Vascular	Vascular	Vascular
	Trauma	Infectious	Neoplasm-related (brain tumors, paraneoplastic syndromes)	Degenerative
		Inflammatory	Inflammatory	Normal Pressure Hydrocephalus
			Infectious (fungal, TB, parasitic, complications of HIV)	Infectious (syphilis, HIV-associated neurocognitive disease)
Systemic				
Organ failure	Cardiac arrest (anoxic-ischemic)	Respiratory (hypoxia, hypercapnia) Hepatic Uremic		
		Severe electrolyte imbalance Glucose metabolism disturbances Cofactor deficiency (Wernicke encephalopathy)		
Endocrine			Thyroid (myxedema coma, thyrotoxicosis) adrenal (Addison disease) Hypothalamic and pituitary failure	
Systemic infection		Septic encephalopathy		
Environmental exposures		Carbon monoxide	Heavy metals	
Pharmacologic	Ozone	Antibiotics Cancer treatments Antidepressants and antipsychotics		
	Contrast medium			
Drugs of abuse		Alcohol Illicit drugs		

Modified from: Ref. [12]

1.2 Main Acquired Encephalopathies

In this chapter, we will focus on the major acquired encephalopathies consequent to indirect brain damage by systemic conditions (see Table 1.4).

1.2.1 Organ Failure

1.2.1.1 Cardiac Arrest and Hypoxic--Ischemic Encephalopathy (HIE)

Cardiac and circulatory arrest, despite successful cardiopulmonary resuscitation (CPR), causes diffuse hypoxic-ischemic brain injury, leading to death, persistent vegetative state, or severe neurological disability. Early prognostication of poor outcome is fundamental to provide correct information to relatives and to avoid inappropriate treatments. In 2014, the European Resuscitation Council and the European Society of Intensive Care Medicine published an advisory statement, reached after a GRADE-based systematic review of predictors based on clinical examination, electrophysiology, biomarkers, and imaging followed by expert consensus achieved using Web-based Delphi methodology [14]. They suggest 72 h after ROSC as a suitable time for prognostication in comatose survivors from cardiac arrest, after having excluded residual sedation, neuromuscular blockade, and other major confounders. The

Table 1.4 Acquired encephalopathies consequent to indirect brain damage by systemic conditions

Organ failure	Cardiac arrest (anoxic-ischemic encephalopathy)
	Respiratory (encephalopathies associated with hypoxia, hypercapnia)
	Hepatic encephalopathy
	Uremic encephalopathy
Metabolic	Severe electrolyte imbalance
	Glucose metabolism disturbances
	Cofactor deficiency (Wernicke encephalopathy)
Endocrine	Thyroid (myxedema coma, thyrotoxicosis)
	Adrenal (Addison disease)
	Hypothalamic and pituitary failure
Systemic infection	Septic encephalopathy
Environmental exposures	Carbon monoxide
	Heavy metals
Pharmacologic	Antibiotics
	Cancer treatments
	Antidepressants and antipsychotics
	Ozone
	Contrast medium
Drugs of abuse	Alcohol
	Illicit drugs

absence of pupillary and corneal reflexes, and/or bilaterally absent N20 Somato Sensory Evoked Potentials (SSEP) wave, indicates a poor outcome that is very likely. If neither of the features is present, reassess after 24 h. A poor outcome is likely if two or more of the following are present: status myoclonus ≤48 h; high neuron-specific enolase values; unreactive Electro Encephalo Graphy (EEG) with burst suppression or status epilepticus; diffuse anoxic injury on brain Computed Tomography (CT) and/or Magnetic Resonance Imaging (MRI). If none of these criteria are met consider continue to observe and re-evaluate. The Authors underlie the need of a multimodal evaluation to increase safety and sensitivity [15].

1.2.1.2 Hypercapnic Encephalopathy Syndrome (HES)

HES presents with a wide spectrum of neurological alterations that range from cognitive defects, psychomotor agitation, and confusion with asterixis to soporous status, delirium, and coma. It is a consequence of acute respiratory failure with severe decompensated respiratory hypercapnic acidosis. Symptoms of HES correlate stronger with the changes in cerebrospinal pH than with those of arterial pH and/or PaCO2 [16].

1.2.1.3 Hepatic Encephalopathy

Hepatic encephalopathy consists of a broad range of neurological, cognitive, and behavioral abnormalities [17]. It is classified according to the type of hepatic insufficiency, and further graded using the West Haven criteria (or Conn score) with a score ranging from grade 0 (no abnormalities) to grade 4 (coma) (see Table 1.5). [18]. In the absence of obvious physical examination findings of hepatic encephalopathy, neuropsychometric tests can be used to identify minimal hepatic encephalopathy among which the most highly recognized are the followings: Number Connection Test Part A and Part B, Portosystemic Encephalopathy (PSE) Syndrome Test, Psychometric Hepatic Encephalopathy Score (PHES), Critical Flicker-Frequency Test (CFF), Stroop test, Inhibitory Control Test (ICT), Repeatable Battery for the Assessment of Neurological Status (RBANS), Continuous Reaction Time (CRT) Test, SCAN Test.

1.2.1.4 Uremic Encephalopathy and Dialysis Disequilibrium Syndrome

Uremic encephalopathy is a syndrome of cognitive and nervous system dysfunction seen in patients with acute (AKI) or chronic kidney disease (CKD). Despite lacking a consensus definition, major proposed characteristics have been proposed (see Table 1.6). Severe encephalopathy is an uncommon occurrence in patients with progressive CKD because the majority of the patients will start planned Kidney Replacement Therapy (KRT) before the onset of Central Nervous System (CNS) manifestations. In these patients, the onset of uremic encephalopathy may be more insidious over weeks or months and may remain unrecognized and require specific psychometric studies for detection. Sleep disorders are very common. Despite multiple dialysis sessions,

Table 1.5 Hepatic encephalopathy nomenclature

Type	Encephalopathy associated with	Subcategory	Subdivision	West Haven criteria for semi-quantitative grading
A	Acute liver failure			
B	Portal-systemic bypass, no intrinsic hepatocellular disease			
C	Cyrrosis and portal hypertension and/ or portal-systemic shunts	Episodic	Precipitated spontaneous recurrent	
		Persistent	Mild (grade 1)	Trivial lack of awareness Euphoria or anxiety Shortened attention span Impaired performance on addition
			Severe (grade 2)	Lethargy or apathy Minimal disorientation Subtle personality changes Inappropriate behavior
			Severe (grade 3)	Somnolence to semi-stupor Confusion Gross disorientation
			Severe (grade 4)	Coma (unresponsive to stimuli)
			Treatment-dependent	
		Minimal		

From: Ref. [18]

Table 1.6 Proposed characteristics of uremic encephalopathy

Definition	Acute or subacute toxic syndrome attributable to the accumulation of solutes that occurs with severely reduced kidney function Other putative etiologies include imbalance of excitatory and inhibitory neurotransmitters in the brain, alterations in the blood–brain barrier, changes in vascular permeability, increased inflammation, and cerebral edema.
Symptoms	Cognitive and nervous system dysfunction associated with acute kidney disease or CKD CNS symptoms are variable and may include loss of memory, impaired concentration, depression, delusions, lethargy, irritability, fatigue, insomnia, psychosis, stupor, catatonia, seizures, and coma. Other related symptoms may include peripheral neuropathies, sleep disorders, restless legs, muscle cramps, and myoclonus. May have associated non-neurological symptoms such as nausea, vomiting, and dysgeusia.
Characteristics	Usually manifested when GFR is <15 ml/min per 1.73 m2 or seen in patients with kidney failure who are receiving inadequate dialysis Symptoms may be milder and more insidious with slowly progressive CKD. Symptoms are more severe when the fall in GFR is acute. No definitive characteristic imaging or EEG findings Symptoms are independent of the etiology of kidney failure Substantial overlap with other conditions. Diagnosis of exclusion with the key distinguishing feature being improvement with the initiation of dialysis, increase of dialysis clearance, or transplantation

From: Ref. [19]

residual neurological symptoms may persist suggesting irreversible neurological disease or other comorbid conditions.

In the setting of AKI, patients present with more severe symptoms of confusion, delirium, tonic-clonic seizures, and coma. Physical examination may reveal the presence of myoclonic jerks, asterixis, restless legs, dysarthria, nystagmus, papilledema, agitation, and tetany. Patients may also refer pruritus and gastrointestinal symptoms such as nausea and vomiting.

Imaging is usually normal or shows nonspecific findings. Case reports describe isolated cortical, centrum semiovale, basal ganglia, and brainstem involvement. The lentiform fork sign characterized by hyperintensity on the basal ganglia in T2/fluid-attenuated inversion recovery (FLAIR) sequences surrounded by a hyperintense rim delineating the lentiform nucleus is described in uremic encephalopathy, but is neither sensitive nor specific, being described in other metabolic encephalopathies.

EEG generally show nonspecific generalized slowing. However, in the setting of AKI, slowing of the posterior dominant alpha rhythm and occasional theta bursts and prolonged bursts of bilateral, synchronous slow and sharp waves or spikes and waves are present. Rarely, generalized or partial seizure activity may be encountered.

Uremic encephalopathy is a diagnosis of exclusion, based mainly on improvement in clinical condition after the initiation of KRT. In patients with delayed, incomplete, or no neurological recovery after the initiation of dialysis, for at least 3–5 sessions, other possible explanations should be considered [19, 20].

Dialysis disequilibrium syndrome (DDS) refers to a variety of neurological manifestations seen during or following dialysis, primarily after the new initiation of dialysis. The symptoms and signs of DDS are consequent to an imbalance in intracellular fluid, causing brain edema and develop sequentially as intracranial pressure rises. Symptoms start with headache, nausea, vomiting, restlessness, and confusion, and progress, if not promptly recognized and managed, to seizures, coma, and even death. They are usually ascribed to excessive or aggressive ultrafiltration, and hyper- or hypotension. However, DDS can occur in patients on chronic dialysis especially when predialysis blood urea nitrogen (BUN) is high and/or other causes for hyperosmolality, such as hyperglycemia or hypernatremia, are present. [21, 22].

1.2.2 Metabolic

1.2.2.1 Electrolitic Derangements

Dysnatremia: Severe dysnatremias are usually defined as serum-sodium <125 mmol/L or > 165 mmol/L. Nausea, falling, and asthenia are common in severe hyponatremia, while decreased consciousness and confusion are common in severe hypernatremia. Other signs and symptoms include headache, dizziness, agitation, and seizures. Among subjects with acute severe hyponatremia, women are overrepresented likely due to less body water compared to men. Main causes of acute dysnatremias are primary polydipsia, water intoxication, ectasy abuse, prolonged physical activity, and salt intoxication.

Severe acute dysnatremias have significant mortality, especially in hypernatremia, and require immediate treatment.

The presence of signs of cerebral edema at head CT supports an acute genesis. Distinguishing between acute and acute-on-chronic hyponatremia in patients with hyponatremic encephalopathy is relevant for therapeutic decision regarding the correction rate. In chronic dysnatremias a slow correction rate (< 10 mmol/L/24 h) is preferred to avoid neurological complications, while expert recommendations [23, 24] suggest that patients with acute dysnatremias have lower risk of complications due to rapid correction [25].

Hypomagnesemia—Magnesium is the second most abundant intracellular ion after potassium and the fourth most abundant ion in plasma. Its serum levels are tightly regulated due to its critical role in cellular homeostasis, vascular tone maintenance, and endothelial integrity. Hypomagnesemia is defined as serum magnesium levels below 0.66 mmol/L or 1.7 mg/dL.

The most frequent clinical manifestations of hypomagnesemia are Hypomagnesemia-Induced Cerebellar Syndrome (HICS) and movement disorders. HICS presents with subacute onset and fluctuating course, often accompanied by cerebellar oculomotor signs such as jerky horizontal or downbeat nystagmus and very rarely ocular flutter. Brain MRI shows a pattern of vasogenic edema characterized by poorly defined T2/FLAIR hyperintensities in unilateral or bilateral cerebellar hemispheres with concomitant increased signal in diffusion-weighted sequences and ADC map. The cerebellar hemispheric swelling can be severe enough to cause distortion of fourth ventricle and hydrocephalus. Hyperintensities have also been observed in the vermis, in the region of nodulus. Unilateral cerebellar clinical involvement has been observed with bilateral cerebellar edema [26, 27]. The commonest movement disorders are tremors, generally postural and intentional and most commonly seen over upper limbs, with a jerky, irregular, or flapping quality. Rest tremors and acute onset of action tremors have been reported in the upper limb, athetosis, myoclonus, chorea, and signs of tetany are relatively rare [28].

In addition, severe hypomagnesemia is an increasingly recognized cause of Posterior Reversible Encephalopathy Syndrome (PRES) [29].

Somnolence and confusion up to deep stupor can be concomitantly seen in hypomagnesemia, with no correlation between the severity of hypomagnesemia and degree of obtundation. Acute cognitive impairment in these patients could manifest in the form of short-term memory loss. Depression, disorientation, and agitation can be associated with visual hallucinations that could be aggravated by the secondary hypocalcemia.

Hypercalcemia is defined as a total serum calcium concentration > 10.4 mg/dL (> 2.60 mmol/L) or ionized serum calcium >5.2 mg/dL (> 1.30 mmol/L). Major causes include hyperparathyroidism (HPT), vitamin D intoxication, and malignancies. HPT may be associated with nonspecific complaints such as decreased concentration, but can also cause neuropsychiatric issues ranging from depression to thoughts of death and suicide, delusions, and hallucinations. To note, HPT can be associated to normocalcemic level, e.g. due to calcium loss secondary to acute kidney injury, highlighting the importance of PTH screening even in normocalcemic patients presenting with acute psychosis [30].

1.2.2.2 Glucose Metabolism Disturbances

Hypoglycemic Encephalopathy (HH). Hypoglycemia is defined as an abrupt diminution in blood glucose level < 50 mg/dl. It is usually observed in chronic alcoholism, severe metabolic disorders, or in patients treated for diabetes. Clinical signs of hypoglycemia depend on the severity and duration of reduced serum glucose levels. Patients with HE usually exhibit with focal signs such as aphasia, hemiplegia, hemianopsia, and convulsions. In addition, numerous hyperkinetic movements disorders have been described, including chorea and ballismus, limb dystonia, jaw closure dystonia, awake bruxism, and stereotypies. Prolonged hypoglycemia leads to a more severe condition with lethargy and coma. The brain areas most vulnerable to hypoglycemia are the temporal lobe, hippocampus, basal ganglia, and corpus callosum, whereas the cerebellum, brainstem, and thalamus are spared in hypoglycemic brain insults.

Robust data on long-term outcome of comatose patients with prolonged hypoglycemic encephalopathy are lacking. Brain imaging has been evaluated as prognostic tool and normal brain imaging have been suggested as factor of good outcome, while a long duration of hypoglycemia as a predictor of poor outcome [31].

Diabetic ketoacidosis is a frequent complication of diabetes, more frequent in patients with type 1 diabetes, that, if not promptly recognized and properly treated, evolves in a severe metabolic encephalopathy. Clinical and imaging characteristics are those of metabolic encephalopathy [32]. Usually associated with hyperglycemia, it has been described in euglycemic patients [33].

1.2.2.3 Cofactor Deficiency

Wernicke encephalopathy (WE) is caused by thiamine (Vitamin B1) deficiency. Despite the most common predisposing factor is alcoholism, WE can also occur in patients with nutritional deficiencies, which occur in hyperemesis gravidarum, intestinal obstruction, bariatric surgery, cancer chemotherapy, hemodialysis, and malignant diseases. The classical clinical syndrome is characterized by mental status changes, ophthalmoplegia, and gait ataxia. Mental status changes range from apathy and mild neurocognitive symptoms to severe symptoms up to coma. Complete ophthalmoplegia occurs rarely, whereas horizontal nystagmus, sixth nerve palsy, ptosis, retinal hemorrhage, papilledema, anisocoria, or miosis are described. To that respect the term "ocular" signs have been suggested to replace ophthalmoplegia. However, the full triad is reported in only 10% of the patients, so it has been proposed that, in known alcoholics, a presumptive diagnosis is made if 2 of the following 4 conditions are present: (1) nutritional deficiency, (2) ocular findings, (3) ataxia, and (4) mental status changes.

There is evidence that dietary deficiency and vomiting are more frequent among nonalcoholics, eye and cerebellar signs are more frequent among alcoholics, and the classical triad is significantly more frequent in alcoholics. [34, 35].

1.2.3 Endocrine

Thyroid storm and myxedema coma are the opposite extremes of severe thyroid dysfunction, which, despite uncommon, have a high mortality rate if not recognized and treated timely [36, 37].

Myxedema coma is defined as decompensated hypothyroidism leading to multiorgan failure. It is often precipitated by an acute illness such as infection, stroke, or myocardial infarction. The neurologic change may present as lethargy and obtundation or an activated state known as "myxedema madness" [38].

Thyroid storm, a life-threatening syndrome of excessive thyroid hormone activity, is defined on the basis a constellation of neurologic, thermoregulatory, gastrointestinal-hepatic, and cardiovascular signs. A set of criteria, and their relative scores, has been defined to help in establishing the severity of thyrotoxicosis. Within this score, CNS involvement is scored 0 if absent, 10 if mild (agitation), 20 if moderate (delirium, psychosis, extreme lethargy), 20 if severe (seizure, coma) [39].

1.2.4 Sepsis-Associated Encephalopathy (SAE)

Sepsis-associated encephalopathy is defined by diffuse cerebral dysfunction that accompanies sepsis in the absence of direct CNS infection, structural abnormality, or other types of encephalopathy [40]. Patients with sepsis and encephalopathy were previously diagnosed as having septic encephalopathy. However, the use of this term is discouraged, because it suggests an active infection within the CNS. The prerequisite to the diagnosis of SAE is the presence of sepsis, according to the seminal definition of the American College of Chest Physicians and the Society of Critical Care Medicine (ACCP/SCCM) [41], updated in 2001 [42]. The key clinical feature is a change in mental status, which is not justified by any kind of sedative medications. The exact incidence and prevalence of SAE is difficult to ascertain due to the absence of specific tests or set of diagnostic criteria to define this condition. Some authors have used clinical assessment of mental status by testing attention, memory, and orientation, others have used Glasgow coma scale (GCS), slowing of the EEG, or abnormalities on cortical sensory evoked potentials to define SAE. In addition, SAE can present in the early phases of infection when criteria for sepsis are not yet fulfilled or in the presence of remote "not septic" infection. Despite these limitations, it is believed that SAE is the most common cause of encephalopathy in the medical-surgical ICUs, and that over half of patients with sepsis have encephalopathy. It can manifest with agitation, confusion, disorientation, and irritability, or hypersomnolence, stupor, and coma. The most common motor sign is paratonic rigidity. Movement disorders such as myoclonus, asterixis, tremor, are quite infrequent in SAE compared to other metabolic encephalopa-

Table 1.7 Laboratory and instrumental features of Sepsis Associated Encephalopathy

CSF analysis
Elevated protein levels
Normal glucose levels and cell culture analysis
EEG
Normal
Theta waves
Delta waves
Triphasic waves
Burst–suppression pattern
SSEP
Increased peak latencies
Brain MRI
Normal
Multiple ischemic strokes
Nonspecific subcortical white matter lesions

thies. Almost 70% of advanced cases of SAE have an associated critical illness neuropathy or myopathy, typically with sparing of cranial nerves and involvement of the phrenic nerves. Focal signs are extremely rare and mandate prompt exclusion of other causes. One of the challenges in studying SAE is that without a specific diagnostic test, it remains a syndrome diagnosed by exclusion. Additional laboratory and instrumental evaluations including cerebrospinal fluid (CSF) analysis, EEG [43], SSEP, brain MR, although nonspecific, support the diagnosis of SAE (See Table 1.7).

1.2.5 Environmental Exposure

1.2.5.1 Carbon Monoxide (CO)

CO is an odorless gas produced from incomplete hydrocarbon combustion, common potential sources of which are poorly functioning heating systems, improperly vented fuel burning systems, hookah use, and exposure to methylene chloride, which is metabolized to CO. Compared to oxygen, CO binds with 200-fold affinity to the heme ring resulting in allosteric changes, which preclude additional oxygen molecule binding and consequent hypoxic tissue injury. Common symptoms include headache (80%), nausea (50%), dizziness (55%), and mild confusion (30%) up to coma, as the carboxyhemoglobin level increases [44], and myocardial injury documented by increased troponin I and/or creatine kinase-MB level and/or diagnostic ECG [45]. Although uncommon, late or evolving cognitive impairments including cognitive disturbances, depression, anxiety, vestibular problems, and motor dysfunction can develop [46].

1.2.5.2 Heavy Metals

Lithium—Toxicity from lithium overdose—acute, acute-on-chronic, or chronic—can be seen at serum concentrations of 1.5 mEq/L to 2.5 mEq/L (therapeutic level 0.6–1.2 mEq/L). Encephalopathy and confusion result from greater CNS concentration, and, if the intoxication is severe, seizures and status epilepticus can occur [47]. Although the symptoms typically are reversible, the syndrome of irreversible lithium-effectuated neurotoxicity (SILENT) can occur, with chronic cerebellar ataxia, extrapyramidal symptoms, and dementia [48]. Common associated findings include ECG changes, especially T-wave flattening and QT prolongation, GI disturbances with nausea, vomiting, and diarrhea, and polyuria, with associated hyponatremia and dehydration.

Aluminum—Acute intoxication, which manifests as encephalopathy eventually progressing to coma with associated seizures, occurs during dialysis that involves exposure to very high concentrations of aluminum in dialysate. The chronic intoxication syndrome, consequent to aluminum-containing phosphate binder ingestion, results in aluminum deposition in multiple tissues resulting in diffuse bone pain and myalgias, proximal muscle weakness, hypercalcemia, microcytic anemia, and progressive dementia [28].

In 1976, the term "dialysis dementia," was coined and linked to aluminum deposition within the cerebral cortex. The dementing illness presented initially with lack of concentration and retrograde amnesia, followed by time disorientation and memory impairment, associated with mood changes as well as psychotic features. [49]. EEG can show a characteristic pattern of diffuse background slowing with superimposed frontal intermittent rhythmic delta and bursts of frontocentral sharp waves.

The Kidney Disease Outcomes Quality Initiative recommends annual serum aluminum level checks for those undergoing hemodialysis and quarterly for those taking aluminum-containing phosphate binders [50].

1.2.6 Pharmacologic

1.2.6.1 Antibiotic-Associated Encephalopathy (AAE)

CNS toxicity has been reported at a frequency up to 15%. Factors associated with increased susceptibility include older age, nutritional status, integrity of the blood brain barrier, rate and route of medication delivery, activation and elimination of the drug and metabolites, and comedication administration. Neurologic symptoms in AAE can occur from the first dose of antibiotic or emerge months after treatment, but the median time of onset to symptoms is 5 days. The time to resolution of encephalopathy after antibiotic discontinuation or change also is approximately 5 days. Retrospective reviews report neurologic toxicity with at least 12 different classes of antibiotics and 54 specific antibiotics. A comprehensive review of reported cases of AAE reveals 3 distinct clinical patterns. A type 1 AEE commonly accompanied by seizures or myoclonus arising within days after antibiotic administration, more typical with penicillin or cephalosporins administration. Cephalosporin-associated encephalopathy was reported most commonly in the setting of renal insufficiency. EEG is frequently abnormal with both nonspecific signs of encephalopathy and epileptiform discharges or seizures. Type 2 AEE, seen in association with procaine penicillin, sulfonamides, fluoroquinolones, and macrolides, is characterized by psychosis arising within days of antibiotic administration, nonspecific EEG and normal MR. Type 3 AEE, seen only with metronidazole, is accompanied by cerebellar signs and MR abnormalities emerging weeks after initiation of antibiotics [51].

1.2.6.2 Cancer Treatments

Since nitrogen mustard—the first chemotherapy drug approved by FDA in1949—over 100 of new agents are currently available. Antineoplastic agents can be first classified according to their therapeutic target; a second level of classification pertains to the mechanism of action [52].

Antineoplastic treatments can result in a wide range of Peripheral (PNS) and CNS disorders and neurotoxicity is second only to myelosuppression as a reason to limit dosing. Although the most common neurologic complication is peripheral neuropathy, CNS dysfunction may occur. Toxic effects are related to premorbid patient conditions, concomitant medications, and exposure to prior or concurrent brain radiation affecting blood-brain-barrier integrity, dose, and route of administration of the chemotherapic drug. Prompt identification of central neurotoxic effects and discerning neurologic toxicity from potential metastatic disease or paraneoplastic syndromes is paramount because early dose reduction and possible drug change are essential components of management. [53–57]. To follow a list, which means to be an exhaustive, despite likely incomplete, guide of the most common chemotherapeutic agents that might cause CNS toxicity manifested as encephalopathy.

Ifosfamide—The neurotoxicity may occur in up to 30% of patients and can manifest with a wide spectrum of clinical presentations (lethargy, somnolence, confusion, hallucinations, irritability, excitement, disorientation, weakness, seizures, movement disorders, coma, etc.) and is known as IFO-induced encephalopathy (IIE). The EEG alterations, comprising epileptiform discharges, background activity attenuation and slowing, and alterations consistent with nonconvulsive status epilepticus (NCSE) appear during the acute phase of the encephalopathy, then gradually disappear according to the clinical improvement. There are no specific neuroradiological findings associated with IIE. There are conflicting results regarding on possible factors increasing the risk of IIE, among which the concomitant administration of drugs metabolized by CYP3A4 and CYP2B6, impaired renal function, low albumin levels; hepatic dysfunction; oral administration, shorter infusion time; CNS metastases, previous CNS irradiation, preexistent neurological disorders; electrolyte imbalance; both young and old age; female sex; obesity. [58, 59].

Platinum compounds includes cisplatin, carboplatin, and oxaliplatin. These medications uncommonly cause CNS adverse effects due to minimal diffusion across the blood–brain barrier. CNS side effects include headache, encephalopathy, ischemic stroke, seizure, and cortical blindness, which are more common with intra-arterial infusion. The mechanism for CNS toxicity is unknown, but the associated encephalopathy may be due, at least in part, to the electrolyte disorders associated with use (ie, hyponatremia and hypocalcemia) [60].

Methotrexate is an antimetabolite chemotherapeutic that interferes with the metabolism of folic acid, commonly used for the treatment of osteosarcoma, acute lymphoblastic leukemia, non-Hodgkin lymphoma, histocytes, and especially in childhood cancers [61]. It can be administered intrathecally, orally (po), intramuscularly (im), or intravenously (iv), at doses ranging from 12 mg intrathecally to 20 mg/m2 per os, im or iv. Both the total dose and route of administration are risk factors for CNS toxicity. Acute toxicity, characterized by fatigue, confusion, and headache, typically develops 2 to 4 h after high dose administration and lasts for 12–72 h. Subacute presentations include stroke-like syndromes, with the evidence, at brain MRI, of T2-weighted hyperintensities and related diffusion restriction. Chronic toxicity is characterized by progressive cognitive impairment, gait disturbance, and aphasia [57]. Although prior reports have demonstrated that many patients can be safely rechallenged with MTX, some have recurrences of neurotoxicity. It has been suggested the polymorphisms in genes related to neurogenesis may contribute to susceptibility to MTX-related neurotoxicity [62]. The progressive leukoencephalopathy, the risk of which is increased with whole-brain radiation, results in progressive development of white matter T2/FLAIR signal hyperintense lesions at MRI [63].

Fludarabine is a purine analog rarely associated with neurotoxicity. However, a severe progressive and delayed encephalopathy consisting of cortical blindness, ataxia, seizures, paralysis, and even coma can be seen with higher doses (usually >90 mg/m2/day) [64].

Cytarabine is a pyrimidine analog that inhibits DNA synthesis and is used to treat leukemias, lymphomas, and leptomeningeal spread of malignancies. Encephalopathy can develop 2–5 days after initiation of iv administration, and typically is followed by cerebellar dysfunction. High total dose (> 30 g/ m2), older age (> 40 years), abnormal liver and renal function, and premorbid neurologic dysfunction increase the risk of cerebellar toxicity, MR in these patients demonstrates cerebellar atrophy and reversible white matter T2/FLAIR hyperintensities [65, 66, 67].

Fluorouracil (5-FU)—Despite being rare, 5FU is the most common among the chemiotherapic drugs to cause leukoencephalopathy with symptoms ranging from dizziness, cognitive dysfunction, impairment of memory, gait disturbances, disorientation, confusion, agitation, to stupor, coma, and death [68]. Subjects with dihydropyridine dehydrogenase deficiency are at greater risk [69]. The commonly used clinical diagnostic criteria are as follows: (a) development of encephalopathy during or shortly after completion of 5FU therapy; (b) exclusion of other metabolic or physical factors that may affect the level of consciousness; and (c) exclusion of drug interactions due to concomitant medications. The common radiological imaging findings include symmetrical periventricular white matter hypointensity on CT scan and diffuse high-intensity signal in the white matter and corpus callosum on T2-weighted sequences with concomitant restriction on diffusion-weighted (DWI) MRI [70].

Vincristine, although rarely, may cause CNS toxicity from hyponatremia due to SIADH, potentially resulting in confusion and seizures [71]. However, encephalopathy and seizures unrelated to SIADH have also been reported [72].

Biological and immunotherapeutic agents—Several of the small molecule inhibitors such as sunitinib and bortezomib (a proteasome inhibitor), and immunotherapeutic agents such as blinatumomab are associated with acute changes in mental status that are usually reversible. At high doses, interferon-α (IFN-α) can cause significant mental status changes. IL-2 may also induce dose-dependent neuropsychiatric symptoms, including depression, hallucinations, and cognitive changes, in 30–50% of patients. Cancer Treatment-Induced Neurotoxicity: A Focus on Newer Treatments. After Cytokine-release syndrome (CRS), neurotoxicity termed CAR-T-cell-related encephalopathy syndrome (CRES) is the second most-common adverse event of immunotherapy using T cells genetically engineered to express a chimeric antigen receptor (CAR-T cell therapy) [73].

Radiation therapy—Acute encephalopathy may develop with large fractions of brain radiation (typically greater than 300 cGy), particularly in patients with elevated intracranial pressure. Acute delayed encephalopathy occurs weeks to months after cranial radiation, resolves over weeks to months, and does not result in permanent disability. Late onset leukoencephalopathy is an irreversible process, often fatal, characterized by slowly progressive cognitive dysfunction and personality change that develops months to years after receiving treatment. Additional chemotherapy increases the risk of developing [53, 74].

1.2.7 Antidepressants and Antipsychotics

Serotonin syndrome and neuroleptic malignant syndrome (NMS) are the most important causes of encephalopathy associated with these medications. Despite it is more frequent in patients taking multiple serotonergic medications or large doses of a single drug, it can occur in patients taking normal doses of single serotonergic antidepressants.

A wide variety of drugs have been associated with serotonin syndrome, primarily SSRIs and SNRIs, but also other antidepressants (bupropion, monoamine oxidase inhibitors [MAOIs], tricyclic antidepressants, and St. John's wort), analgesics (tramadol, meperidine, and fentanyl), antiemetics (metoclopromide), antiepileptics (valproate and carbamazepine), antibiotics (linezolid), antitussives (dextromethorphan), and muscle relaxants (cyclobenzaprine) [75]. The onset of serotonin syndrome typically is rapid, usually taking place within hours after starting a serotoninergic drug, either new or overdosed, or after modification the dose of a chronically taken serotonergic drug. Delayed presentation, however, can occur in patients taking both serotonergic and antiserotonergic medications. The typical syndrome is the triad of encephalopathy, neuromuscular excitability, and autonomic hyperactivity. The Sternbach criteria and the Hunter criteria are used to assess for the presence of serotonin syndrome [76]. (See Table 1.8).

Table 1.8 Clinical criteria used to evaluate serotonin syndrome

	Sternbach criteria	Hunter criteria
Medication	Recent addition or increase inknown serotonergic medication No recent addition of or increase in known neuroleptic medication	The presence of a known serotonergic medication
Exclusion	Absence of other possible causes	
Clinical findings	Any 3 of the following: Altered mental status Myoclonus Hyperreflexia Diaphoresis Shivering Tremo Diarrhea. Incoordinatio Fever	One of the following: Spontaneous clonus Inducible clonus OR ocular clonus WITH either - diaphoresis OR agitation - fever AND hypertonicity - tremor AND hyperreflexia

From: Ref. [76]

NMS is the most severe adverse reaction associated with antipsychotic medications. NMS most commonly presents as the tetrad of encephalopathy, rigidity, fever, and dysautonomia. In most cases, encephalopathy is the first symptom of NMS and can have multiple phenotypes, including agitation, psychosis, catatonia, and, when severe, coma. Fever can be severe and take the form of dangerous hyperthermia. Dysautonomia most frequently consists of tachycardia and labile hypertension, but dysrhythmias can occur. Rigidity is a prominent feature, causing elevation of serum creatine kinase, present in approximately 75% of cases, and rhabdomyolysis in approximately one-third of patients. In subjects taking first generation antipsychotics, NMS typically evolves over several days. The syndrome may have different onset and clinical features in subjects on atypical antipsychotics or antidopaminergic antiemetics. In these patients, onset is more insidious, hyperpyrexia, and rigidity may be absent [77].

1.2.7.1 Ozone-Induced Encephalopathy (OIE)

Despite the absence of robust efficacy and safety data, OT is a worldwide practice for a wide spectrum of diseases including spinal disk herniation. A few patients have been described in literature experiencing CNS toxicity, characterized by cortical visual impairment, altered mental status, headache, focal neurological deficits, seizures, dizziness, and nausea and vomiting. All patients exhibited hyperintensities in T2-weighted and/or FLAIR imaging in the territory of the posterior cerebral circulation. DWI was positive in most of the patients, totally or partially corresponding with T2/ FLAIR hyperintensities [78].

1.2.7.2 Contrast-Induced Encephalopathy (CIE)

Along with the increased use of iodinated contrast medium, contrast-induced encephalopathy (CIE), also known as contrast-induced neurotoxicity (CIN), has become a more frequently observed complication. It presents as a spectrum of neurological symptoms ranging from focal signs such as cortical blindness, aphasia, focal motor deficits, and seizures to reduced consciousness. Because of the absence of formal diagnostic criteria, a panel of Australian neurovascular specialists with clinical experience in CIE reached a consensus for a 14-item diagnostic criteria for CIE (see Table 1.9) [79]. A diagnosis of possible CIE is formulated when all absolute criteria are met and of probable CIE when all absolute criteria and ≥ 3 supporting criteria are met. However, this proposal needs validation and confirmation in multicenter and extended cohorts.

Table 1.9 The Australian diagnostic criteria for contrast-induced neurotoxicity

Absolute criteria
1. Presentation is <24 h after contrast administration
2. Neurological signs cannot be explained by the presence of vessel occlusion or vascular territory ischaemia, noting: a. Punctate diffusion restriction on diffusion-weighted MRI, not correlating to symptoms, does not necessarily represent significant vascular territory ischaemia for the purpose of this exclusionary criteria, clinical discretion is advised b. Perfusion abnormality on CT or MR perfusion, without vessel occlusion, does not necessarily represent significant vascular territory ischaemia for the purpose of this exclusionary criteria, clinical discretion is advised
3. Neurological signs cannot be explained by intracranial hemorrhage
4. Neurological signs cannot be explained by a pre-existing seizure pattern in patients with known epilepsy
5. Neurological signs cannot be explained by biochemical derangement
6. Neurological signs cannot be explained by the presence of intracranial malignancy
7. Neurological signs cannot be explained by recent head trauma
Supporting criteria
1. Neurological signs are reversible
2. Neurological signs correlate to the vascular territory of direct contrast injection (in neurointervention)
3. There is contrast staining, that subsequently resolves
4. There is cerebral oedema, that subsequently resolves
5. There is cortical or subcortical MR signal changes, that subsequently resolves

From: Ref. [79]

1.2.8 Drugs of Abuse

1.2.8.1 Alcohol

In addition to classical complications of chronic alcoholism such as Wernicke's encephalopathy (see Sect. 1.2.2.3), alcohol withdrawal syndrome (AWS) or delirium tremens, it deserves mention coined the subacute encephalopathy with seizures in alcoholics (SESA syndrome) [80, 81].

1.2.8.2 Illicit Drugs

Case reports of drug-induced encephalopathy have been described for almost all drug categories [82, 83].

References

1. American Psychiatric Association. Diagnostic and statistical manual of mental disorders. 5th ed. Arlington: American Psychiatric Association; 2013.
2. Liptzin B, Levkoff SE. An empirical study of delirium subtypes. Br J Psychiatry. 1992;161:843–84. https://doi.org/10.1192/bjp.161.6.843.
3. Teasdale G, Jennett B. Assessment of coma and impaired consciousness. A practical scale. Lancet. 1974;7872:81–4. https://doi.org/10.1016/s0140-6736(74)91639-0.
4. Wijdicks EF, Bamlet WR, Maramattom BV, Manno EM, McClelland RL. Validation of a new coma scale: the FOUR score. Ann Neurol. 2005;58:585–93. https://doi.org/10.1002/ana.20611.
5. Khan BA, Zawahiri M, Campbell NL, Fox GC, Weinstein EJ, Nazir A, Farber MO, Buckley JD, MacLullich A, Boustani MA. Delirium in hospitalized patients: implications of current evidence on clinical practice and future avenues for research—a systematic evidence review. J Hosp Med. 2012;7(7):580–9. https://doi.org/10.1002/jhm.1949.
6. Inouye SK, Van Dyck CH, Alessi CA, Balkin S, Siegal AP, Horwitz RI. Clarifying confusion: the confusion assessment method: a new method for detection of delirium. Ann Intern Med. 1990;113(12):941–8. https://doi.org/10.7326/0003-4819-113-12-941.
7. Reade MC, Eastwood GM, Peck L, Bellomo R, Baldwin I. Routine use of the Confusion Assessment Method for the Intensive Care Unit (CAM-ICU) by bedside nurses may underdiagnose delirium. Crit Care Resusc. 2011;13:217–24.
8. van Eijk MM, van den Boogaard M, van Marun RJ, Benner P, Eikelenboom P, Honing ML, van der Hoven B, Horn J, Izaks GJ, Kalf A, Karakus A, Klijn IA, Kuiper MA, de Leeuw F-E, de Man T, van der Mast RC, Osse R-J, de Rooij SE, Spronk PE, van der Voort PH, van Gool WA, Slooter AJ. Routine use of the confusion assessment method for the intensive care unit: a multicenter study. Am J Respir Crit Care Med. 2011;184:340–4. https://doi.org/10.1164/rccm.201101-0065OC.
9. De Jonghe B, Cook D, Griffith L, Appere-de--Vecchi C, Guyatt G, Théron V, Vagnerre A, Outin H. Adaptation to the intensive care environment (ATICE): development and validation of a new sedation assessment instrument. Crit Care Med. 2003;31(9):2344–54. https://doi.org/10.1097/01.CCM.0000084850.16444.94.
10. Bergeron N, Dubois M-J, Dumont M, Dial S, Skrobik Y. Intensive care delirium screening checklist: evaluation of a new screening tool. Intensive Care Med. 2001;27(5):859–64. https://doi.org/10.1007/s001340100909.
11. Tomasi CD, Grandi C, Salluh J, Soares M, Giombelli VR, Cascaes S, Macedo RC, de Souza CL, Biff D, Ritter C, Dal Pizzol F. Comparison of CAMICU and ICDSC for the detection of delirium in critically ill patients focusing on relevant clinical outcomes. J Crit Care. 2012;27(2):212–7. https://doi.org/10.1016/j.jcrc.2011.05.015.
12. Erkkinen MG, Berkowitz AL. A clinical approach to diagnosing encephalopathy. Am J Med. 2019;132(10):1142–7. https://doi.org/10.1016/j.amjmed.2019.07.001.
13. Stevens RD, Pustavoitau A, Sharshar T. Bhardwaj A, Mirski MA, editors. Handbook of neurocritical care. 2nd ed. p. 287. https://doi.org/10.1007/978-1-4419-6842-5_17.
14. Sandroni C, Cariou A, Cavallaro F, Cronberg T, Friberg H, Hoedemaekers C, Horn J, Nolan JP, Rossetti AO, Soar J. Prognostication in comatose survivors of cardiac arrest: an advisory statement from the European Resuscitation Council and the European Society of Intensive Care Medicine. Intensive Care Med. 2014;40:1816–31. https://doi.org/10.1007/s00134-014-3470-x.
15. Rossetti AO, Rabinstein AA, Oddo M. Neurological prognostication of outcome in patients in coma after cardiac arrest. Lancet Neurol. 2016;15(6):597–609. https://doi.org/10.1016/S1474-4422(16)00015-6.
16. Scala R. Hypercapnic encephalopathy syndrome: a new frontier for non-invasive ventilation? Respir Med. 2011;105(8):1109–17. https://doi.org/10.1016/j.rmed.2011.02.004).
17. Vilstrup H, Amodio P, Bajaj J, Cordoba J, Ferenci P, Mullen KD, Weissenborn K, Wong P. Hepatic encephalopathy in chronic liver disease: 2014 practice guideline by the American Association for the Study of Liver Diseases and the European Association for the Study of the liver. Hepatology. 2014;60:715–35. https://doi.org/10.1002/hep.27210.
18. Ferenci P, Lockwood A, Mullen K, Tarter R, Weissenborn K, Blei AT. Hepatic encephalopathy—definition, nomenclature, diagnosis, and quantification: final report of the working party at the 11th World Congresses of Gastroenterology, Vienna, 1998. Hepatology. 2002;35:716–21. https://doi.org/10.1053/jhep.2002.31250.

19. Rosner MH, Husain-Syed F, Reis T, Ronco C, Vanholder R. Uremic encephalopathy. Kidney Int. 2022;101:227–41. https://doi.org/10.1016/j.kint.2021.09.025.
20. Seifter JL, Samuels MA. Uremic encephalopathy and other brain disorders associated with renal failure. Semin Neurol. 2011;31(2):139–43. https://doi.org/10.1055/s-0031-1277984.
21. Bhandari B, Komanduri S. Dialysis disequilibrium syndrome. In: StatPearls [Internet]. Treasure Island (FL): StatPearls Publishing; 2025.
22. Mistry K. Dialysis disequilibrium syndrome prevention and management. Int J Nephrol Renov Dis 2019:12 69–77. ohttps://doi.org/10.2147/IJNRD.S165925.
23. Verbalis JG, Goldsmith SR, Greenberg A, Korzelius C, Schrier RW, Sterns RH, Thompson CJ. Diagnosis, evaluation, and treatment of hyponatremia: expert panel recommendations. Am J Med. 2013;126(10 Suppl 1):S1–42. https://doi.org/10.1016/j.amjmed.2013.07.006.
24. Sterns RH. Disorders of plasma sodium—causes, consequences, and correction. N Engl J Med. 2015;372(1):55–65. https://doi.org/10.1056/NEJMra140448.
25. Joergensen D, Tazminicand K, Jacobsen D. Acute Dysnatremias—a dangerous and overlooked clinical problem. Scand J Trauma Resusc Emerg Med. 2019;27:58. https://doi.org/10.1186/s13049-019-0633-3.
26. Wahane M, Kaushal H, Goyal G, Sarna M. An atypical case of hypomagnesemia- induced cerebellar syndrome with literature review. J R Coll Physicians Edinb. 2023;53(4):272–7. https://doi.org/10.1177/14782715231209776.
27. Olmedo-Saura G, Pérez-Pérez J, Xuclà-Ferrarons T, Collet R, Martínez-Viguera A, Kulisevsky J. Cerebellar syndrome induced by hypomagnesemia: a treatable cause of ataxia not to be missed. Report of three cases and a review of the literature. Mov Disord Clin Pract. 2023;10(6):1004–12. https://doi.org/10.1002/mdc3.13739.
28. Ray S, Park KW. Movement disorders and other neurologic impairment associated with hypomagnesemia A systematic review. Neurology: clinical Practice. 2023;13(6):e200202. https://doi.org/10.1212/CPJ.0000000000200202.
29. Naya Rosato M, Núñez Calvo ML, Barrera López L. Posterior reversible encephalopathy syndrome related to severe hypomagnesemia. Eur J Case Rep Intern Med. 2025;12(2):005098. https://doi.org/10.12890/2025_005098.
30. El-Husari A, Phrathep D, Ibrahim M, et al. Acute psychosis in the setting of undiagnosed Normocalcemic hyperparathyroidism: a case report. Cureus. 2023;15(3):e35840. https://doi.org/10.7759/cureus.35840.
31. Barbara G, Mégarbane B, Argaud L, Louis G, Lerolle N, Schneider F, Gaudry S, Barbarot N, Jamet A, Outin H, Gibot S, Bollaert P-E. Functional outcome of patients with prolonged hypoglycemic encephalopathy. Ann Intensive Care. 2017;7:54. https://doi.org/10.1186/s13613-017-0277-2.
32. Tomkins M, McCormack R, O'Connell K, Agha A, Merwick Á. Metabolic encephalopathy secondary to diabetic ketoacidosis: a case report. BMC Endocr Disord. 2019;19(1):71. https://doi.org/10.1186/s12902-019-0398-8.
33. Chu L, Xi Z, Ma R, Shi W, Yu G. Euglycemic diabetic ketoacidosis associated metabolic encephalopathy caused by dapagliflozin: a rare case report. BMC Neurol. 2025;25:20. https://doi.org/10.1186/s12883-025-04027-5.
34. Sinha S, Kataria A, Kolla BP, Thusius N, Loukianova LL. Wernicke Encephalopathy-Clinical Pearls. Mayo Clin Proc. 2019;94(6):1065–72. https://doi.org/10.1016/j.mayocp.2019.02.018.
35. Galvin R, Bra°then G, Ivashynka A, Hillbom M, Tanasescu R, Leone MA. EFNS guidelines for diagnosis, therapy and prevention of Wernicke encephalopathy. Eur J Neurol. 2010;17:1408–18. https://doi.org/10.1111/j.1468-1331.2010.03153.
36. Cruz-Flores S. Neurological complications of endocrine emergencies. Curr Neurol Neurosci Rep. 2021;21(5):21. https://doi.org/10.1007/s11910-021-01105-2.
37. Waheed A, Awais SB, Kamboj S, Mahmud H. Endocrine Emergencies. Prim Care. 2024;51(3):495–510.
38. Wiersinga WM. Myxedema and coma (severe hypothyroidism). Endotext; 2018. Available at: https://www.ncbi.nlm.nih.gov/books/NBK279007/. Accessed 22 Nov 2023
39. Burch HB, Wartofsky L. Life-threatening thyrotoxicosis. Thyroid storm. Endocrinol Metab Clin N Am. 1993;22(2):263–77.
40. Gofton TE, Young GB. Nat Rev Neurol. 2012;8:557–66. https://doi.org/10.1038/nrneurol.2012.183.
41. Bone RC, Sprung CL, Sibbald WJ. Definitions for sepsis and organ failure. Crit Care Med. 1992;20:724–6. https://doi.org/10.1097/00003246-199206000-00002.
42. Levy MM, Fink MP, Marshall JC, Abraham E, Angus D, Cook D, Cohen J, Opal SM, Vincent JL, Ramsay G. SCCM/ESICM/ACCP/ATS/SIS. 2001 SCCM/RSICM/ACCP/ATS/SIS international sepsis definition conference. Crit Care Med. 2003;31(4):1250–6. https://doi.org/10.1097/01.CCM.0000050454.01978.3B.
43. Young GB, Bolton CF, Archibald YM, Austin TW, Wells GA. The electroencephalogram in sepsis-associated encephalopathy. J Clin Neurophysiol, 1992(9);1:145–152. doi:https://doi.org/10.1097/00004691-199201000-00016.
44. Ernst A, Zibrak JD. Carbon monoxide poisoning. N Engl J Med. 1998;339:1603. https://doi.org/10.1056/NEJM199811263392206.
45. Satran D, Henry CR, Adkinson C, Nicholson CI, Henry TD. Cardiovascular injury and long-term mortality following moderate to severe carbon monoxide

poisoning. JAMA. 2006;295(4):398–402. https://doi.org/10.1001/jama.295.4.398.
46. Hampson NB, Piantadosi CA, Thom SR, Weaver LK. Practice recommendations in the diagnosis, management, and prevention of carbon monoxide poisoning. Am J Respir Crit Care Med. 2012;186(11):1095–101. https://doi.org/10.1164/rccm.201207-1284CI.
47. Strobusch AD, Jefferson JW. The checkered history of lithium in medicine. Pharm Hist. 1980;22:72.
48. Adityanjee, Munshi KR, Thampy A. The syndrome of irreversible-lithium effectuated neurotoxicity. Clin Neuropharmacol. 2005;28:38–49. https://doi.org/10.1097/01.wnf.0000150871.52253.b7.
49. Alfrey AC, LeGendre GR, Kaehny WD. The dialysis encephalopathy syndrome—possible aluminum intoxication. N Engl J Med. 1976;294:184–8. https://doi.org/10.1056/NEJM197601222940402.
50. National Kiney Foundation. K/DOQI clinical practice guidelines for bone metabolism and disease in chronic kidney disease. Am J Kidney Dis. 2003;42(4 suppl 3):S1–201.
51. Bhattacharyya S, Darby RR, Raibagkar P, Gonzalez Castro LN, Berkowitz AL. Antibiotic-associated encephalopathy. Neurology. 2016;86(10):963–71. https://doi.org/10.1212/WNL.0000000000002455.
52. Ostios-Garcia L, Perez DM, Castelo B, Herradon NH, Zamora P, Feliu J, Espinosa E. Classification of anticancer drugs: an update with FDA and EMA-approved drugs. Cancer Metastasis Revws. 2024;43:1561–71. https://doi.org/10.1007/s10555-024-10188-5.
53. Stone JB, DeAngelis LM. Cancer treatment-induced neurotoxicity: A focus on newer treatments. Nat Rev Clin Oncol. 2016;13(2):92–105. https://doi.org/10.1038/nrclinonc.2015.152.
54. Ly KI, Arrillaga-Romany IC. Neurologic complications of systemic anticancer therapy. Neurol Clin. 2018;36(3):627–51. https://doi.org/10.1016/j.ncl.2018.04.013.
55. Magge RS, DeAngelis LM. The double-edged sword: neurotoxicity of chemotherapy. Blood Rev. 2015;29(2):93–100. https://doi.org/10.1016/j.blre.2014.09.012.
56. Sioka C, Kyritsis AP. Central and peripheral nervous system toxicity of common chemotherapeutic agents. Cancer Chemother Pharmacol. 2009;63:761–7. https://doi.org/10.1007/s00280-008-0876-6.
57. Verstappen CC, Heimans JJ, Hoekman K, Postma TJ. Neurotoxic complications of chemotherapy in patients with cancer: clinical signs and optimal management. Drugs. 2003;63:1549–63. https://doi.org/10.2165/00003495-200363150-00003.
58. Torchia A, Vari S, Onesti CE, Ceddia S, Maschio M, Maggi G, Riva F, Faltyn W, Russillo M, Ferraresi V. A narrative review on diagnosis and treatment of ifosfamide-induced encephalopathy, the perspective of a EURACAN reference center for sarcomas. Front Pharmacol. 2025;16:1512966. https://doi.org/10.3389/fphar.2025.1512966.
59. Idle JR, Beyoğlu D. Ifosfamide—history, efficacy, toxicity and encephalopathy. Pharmacol Ther. 2023;243:108366. https://doi.org/10.1016/j.pharmthera.2023.108366.
60. Lyass O, Lossos A, Hubert A, Gips M, Peretz T. Cisplatin-induced non-convulsive encephalopathy. Anti-Cancer Drugs. 1998;9(1):100–4. https://doi.org/10.1097/00001813-199801000-00013.
61. Mshaymesh S. Neurotoxic effects of the chemotherapeutic drug "methotrexate": a literature review. Ann Med Surg. 2025;87:1394–405. https://doi.org/10.1097/MS9.0000000000002863.
62. Bhojwani D, Sabin ND, Pei D, Yang JJ, Khan RB, Panetta JC, Krull KR, Inaba H, Rubnitz JE, Metzger ML, Howard SC, Ribeiro RC, Cheng C, Reddick WE, Jeha S, Sandlund JT, Evans WE, Pui CH, Relling MV. Methotrexate-induced neurotoxicity and leukoencephalopathy in childhood acute lymphoblastic leukemia. J Clin Oncol. 2014;32:949–59. https://doi.org/10.1200/JCO.2013.53.0808.
63. Oka M, Terae S, Kobayashi R, Sawamura Y, Kudoh K, Tha KK, Yoshida M, Kaneda M, Suzuki Y, Miyasaka K. MRI in methotrexate-related leukoencephalopathy: disseminated necrotising leukoencephalopathy in comparison with mild leukoencephalopathy. Neuroradiology. 2003;45:493–7. https://doi.org/10.1007/s00234-003-0983-3.
64. Cheson BD, Vena DA, Foss FM, Sorensen JM. Neurotoxicity of purine analogs: a review. J Clin Oncol. 1994;12:2216–28. https://doi.org/10.1200/JCO.1994.12.10.2216.
65. Chun HG, Leyland-Jones BR, Caryk SM, Hoth DF. Central nervous system toxicity of fludarabine phosphate. Cancer Treat Rep. 1986;70:1225–8.
66. Casasnovas NM, Manzaneque A, Muntañola A, Castells GJ. Retreatment with full-dose cytarabine in a patient with previous neurological toxicity. Oncol Pharm Pract. 2022;28(7):1634–6. https://doi.org/10.1177/10781552221076777.
67. Lenfant C, Greiner N, Duprez TJ. Cytarabine-induced encephalitis. Belg Soc Radiol. 2021;105(1):46. https://doi.org/10.5334/jbsr.2492.
68. Manikandan M, Azariah B, Sharma R. 5-Fluorouracil--induced leukoencephalopathy. J Cancer Res Ther. 2023;19(7):2076–8. https://doi.org/10.4103/jcrt.jcrt_2165_21.
69. Takimoto CH, Lu ZH, Zhang R, Liang MD, Larson LV, Cantilena LR Jr, Grem JL, Allegra CJ, Diasio RB, Chu E. Severe neurotoxicity following 5-fluorouracil based chemotherapy in a patient with dihydropyrimidine dehydrogenase deficiency. Clin Cancer Res. 1996;2:477–81.
70. Tha KK, Terae S, Sugiura M, Nishioka T, Oka M, Kudoh K, Kaneko K, Miyasaka K. Diffusion--weighted magnetic resonance imaging in early stage of 5-fluorouracil-induced leukoencephalopathy. Acta Neurol Scand. 2002;106:379–86. https://doi.org/10.1034/j.1600-0404.2002.01253.x.

71. Escuro RS, Adelstein DJ, Carter SG. Syndrome of inappropriate secretion of antidiuretic hormone after infusional vincristine. Cleve Clin J Med. 1992;59(6):643–4. https://doi.org/10.3949/ccjm.59.6.643.
72. Scheithauer W, Ludwig H, Maida E. Acute encephalopathy associated with continuous vincristine sulfate combination therapy: case report. Investig New Drugs. 1985;3(3):315–8. https://doi.org/10.1007/BF00179439.
73. Velasco R, Mussetti A, Villagrán-García M, Sureda A. CAR T-cell-associated neurotoxicity in central nervous system hematologic disease: is it still a concern? Front Neurol. 2023;14:1144414. https://doi.org/10.3389/fneur.2023.1144414.
74. Moretti R, Caruso P. An iatrogenic model of brain small-vessel disease: post-radiation encephalopathy. Int J Mol Sci. 2020;21:6506. https://doi.org/10.3390/ijms21186506.
75. Boyer EW, Shannon M. The serotonin syndrome. N Engl J Med. 2005;352(11):1112–20. https://doi.org/10.1056/NEJMra041867.
76. Dunkley EJ, Isbister GK, Sibbritt D, Dawson AH, Whyte IM. The hunter serotonin toxicity criteria: simple and accurate diagnostic decision rules for serotonin toxicity. QJM. 2003;96(9):635–42. https://doi.org/10.1093/qjmed/hcg109.
77. Rosebush PI, Anglin RE, Richards C, et al. Neuroleptic malignant syndrome and the acute phase response. J Clin Psychopharmacol. 2008;28(4):459–61. https://doi.org/10.1097/JCP.0b013e31817ea9c1.
78. Haggiag S, Prosperini L, Stasolla A, Gerace C, Tortorella C, Gasperini C. Ozone-induced encephalopathy: A novel iatrogenic entity. Eur J Neurol. 2021;28:2471–8. https://doi.org/10.1111/ene.14793.
79. Mariajoseph FP, Lai LT, Praeger A, Chandra RV, Moore J, Asadi H, de Villiers L, Goldschlager T, Gan C, Zhou K, Chiu AHY, Miteff F, Banez RM, Phan T, Pavlin-Premrl D, Chong W, Dunkerton S, Madan A, Slater LA. The Australian diagnostic criteria for contrast-induced encephalopathy. Neuroradiology. 2025; https://doi.org/10.1007/s00234-025-03601-).
80. Niedermeyer E, Freund G, Krumholz A. Subacute encephalopathy with seizures in alcoholics: a clinical-electroencephalographic study. Clin Electroencephalogr. 1981;12:113–29. https://doi.org/10.1177/155005948101200304.
81. Fernández-Torre JL, Kaplan PW. Subacute encephalopathy with seizures in alcoholics (SESA syndrome) revisited. Seizure. 2014;23:393–6. https://doi.org/10.1016/j.seizure.2014.02.002.
82. Humayun M, Suarez JI, Shah VA. Neurological complications of cannabinoids. Semin Neurol. 2024;44(4):430–40. https://doi.org/10.1055/s-0044-1787570.
83. Macchi ZA, Carlisle TC, Filley CM. Prognosis in substance abuse-related acute toxic leukoencephalopathy: A scoping review. J Neurol Sci. 2022;442:120420. https://doi.org/10.1016/j.jns.2022.120420.

2 Encephalopathy: MRI Aspects

Simonetta Gerevini

2.1 Nomenclature and Classification

Specific etiological clues exist according to different pathologic mechanisms.

Symptoms are often nonspecific and range from seizures, focal neurological deficits, and movement disorders, to coma, permanent sequelae, and death. Distinctive MRI patterns, such as diffusion restriction or enhancement patterns, can suggest the underlying cause, such as toxic, metabolic, or autoimmune encephalopathies.

Recognition of distinct MRI enhancement patterns concerning symmetry and topographic distribution can help identify the underlying pathology.

In some cases, focal or diffuse MRI alterations can be reversible. A review of literature offers different classification schemes of the most common toxic, autoimmune, and metabolic encephalopathies to foster an understanding and awareness of typical imaging appearances the radiologist may encounter (Table 2.1) [1, 2].

Table 2.1 Classical differentiation of acquired encephalopathies by mechanisms of brain damage

Mechanisms		
Autoimmune	Toxic	Metabolic
Anti-NMDA R encephalopathy Limbic encephalopathy Hashimoto's encephalopathy	Heroin Methanol Tacrolimus Thermatrim Carbon-monoxide	Osmotic demyelination Wernicke encephalopathy Diabetic striatopathy Hypoglycemic Hepatic Hyperammoniemic Hypoxic

2.1.1 Organ Failure

2.1.1.1 Cardiac Arrest and Hypoxic-Ischemic Encephalopathy (HIE)

Hypoxic–ischemic brain injury (HIBI) or Hypoxic-ischemic encephalopathy (HIE) occurs following cardiac arrest in patients who are revived by cardiac resuscitation. Imaging is performed to assess the extent of damage and to prognosticate the outcome.

CT scan has a limited role in diagnosing the extent of brain injury. Loss of cortical gray–white matter differentiation, reduced delineation of deep gray matter, and effacement of cortical sulci may be the only signs of global hypoxia seen on CT, which do not sufficiently help in assessing the severity and determining the patient's prognosis.

Signs of HIE on CT include both early cytotoxic (i.e. ionic) edema seen as a reduced distinc-

S. Gerevini (✉)
Neuroradiology Unit, Azienda Socio Sanitaria Territoriale (ASST) Papa Giovanni XIII, Bergamo, Italy
e-mail: sgerevini@asst-pg23.it

M. Zedde, R. Pascarella (eds.), *Neuroimaging of Treatment-Related Conditions in the Brain*,
https://doi.org/10.1007/978-3-032-23618-0_2

tion between the gray and white matter radiodensity, and later vasogenic edema with displacement of cerebrospinal fluid/effacement of sulci and basal cisterns (Fig. 2.1). Other signs associated with HIE are high radiodensity along sulci and cisterns from distension of superficial veins (**"the Pseudo Subarachnoid Hemorrhage Sign"**), decreased radiodensity in the supratentorial brain in comparison to the cerebellum ("**the White Cerebellum Sign**"), and higher radiodensity in white matter in comparison to gray matter "the Reversal Sign" (Fig. 2.1).

Diffusion-weighted MR imaging is the earliest imaging modality to become positive, usually within the first few hours after a hypoxic-ischemic event, due to early cytotoxic edema. During the first 24 h, restricted diffusion may be present in the cerebellar hemispheres, basal ganglia, or cerebral cortex (particularly the perirolandic and occipital cortices). Thalami, brainstem, or hippocampi may also be involved. Diffusion-weighted imaging abnormalities usually pseudonormalize by the end of the first week. As in younger patients, conventional T1 and T2 weighted images are often normal or demonstrate only subtle abnormalities. In the early subacute period (24 h to 2 weeks), conventional T2 weighted images typically become positive showing increased signal intensity and swelling of the injured gray matter structures. T1 hyperintensities, indicating cortical laminar necrosis become evident after 2 weeks. This hyperintense signal does not represent hemorrhage; it is believed to be caused by the accumulation of denatured proteins in dying cells. This hyperintensity can also be seen within a few days on FLAIR and T2 (Fig. 2.2).

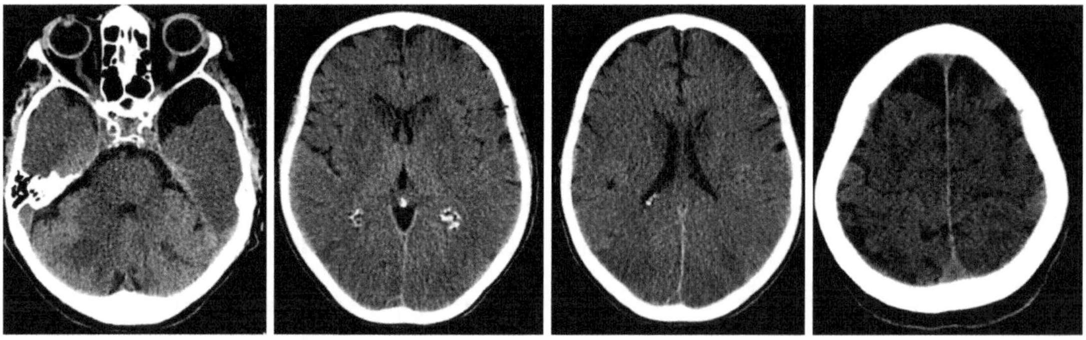

Fig. 2.1 CT scan: cardiocirculatory arrest (CCA); patient in coma. Reduced differentiation between white matter and gray matter, with associated bilateral and symmetric hypodensities of the lenticular and caudate nuclei; subtle hypodensities also in the bilateral parietal and occipital regions and at the level of both cerebellar hemispheres. The thalami are recognizable, normal. Diffuse and global, nuanced hyperdensity of the cerebellum also appears to be recognized (so called "white cerebellum sign" or reversal sign or dense cerebellum sign).

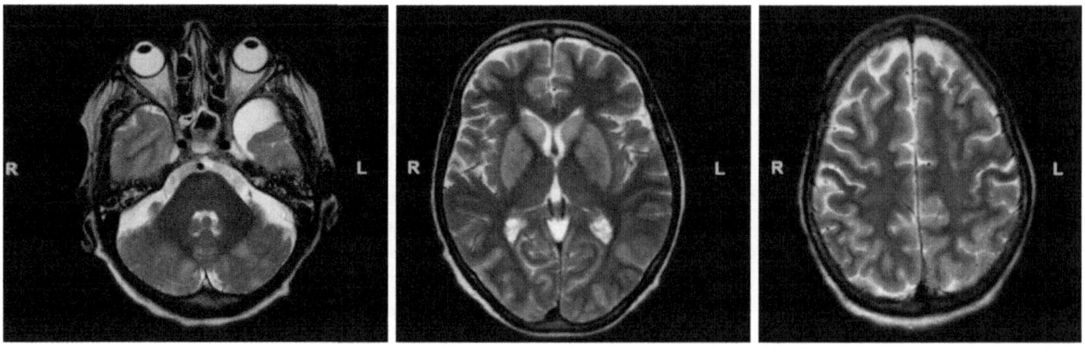

Fig. 2.2 MRI: Axial T2 at different levels (cerebellar, periventricular, and at the level of centrum semiovale)

MR imaging is modality of choice due to its inherent ability to delineate the gray and white matter differentiation and identify the cytotoxic edema, which aids not only in assessing severity but also in predicting prognosis. MR findings in HIBI depend on the duration and severity of the insult, and the period of time after which MRI is performed [3–11].

Figures 2.2 and 2.3: Diffuse T2 and FLAIR hyperintensity consisting of multiple small confluent alterations, with minimal to moderate diffusion restriction, in the cerebellar hemispheres and in posteriorly in temporo-pareto-occipital cortical–subcortical regions. Diffuse hypoxic-ischemic alterations are observed in the basal ganglia, particularly the caudates, putamen, and lenticular nuclei, with diffusion restriction in the globus pallidus. Marked diffusion restriction due to cytotoxic edema involves the hemispheric subcortical white matter, particularly the corona radiata and in the bilateral posterior periventricular area, with a symmetrical distribution and extensive involvement of the splenium of the corpus callosum. A mild spontaneous cortical hyperintensity is observed in the left Rolandic level on the T1 sequence (initial laminar necrosis). A mild T2/FLAIR signal alteration with mild diffusion restriction is also evident in the corticospinal tracts in the posterior capsular region and in the cerebral peduncles (hypoxic-initial Wallerian degeneration). The right optic radiation is also partially involved. No hemorrhagic lesions are visible (SWI) (Figs. 2.3, 2.4 and 2.5).

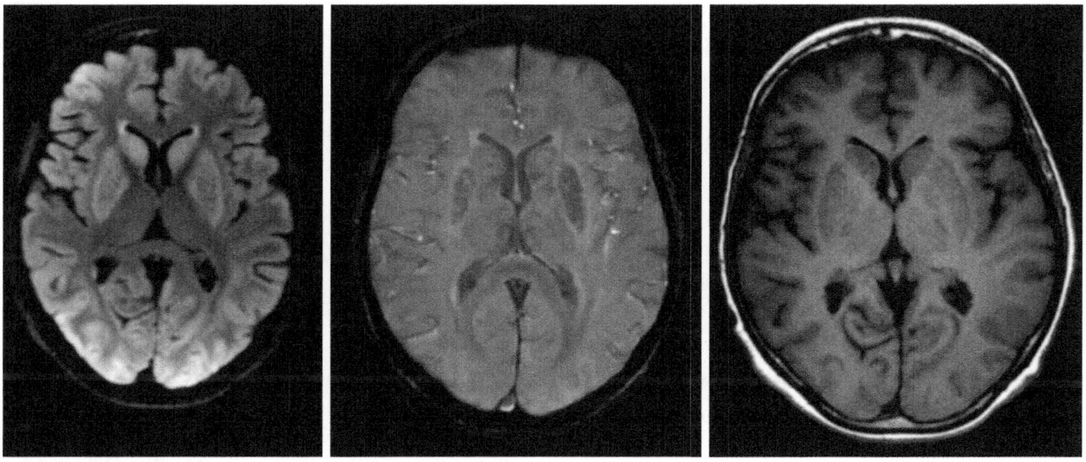

Fig. 2.3 MRI: Axial DWI, Axial SWI, and Axial T1

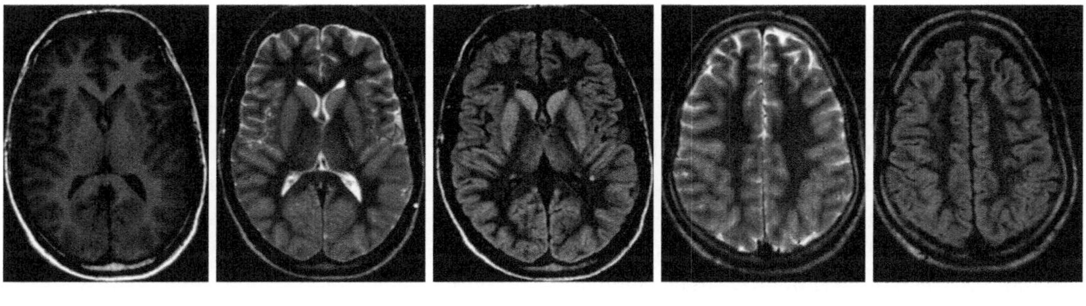

Fig. 2.4 MRI. Axial T1, T2, and FLAIR images at the level of periventricular and centra semiovalia region showing diffuse symmetric hyperintense signal alteration on T2 and FLAIR, without significant diffusion alterations, of the basal ganglia, especially the caudate and lenticular nuclei. There is lesser involvement in the thalami and in part of the capsulopeduncular portion of the corticospinal tracts. Minimum mass effect on the ventricular system. No hemorrhagic components.

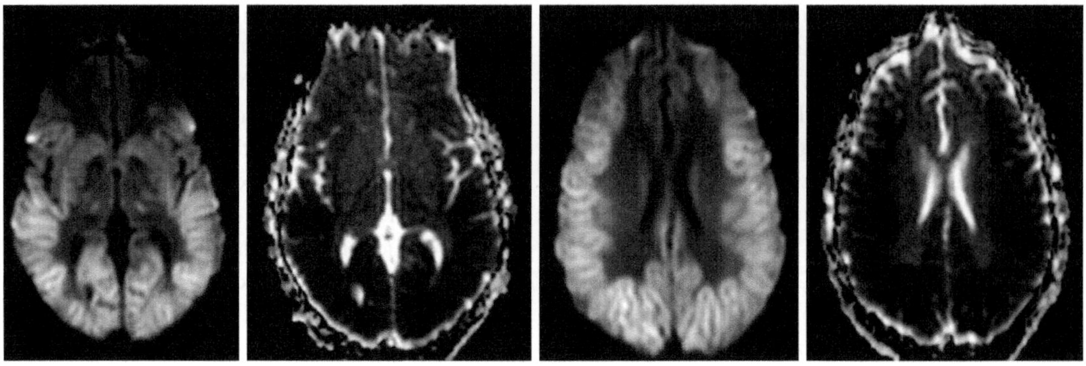

Fig. 2.5 Axial DWI and ADC (paired) at the temporo-occipital and periventricular region showing cortical restriction

2.1.1.2 Hypercapnic Encephalopathy Syndrome (HES)

Hypercapnic encephalopathy develops from the combined effects of hypoxia and hypercapnia in patients with pulmonary insufficiency, leading to carbon dioxide ($C0_2$) retention. The neurological symptoms are directly proportional to the degree of carbon dioxide accumulation/storage; patients may exhibit lethargy, memory loss, confusion, and stupor.

The results in cerebral vasodilatation and increased CBF that might lead to increased intracranial pressure.

2.1.1.3 Hepatic Encephalopathy

Hepatic encephalopathy, also known as acute hyperammonemic encephalopathy or portosystemic encephalopathy, refers to a spectrum of neuropsychiatric abnormalities occurring in patients with liver dysfunction and portal hypertension. It results from the exposure of the brain to excessive amounts of ammonia.

MR imaging features of acute hyperammonemia include high signal on T1 sequences within the caudate nucleus, globus pallidus, putamen, and anterior midbrain due to deposition of manganese (Fig. 2.6).

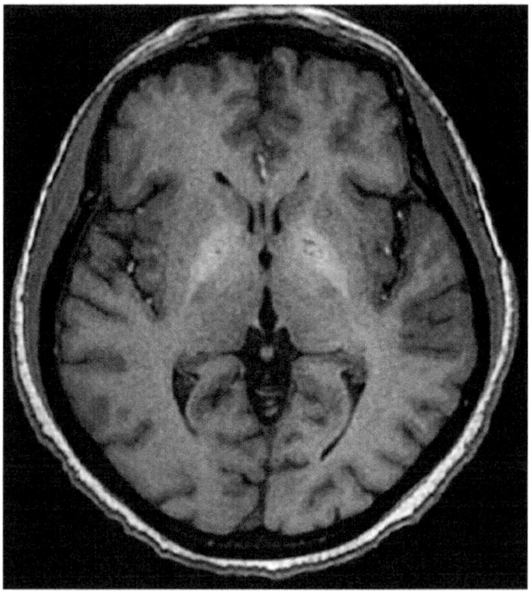

Fig. 2.6 Encephalopathy in Liver Transplant (Cirrhosis HCV +). Bilateral globus pallidus T1-weighted hyperintensity, consistent with accumulation of paramagnetic substances (manganese) in a patient with chronic liver disease

On T2/FLAIR/DWI there can be smooth or marked presence of symmetric hyperintensity within the insula (most common), thalamus, and posterior limbs of the internal capsule, and cingulate gyrus, often reversible with appropriate therapy [12–16]. If severe, the disease can be associated with diffuse cortical edema. The perirolandic and occipital regions are typically spared (Fig. 2.7).

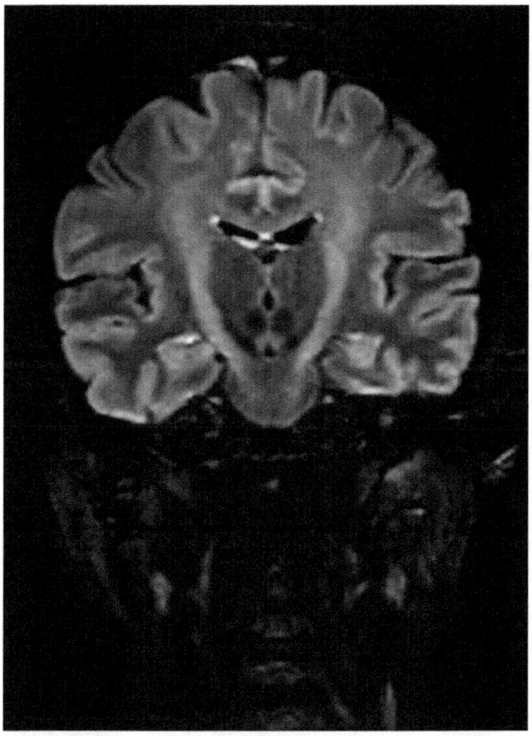

Fig. 2.7 The hyperintensity along the bilateral corticospinal tracts on long-TR sequences is also consistent with typical manifestations of chronic liver disease (coronal view is showed)

On Susceptibility-Weighted Imaging (SWI), microhemorrhages may be present, which do not affect the outcome. MR spectroscopy may show an elevated glutamine/glutamate peak coupled with decreased myoinositol and choline signals on proton MR spectroscopy [17–20].

2.1.1.4 Uremic Encephalopathy (UE) and Dialysis Disequilibrium Syndrome

UE is a neurological complication associated with Acute Renal Failure (ARF) or Chronic Renal Failure. It is likely caused by the effects of neurotoxic compounds.

Accumulation of uremic toxins might stimulate the neurotoxic effect of excitatory N-methyl-D-aspartate receptors, and concomitant inhibition of inhibitory-aminobutyric acid receptors may play an important role in the etiology of UE.

MR imaging can show bilateral, symmetric basal ganglia lesions with hyperintensity on T2WI, FLAIR, and/or ADC maps, compatible with vasogenic edema. More frequently diffuse mildly increased signal intensity can be seen on deep with matter, both supra and infratentorially [21–23] (Fig. 2.8).

Focal hypointense areas are also evident in the gradient-echo sequence.

2.1.2 Metabolic

2.1.2.1 Electrolytic Derangements

Brain MRI shows the imaging consequences of electrolyte derangements, such as brain swelling or shrinkage (seen with hyponatremia or hypernatremia), or specific lesions such as those in **Osmotic Demyelination Syndrome (ODS),** which appear as demyelinated areas in the brainstem or other regions. While MRI does not directly measure electrolyte levels, it reveals the resulting damage, which can be widespread and symmetric in metabolic encephalopathies or localized in conditions like ODS, helping to diagnose the cause and assess the severity of neurological dysfunction.

2.1.2.2 Glucose Metabolism Disturbances

Brain MRI findings in glucose metabolism disturbances often show changes in signal intensity, particularly in the cortex and underlying white matter, and may include cortical swelling. These changes can be transient and may resolve with correction of the glucose imbalance, although some cases can show gliosis. Specific patterns of involvement can vary, with some toxic and metabolic disorders showing **bilateral and symmetric involvement** of deep gray nuclei, cortical gray matter, and periventricular white matter.

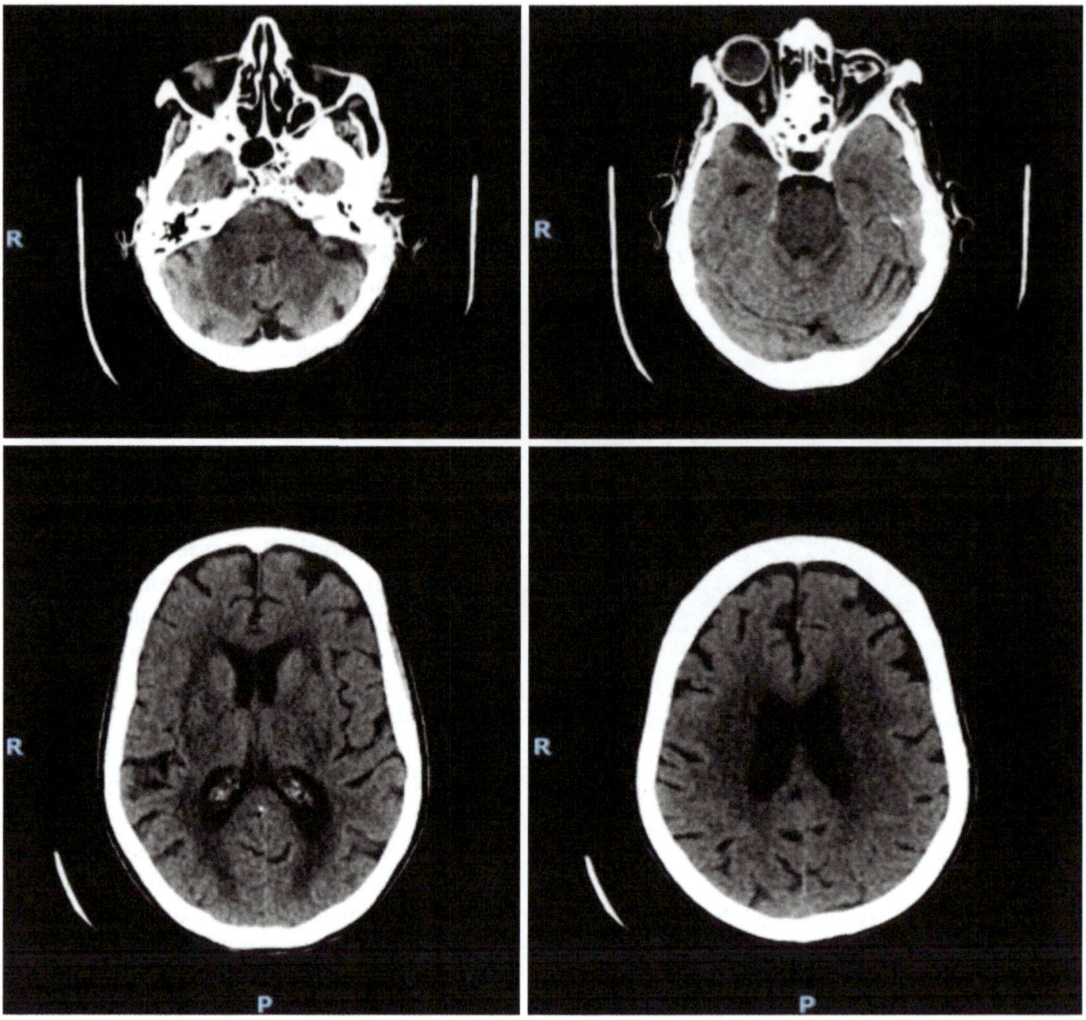

Fig. 2.8 Female, 68 y.o, presenting with headache for a week, hypertension, and chronic kidney disease, with a history of maculopathy. CT scan shows high and diffuse hypodensity involving the pons and the middle cerebellar peduncles and the white dentate nuclei of both cerebellar hemispheres. Symmetrical, smoother hypodensity is also evident in the supratentorial area of the internal capsules (Fig. 2.9)

Signal alteration can be seen as hypointensity on T1, and smooth to intense hyperintensity on T2/FLAIR. DWI and ADC map can help in defining the complete pattern of involvement. Since the signal modification can be reversible, transiently reduced ADC values can be seen in affected areas [24–27] (Fig. 2.10).

Spectroscopy shows widespread lactate peaks with reduction in normal cerebral metabolites. The cortical mantle appears likely spared from the described alterations, with only mildly reduced perfusion and subtle early FLAIR changes at the cortico-subcortical interface.

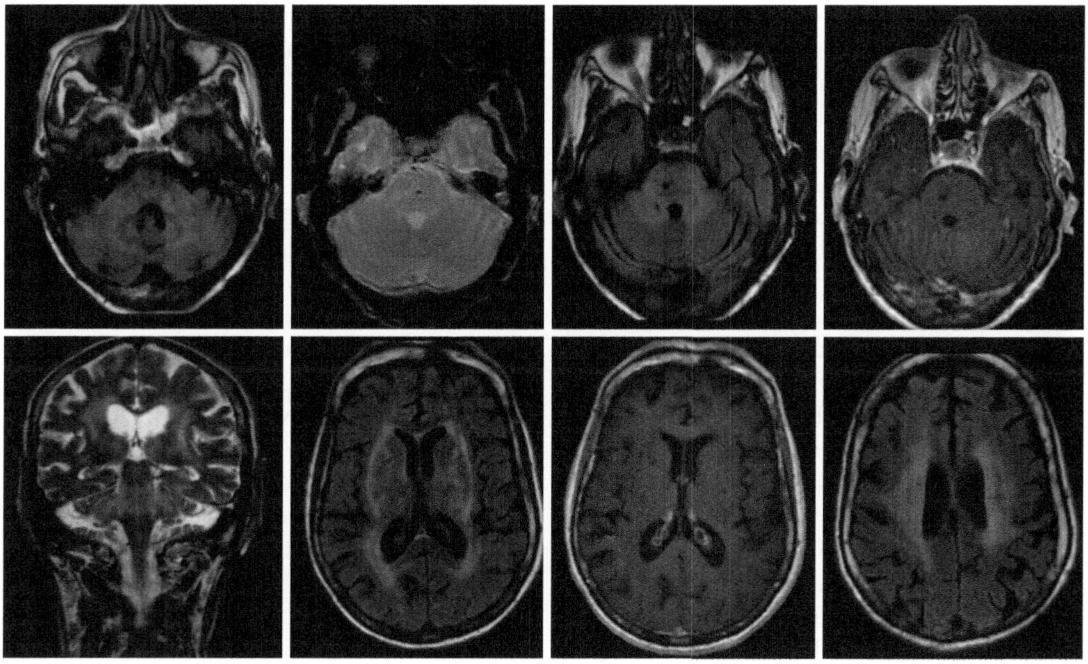

Fig. 2.9 MRI images in the upper panel: acquisition obtained at the infratentorial level. Sequences include axial FLAIR, GE (Gradient Echo), and postcontrast T1-weighted. MRI images in the lower panel: coronal T2, axial FLAIR and axial T1-weighted images acquired at the deep periventricular level, as well as FLAIR images at the periventricular and centrum semiovale regions. The images demonstrate extensive and symmetric T2/FLAIR hyperintensity involving both the brainstem (predominantly the pons and middle cerebellar peduncle) and the supratentorial compartment (including thalami, basal ganglia, and periventricular white matter)

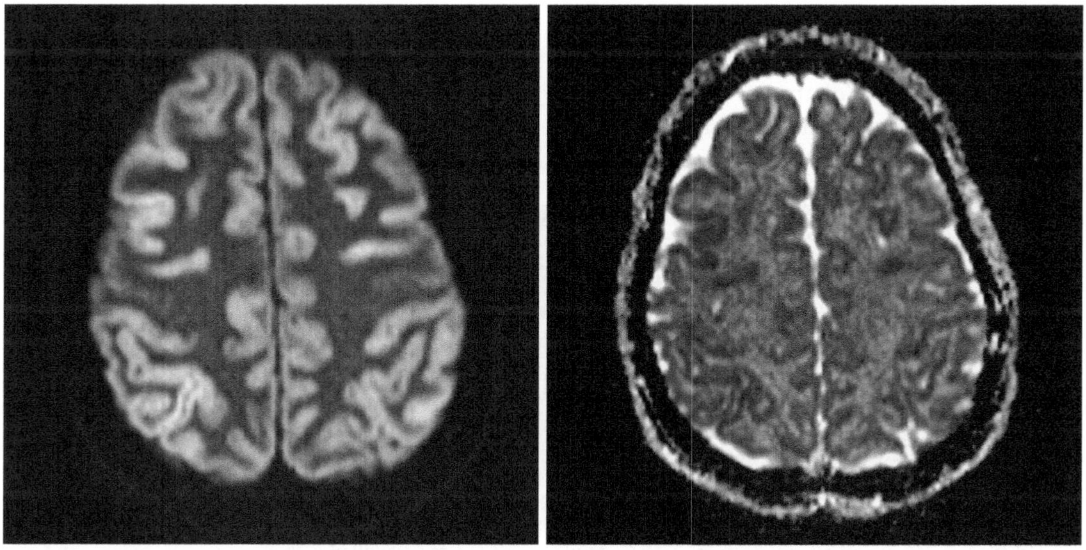

Fig. 2.10 On DWI/ADC: Diffuse, bilateral, and symmetric diffusion-weighted alteration due to cytotoxic edema involving the subcortical white matter of both hemispheres, the cortico-subcortical interface, and the U-fibers, with a posterior-to-anterior gradient and corresponding hypoperfusion. This alteration is not (yet) visible on the other sequences

The cerebellum and brainstem are essentially normal. Minimal early involvement of the deep basal ganglia and thalami is observed, with subtle hyperintense changes in T2/FLAIR and T1 sequences. Ventricles appear small, likely due to the described subcortical edema.

No pathological contrast enhancement areas are seen. No hemorrhagic components are detected (Fig. 2.11).

2.1.2.3 Cofactor Deficiency

Wernicke encephalopathy (WE) or Wernicke Korsakoff syndrome (WKS) is spectrum of neurological disorders resulting from thiamine (vitamin B_1) deficiency, most commonly associated with chronic alcoholism, malnutrition, or malabsorption. MRI is the gold standard for early diagnosis, often demonstrating characteristic bilateral symmetrical signal abnormalities involving the medial thalami, mammillary bodies, tectal plate, and periaqueductal gray matter on T2-weighted and FLAIR sequences. In the acute Wernicke phase, these regions appear hyperintense on T2/FLAIR and may show restricted diffusion on DWI; contrast enhancement of the mammillary bodies is also frequent.

Chronic Korsakoff changes include mammillary body atrophy and volume loss of the thalami and cerebellar vermis, reflecting irreversible neuronal damage.

Early recognition of these MRI features is critical, as timely thiamine supplementation may effectively reverse the acute radiological and clinical manifestations (Figs. 2.12, 2.13, and 2.14).

2.1.3 Endocrine

Endocrine encephalopathy is a neurological manifestation of brain dysfunction caused by hormonal or related metabolic disorder (autoimmune thyroid disease, severe hypoglycemia, electrolyte/ adrenal derangements and malnutrition) which often presents with altered mental status, seizures, or focal deficits.

Magnetic Resonance is the gold standard for evaluating these scenarios.

MRI findings are heterogeneous and largely range from normal to nonspecific abnormalities. The most important sequences used for the assessment are T2-W images, T1-w, FLAIR, and DWI/ADC.

The following common conditions can manifest clinically and radiologically as distinctive disorders (some of them can overlap): Hashimoto Encephalopathy (also known as Steroid responsive encephalopathy-SREAT), Hypoclycemic Encephalopathy, Adrenal hyperplasia, Nonketotic hyperglycemia, Hepatic encephalopathy, Hyperammonemic encephalopathy and Uremic encephalopathy [1] (Figs. 2.15, 2.16, and 2.17).

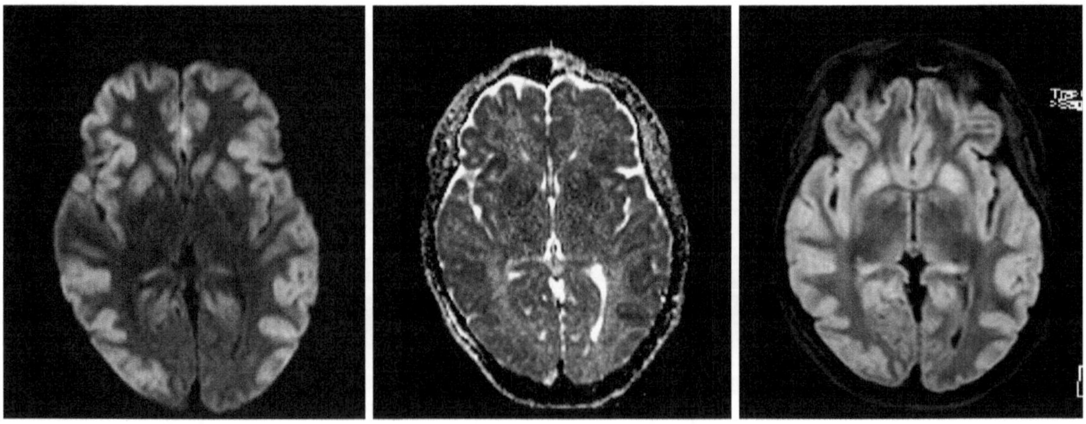

Fig. 2.11 DWI, ADC, and FLAIR: Involvement of the deep basal ganglia(caudate and putamen) is observed also in FLAIR sequences

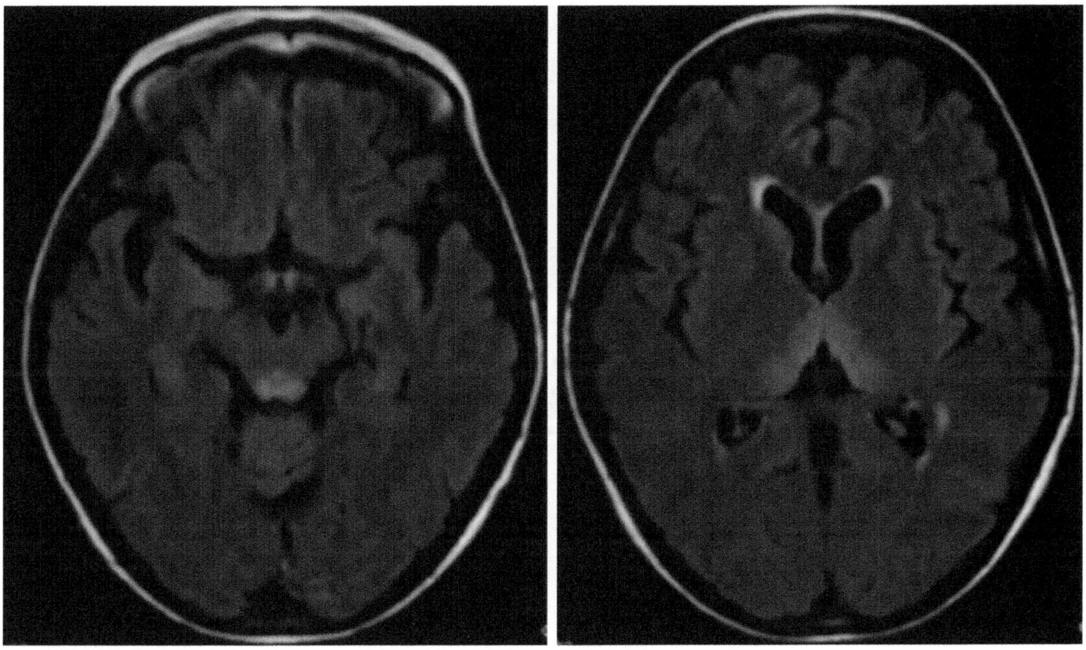

Fig. 2.12 Axial Flair Wernicke's encephalopathy in alcoholic abuse

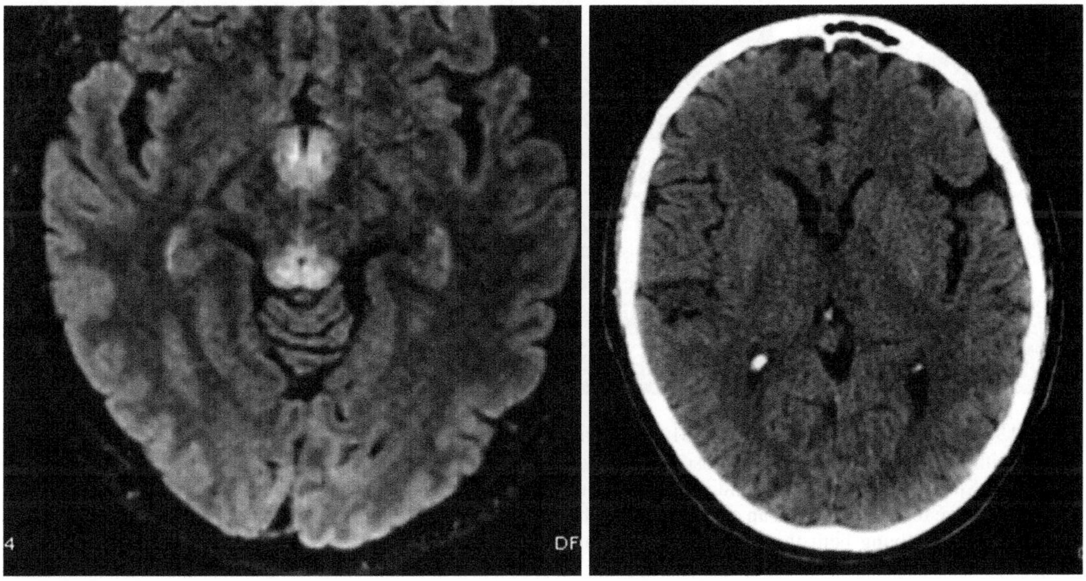

Fig. 2.13 Axial Flair and axial CT scan Wernicke's encephalopathy in Crohn's disease

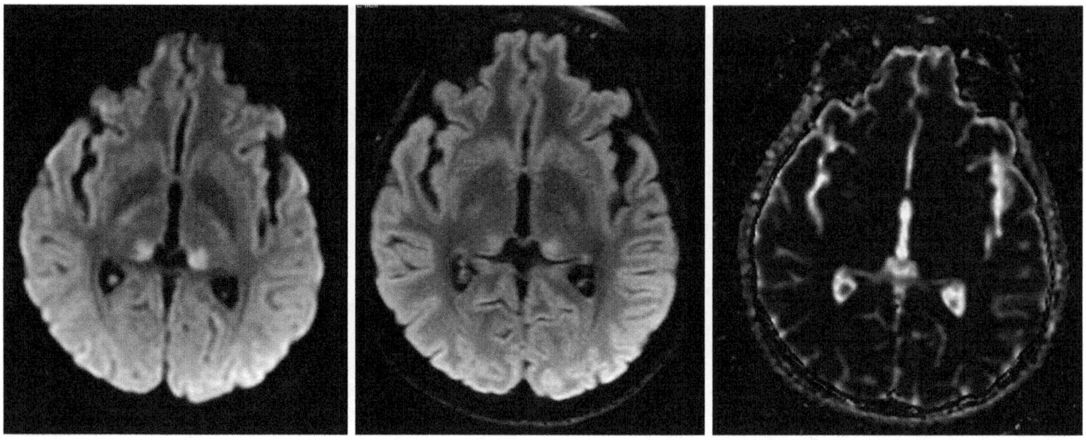

Fig. 2.14 Female 35 y.o 24 weeks pregnant, with undernourishment and repeated vomiting (Hyperemesis Gravidarum) presenting with visual impairment and confusion. Hyperintense signal alteration on DWI and T2-FLAIR (though without true diffusion restriction on ADC) involving both thalami, particularly the posterior mesial portions, and extending superiorly and anteriorly around the third ventricle. There is possible mild involvement of the caudate nucleus and putamen bilaterally. The findings described are most compatible, as a first hypothesis, with a nutritional encephalopathy (Wernicke's encephalopathy)

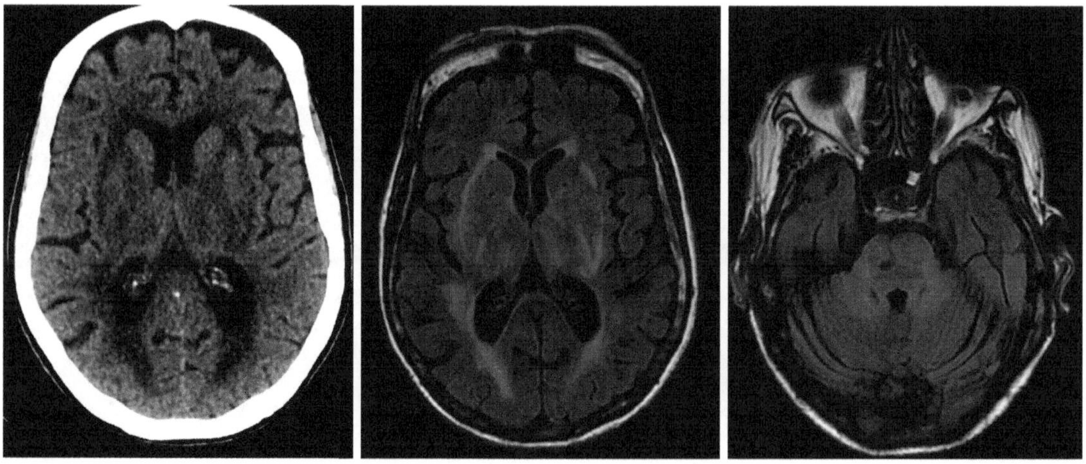

Fig. 2.15 Uremic Encephalopathy in a 61 y.o female patient with Systemic Lupus Erythematosus (SLE) with secondary Sjögren syndrome and kidney involvement (Biopsy positive for SLE). Here is an extensive parenchymal alteration involving both the brainstem particularly the pons, with extension to the cerebellopontine angles (picture on the right) and the supratentorial compartment including the thalami, basal ganglia, and periventricular white matter. The image in the middle depicts a distinctive sign called "Lentiform sign": bilateral and symmetrical hyperintensities in the basal ganglia surrounded by a hyperintense rim delineating the lentiform nucleus

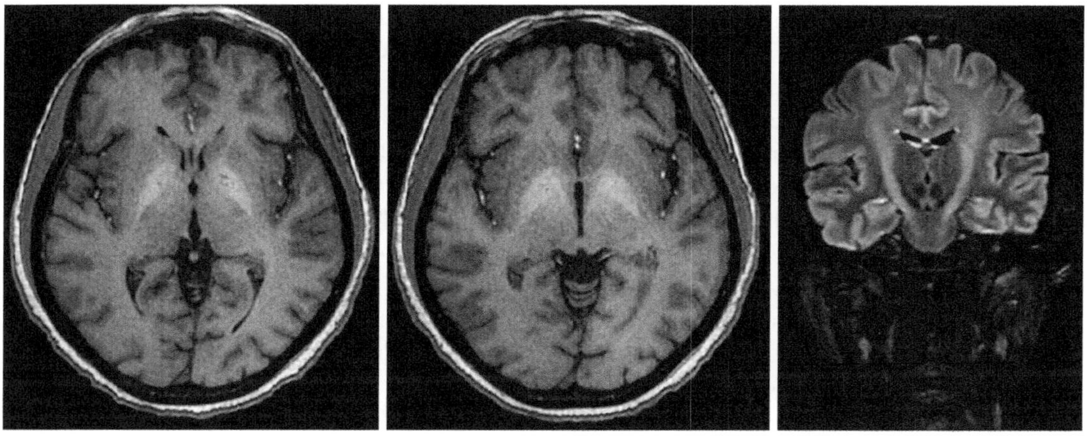

Fig. 2.16 Hepatic Encephalopathy in Liver Transplant in a cirrhotic patient. The first images show bilateral globus pallidus T1-weighted hyperintensity, consistent with accumulation of paramagnetic substances (manganese) in a patient with chronic liver disease. On the right: clear depiction of the extension of the hyperintensity along the bilateral corticospinal tracts on long-TR sequences also consistent with typical manifestations of chronic liver disease

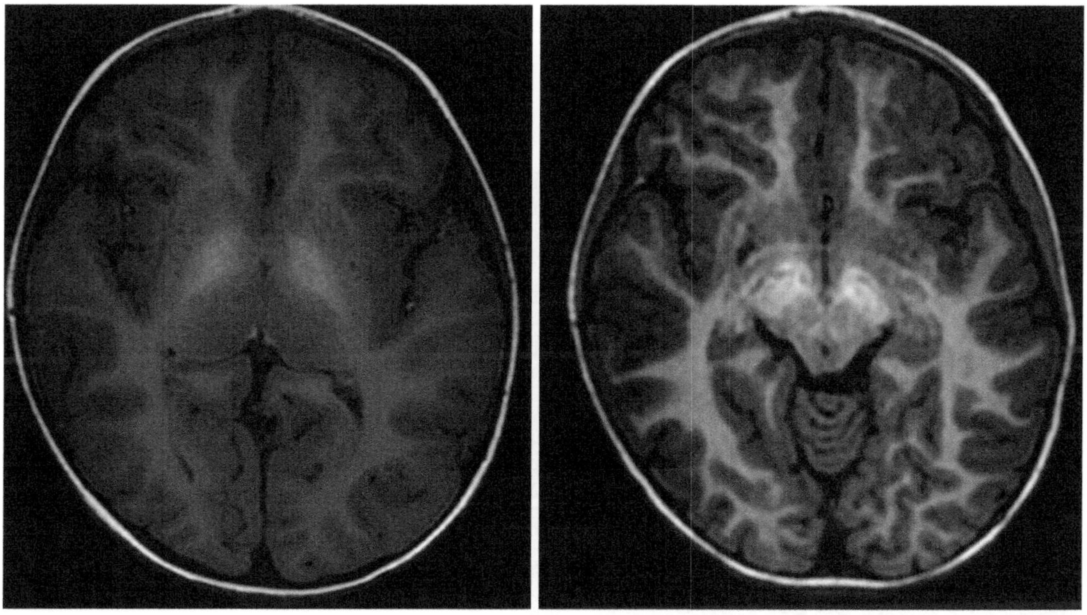

Fig. 2.17 3 y.o patient with biliary atresia with delayed psychomotor development, underwent KASAI procedure (Hepato-portoenterostomy), T1 SE (left) and T1-3D (right) hyperintensity of the globus pallidus and cerebral peduncles, related to metabolic conditions of hepatic insufficiency

2.1.4 Sepsis-Associated Encephalopathy (SAE)

Sepsis is defined as an excessive inflammatory reaction of the organism to an infection.

Septic Encephalopathy is diffuse cerebral dysfunction that occurs due to the considerable susceptibility of the CNS to any pathological factor affecting the body.

It is a frequent but underappreciated complication of sepsis, especially among patients in intensive care units, ranging clinically from mild delirium to deep coma.

The mechanisms driving SAE are multifactorial and include: Neuroinflammation, Blood Brain Barrier dysfunction, Cytotoxic Injury, altered cerebral perfusion (with microcirculatory failure with eventually DIC—Disseminated Intravascular Coagulation, microthrombi, or ischemia) (Fig. 2.18).

These alterations are aligned along the course of the medullary–periventricular veins.

Similar alterations are also observed in the more superficial subcortical regions of the left posterior parasagittal parietal lobe and the right posterolateral temporal lobe (Fig. 2.19).

On the right, after contrast administration, a mild leptomeningeal enhancement is observed in some cortical sulci on postcontrast FLAIR sequences.

2.1.5 Environmental Exposure

2.1.5.1 Carbon Monoxide (CO)

Patients with CO poisoning show various neuropsychiatric manifestations and magnetic resonance imaging (MRI) findings. Clinically, patients present with mild symptoms such as headache and nausea and may progress to coma or even death. Although CO poisoning usually causes ischemic lesions involving the bilateral globus pallidi within the basal ganglia, additional cortical and subcortical structures may also be affected.

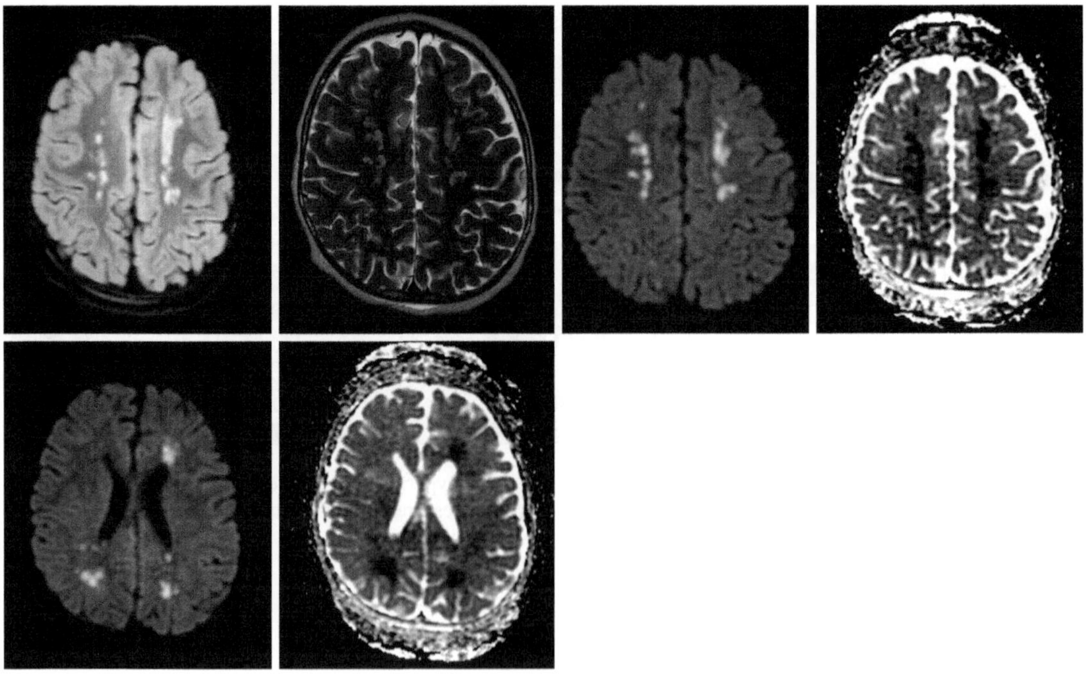

Fig. 2.18 Salmonella B Sepsis in a 3 y.o patient. Multiple hyperintense signal alterations on FLAIR and T2 sequences with reduced diffusion coefficient (white on DWI black on ADC map), without hemorrhagic components, affecting the deep subcortical and periventricular white matter bilaterally, with a symmetrical distribution, predominantly in the bilateral posterior periventricular regions

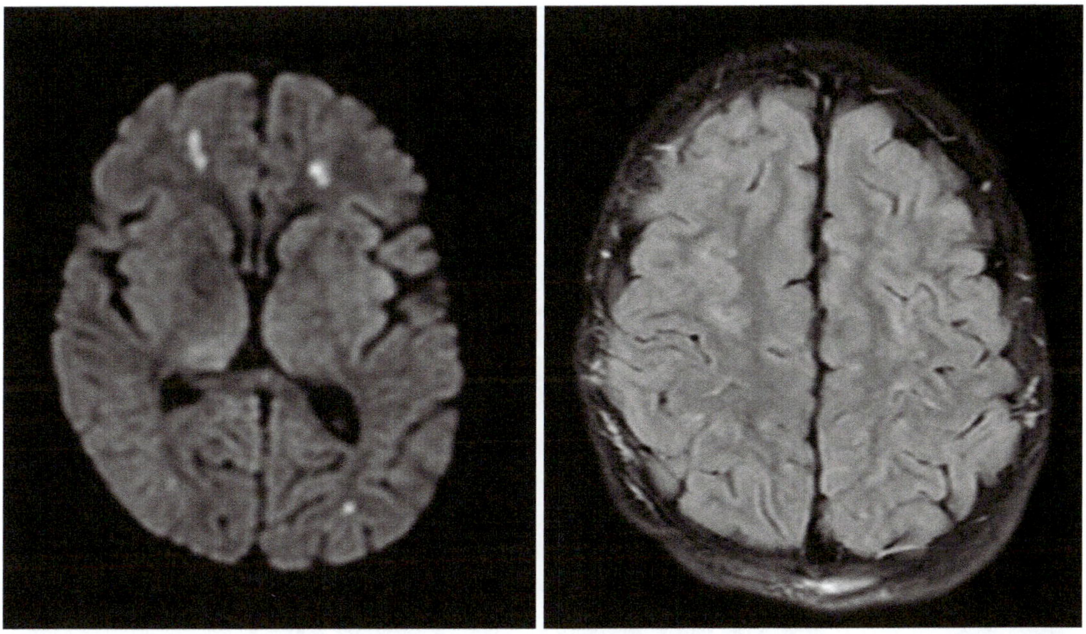

Fig. 2.19 On the left: A very subtle signal alteration is noted in both thalami /pulvinar

On MRI, the globus pallidi tipicallt demonstrate low signals on T1-weighted images and high signal on T2-weighted images, accompanied by restricted diffusion.

In some cases, T1 hyperintensity and a peripheral rim of low T2 signal may be observed, consistent with hemorrhagic necrosis.

Patchy or peripheral contrast enhancement may occasionally be seen during the acute phase. Similar MRI abnormalities may also be identified in the substantia nigra, hippocampi, and cerebral cortex. In patients who develop delayed leukoencephalopathy, bilateral and symmetric confluent areas of high T2 signal are evident in the periventricular white matter and centrum semiovale, often associated with mildly reduced diffusion. Diffuse white matter involvement may also occur in more severe cases [28–31] (Figs. 2.20, 2.21, and 2.22).

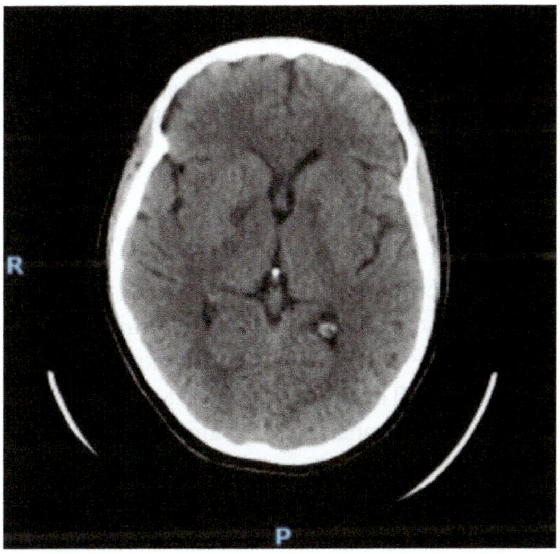

Fig. 2.20 Axial CT scan: bilateral globus pallidus hypodensity in a patient with personality disorder

2.1.5.2 Heavy Metals

Lithium

Lithium can induce reversible splenial lesions in the context of neuroleptic malignant syndrome–like symptoms. Several case reports have described mild encephalitis or encephalopathy associated with reversible splenial lesions, referred to as MERS. Additionally, acute lithium carbonate intoxication may lead to cerebellar degeneration [32, 33].

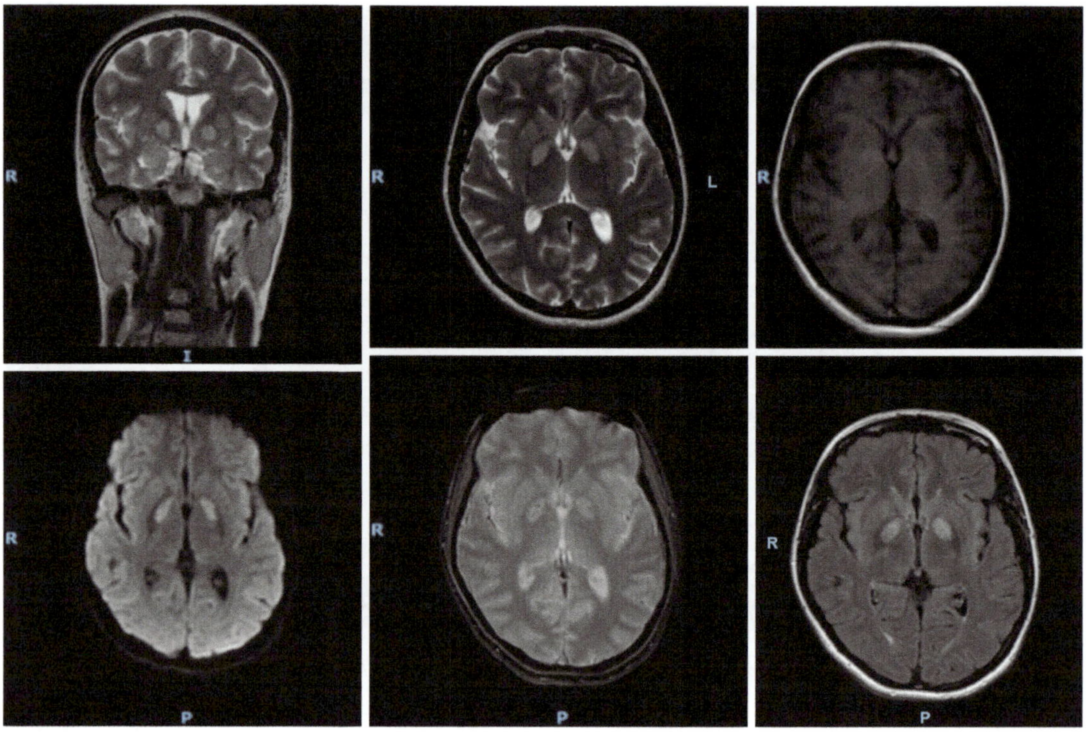

Fig. 2.21 MRI (coronal T2, axial T2, T1, DWI, GRE*, and FLAIR sequences): Bilateral T2/FLAIR hyperintensity is observed in the globus pallidus. No focal T2 *hypointensities suggestive of hemosiderin deposition are detected. No true diffusion restriction is evident on DWI; the observed hyperintensity corresponds to a T2 shine-true effect

2.1.6 Pharmacological

Drug-induced encephalopathy refers to reversible or irreversible damage to the brain function caused by exposure to various medications at toxic levels. The key pathological mechanisms depend on the pharmacodynamics of each distinctive drug. The broad spectrum of mechanisms, which cause pharmacological encephalopathy, includes toxin accumulation, neurotransmitter dysregulation, Blood–Barrier Dysfunction, astrocyte and glial dysfunction, oxidative stress/mitochondrial dysfunction (e.g Linezolid and Chloramphenicol), neuroinflammation, electrolyte imbalance and synaptic plasticity impairment.

Clinical manifestations vary widely and include confusion, distress, seizures, hallucinations or coma, based on the underlying agent and patient susceptibility. Pharmacological encephalopathy causes considerable concern in clinical practice, particularly in elderly patients with multiple comorbidities (e.g hepatic or renal impairment).

An early and rapid identification of the triggering event should be suspected clinically and radiologically.

Generally, MRI patterns are T2/FLAIR and DWI (with restricted diffusion) white matter hyperintensity abnormalities, typically confluent and symmetric.

Microhemorrhages along the periventricular white matter may be present and T1 with Gadolinium could also show pathological contrast enhancement.

2.1.6.1 Antibiotic-Associated Encephalopathy (AAE)

AAE encloses distinct syndromes linked to specific antibiotic classes and mechanisms: excit-

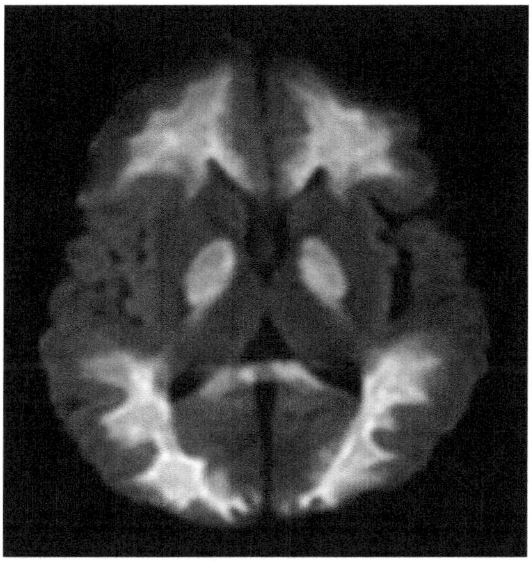

Fig. 2.22 Axial diffusion-weighted MRI (DWI) demonstrating bilateral and symmetric hyperintensity in the subcortical white matter and cortico-subcortical junction of both hemispheres, with involvement of U-fibers. These findings are consistent with cytotoxic edema, displaying a posterior-to-anterior gradient. Corresponding apparent diffusion coefficient (ADC) maps confirm restricted diffusion. The cortical mantle is relatively spared

atory (β-lactams), psychotic (quinolones/macrolides), and cerebellar (metronidazole). Recognition of these patterns is essential for timely diagnosis and management of antibiotic-related neurotoxicity.

Antibiotic-associated encephalopathy (AAE) can be categorized into three distinct types, based on the clinical syndrome, the pharmacologic class of the implicated antibiotic, the temporal pattern of symptom onset and MRI findings.

- **Type 1 = Excitatory/seizure type** (β-lactams, fast onset, EEG abnormal).
- **Type2 = Psychotic type** (quinolones/macrolides, fast onset, MRInormal).
- **Type 3 = Cerebellar type** (metronidazole, delayed onset, MRI abnormal).

The third subtype is characterized by the potential presence of positive MRI findings, reflecting structural or signal abnormalities associated with metronidazole-induced neurotoxicity [34, 35] (Fig. 2.23).

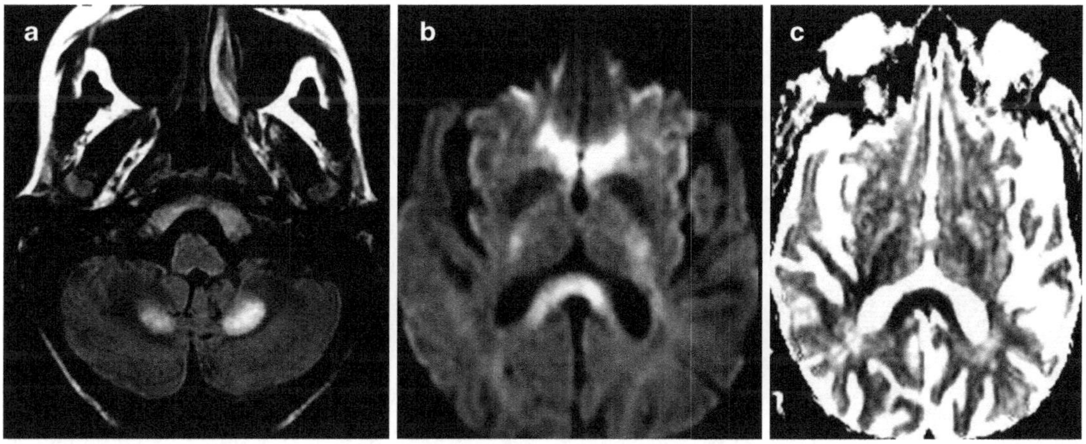

Fig. 2.23 (**a**) The fluid-attenuated inversion recovery (FLAIR) sequence demonstrates bilateral hyperintensities in the deep cerebellar nuclei. In cases of metronidazole toxicity, restricted diffusion within the splenium of the corpus callosum is evident on diffusion-weighted imaging (**b**) and apparent diffusion coefficient (**c**) maps

2.1.6.2 Cancer Treatments

Advances in oncology therapies have substantially improved the overall survival of cancer patients across a broad spectrum of malignancies.

However, these different approaches are frequently associated with neurotoxic complications, making cancer-treatment-related encephalopathy significantly challenging from a clinical and radiological standpoint. Early recognition and identification are crucial.

Cancer treatment-related encephalopathy manifests radiologically in different forms such as: **Acute–Subacute Leukoencephalopathy** (Reversible DWI Pattern)**, Acute Cerebellar Syndrome** and REACT (Reversible Acute Cerebellar Toxicity), **Posterior Reversible Encephalopathy Syndrome (PRES)**, **Neurovascular Complications** (manifested with arterial ischemia, intracranial hemorrhage, and reversible cerebral vasoconstriction syndrome -RCVS-), **Progressive Multifocal Leukoencephalopathy (PML)**, **Immune Checkpoint Inhibitor (ICI)-Related Neurotoxicity, and Spinal Cord Toxicity** [36].

Among these conditions, **posterior reversible encephalopathy syndrome (PRES)** stands as one of the most prototypical manifestations.

Posterior reversible encephalopathy syndrome (PRES) is a neurological disorder presenting with variable symptoms, including visual disturbances, headache, vomiting, seizures, and altered consciousness.

Although the exact pathophysiology of PRES remains incompletely understood, hypertension, and endothelial injury are frequently observed.

Vasoconstriction leading to vasogenic and cytotoxic edema is believed to underline both the clinical manifestations and the neuroradiological findings.

PRES is closely associated with various chemotherapeutic regimens (for example: Rituximab, Cytarabine, Methotraxate) and immunosuppressive therapies.

Imaging studies typically reveal symmetrical white matter abnormalities indicative of edema on Computed Tomography (CT) and Magnetic Resonance Imaging (MRI), most commonly—but not exclusively—in the posterior parieto-occipital regions of the cerebral hemispheres [36–48]. (Figs. 2.24 and 2.25).

DWI is usually positive at the onset. No associated hemorrhagic foci are observed (Fig. 2.26).

Radiation Therapy

Late effects of radiation therapy encompass white matter changes, radionecrosis, and vascular lesions, including lacunar infarcts and parenchymal calcifications. The latency period between radiation exposure and manifestation of these

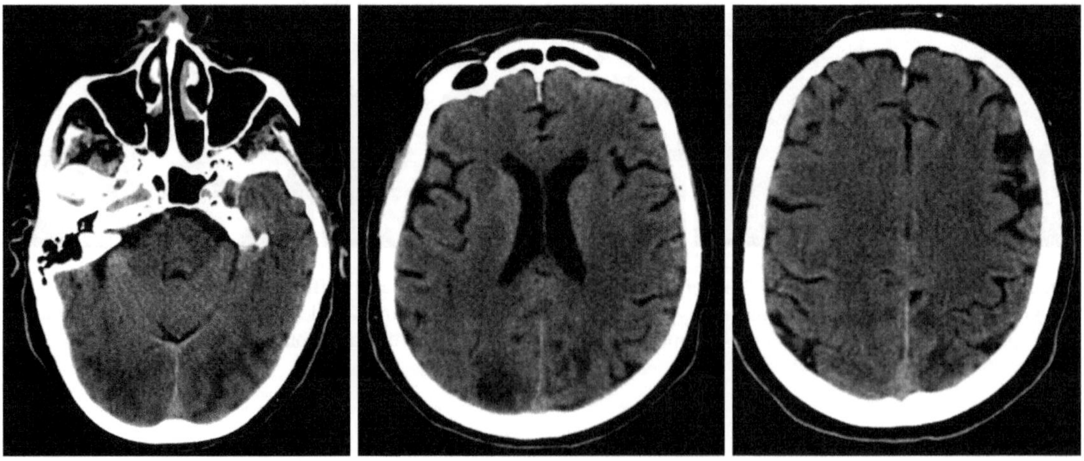

Fig. 2.24 Axial CT scan: PRES in B-cell Lymphoma treated with chemotherapy. Bilateral diffuse hypodensity at the cortico-subcortical junction in the posterior occipito-temporo-parietal regions

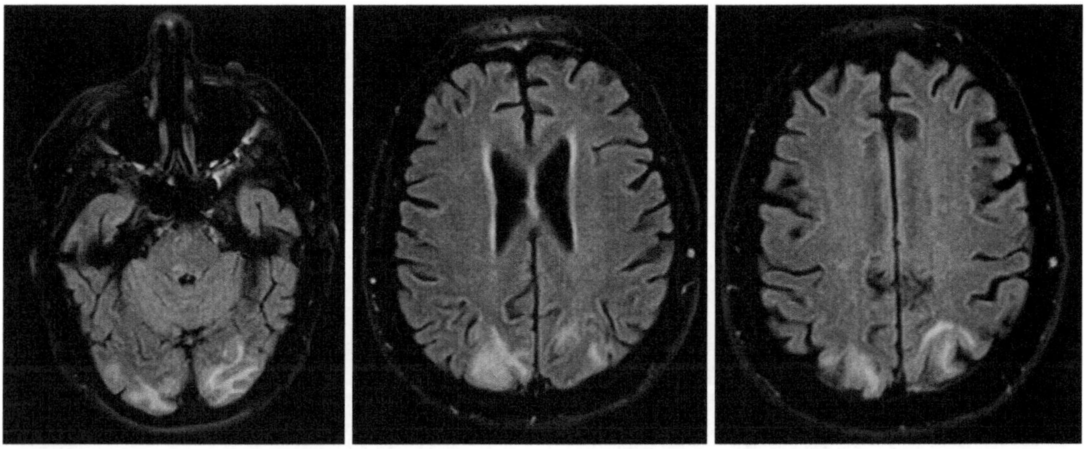

Fig. 2.25 FLAIR axial images: symmetrical signal alteration, with FLAIR and T2 hyperintensity (not shown) at the cortico-subcortical junction in the posterior occipito-temporo-parietal regions bilaterally, extending up to the vertex, particularly in the left postcentral region. At this moment no corresponding diffusion restriction signs are suggestive of ischemic injury or cytotoxic edema

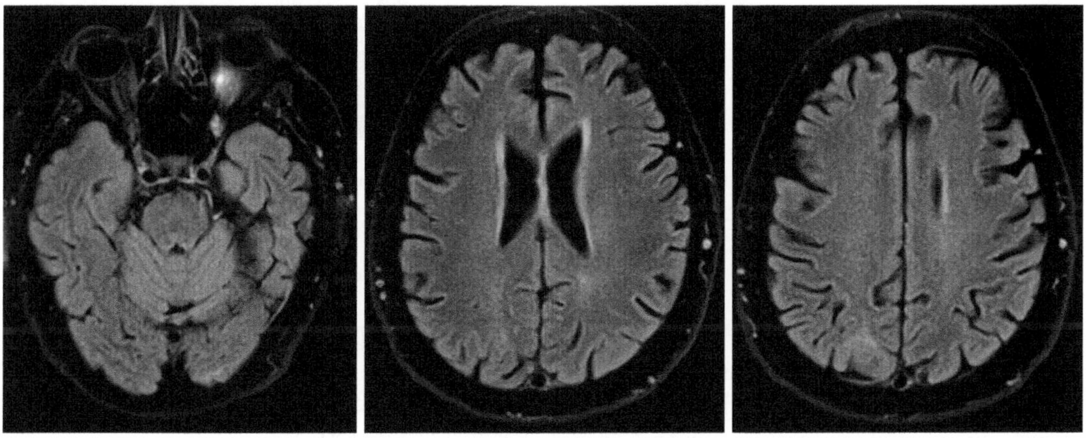

Fig. 2.26 FLAIR axial images: reduction in the extent of signal alterations involving the subcortical white matter in the previously reported areas after treatment, some of which have nearly resolved

changes can range from several months to multiple years [49] (Fig. 2.27).

MRI findings in radiotherapy-induced encephalopathy. Axial brain MRI images demonstrate diffuse white matter changes, predominantly in the periventricular and subcortical regions.

The upper panel shows T1-weighted, T2-weighted, and FLAIR sequences, highlighting hypointense signals on T1 and hyperintense signals on T2/FLAIR consistent with white matter injury. The lower panel shows additional axial SWI and DWI/ADC, illustrating symmetric white matter hyperintensities without mass effect nor restricted diffusion, compatible with radiation-induced leukoencephalopathy.

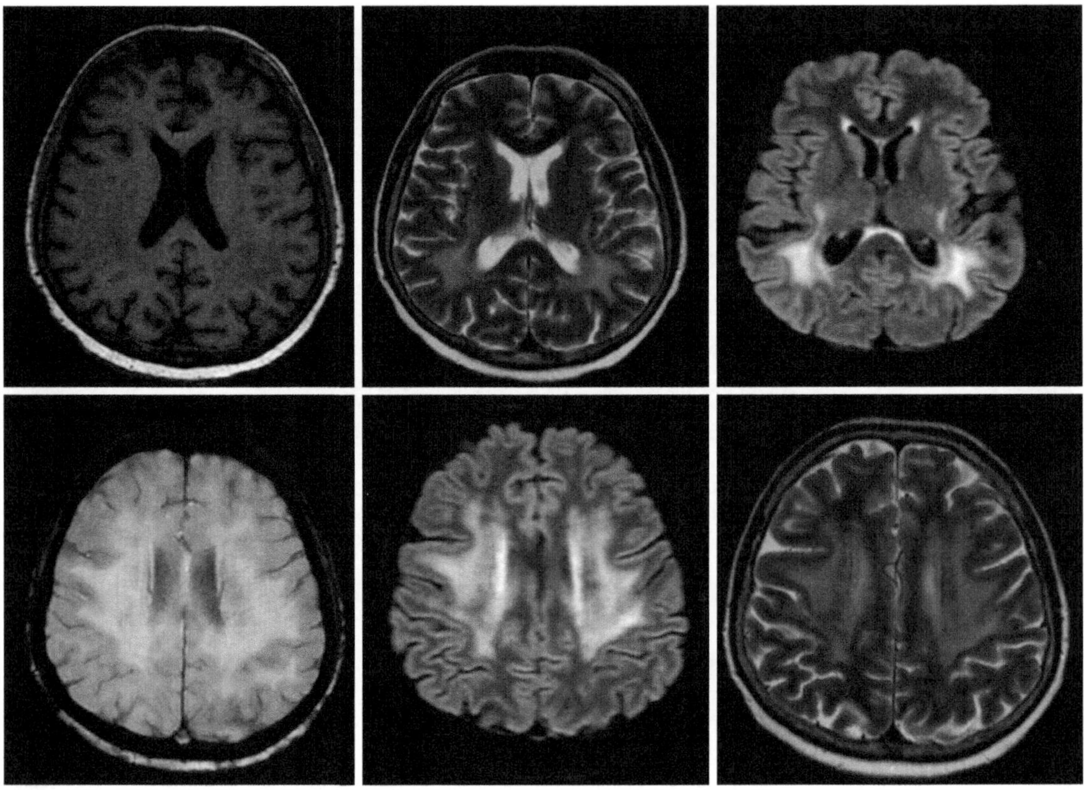

Fig. 2.27 MRI after 2 years of radiotherapy; patient with cognitive impairment (T1, T2, FLAIR, SWI, DWI, ADC maps are shown)

2.1.6.3 Antidepressants and Antipsychotics

In cases of encephalopathy induced by antidepressants and antipsychotics, MRI findings are related to several scenarios; acute, severe antipsychotic-related syndromes (NMS, malignant catatonia) can show reversible MRI abnormalities (often diffuse or focal white matter/ vasogenic changes).

Antidepressant-related encephalopathy is most reported as PRES or PRES-like syndromes in the context of overdose or serotonin syndrome MRI shows classic vasogenic edema (parieto-occipital FLAIR hyperintensities). Examples include duloxetine and mirtazapine in case reports.

Chronic antipsychotic exposure produces measurable MRI structural changes (volume loss / microstructural change) but this is different from acute encephalopathy and reflects longer-term neuroplastic or neurotoxic effects.

Sometimes, cases of drug-induced encephalopathy may present with reversible splenial lesions (RSL) in the context of MERS (Mild encephalitis/encephalopathy with a reversible splenial lesion) [50–52].

However, available literature on this subject remains limited.

2.1.6.4 Ozone-Induced Encephalopathy (OIE)

Oxygen–ozone therapy has been increasingly employed as an alternative treatment for musculoskeletal and pain-related conditions.

Despite its perceived safety and minimally invasive nature, an increased number of case reports have highlighted serious central nervous system complications, including encephalopathy, cerebral ischemia, and posterior reversible encephalopathy syndrome (PRES) following intradiscal, paravertebral, or intravenous ozone administration.

From a radiological standpoint, magnetic resonance imaging (MRI) plays a pivotal role in the diagnosis and characterization of these adverse events. Reported MRI findings range from normal early scans to **multifocal diffusion-restricted infarcts** suggestive of gas embolic ischemia, **vasogenic edema in PRES-like patterns**, and **occasional cerebellar or cortical T2/FLAIR hyperintensities**. The underlying mechanisms are thought to involve gas embolism, vascular endothelial injury, or toxic-inflammatory responses [53, 54].

2.1.6.5 Contrast-Induced Encephalopathy (CIE)

Contrast-induced encephalopathy is a short-term, potentially reversible neurotoxic reaction that occurs following the administration of iodinated contrast media during angiographic or interventional radiologic procedures. The pathophysiology of CIE supposedly involves **breakdown of the blood–brain barrier (BBB)**, which leads to leakage of contrast material into the cerebral parenchyma and subarachnoid space. Hyperosmolarity, direct endothelial toxicity, and impaired cerebral autoregulation are the key factors which contribute to short-term cerebral edema and cortical dysfunction.

Image findings more often **include cortical and subcortical T2/FLAIR hyperintensities, cortical swelling, and transient contrast enhancement**. Diffusion-weighted imaging may show mild restricted diffusion that resolves on follow-up, helping distinguish CIE from acute ischemia especially in hemorrhagic infarction in ischemic stroke scenarios.

In some cases, MRI may show a PRES-like pattern, reflecting the shared mechanisms of vasogenic edema [55–57].

2.1.7 Drugs of Abuse

2.1.7.1 Alcohol

The broad spectrum of alcohol related encephalopathy includes Wernicke's encephalopathy (WE), Marchiafava–Bignami disease (MBD), and diffuse alcohol-induced neurotoxicity, each associated with characteristic clinical and radiologic findings. Sometimes in some distinctive settings image findings can overlap (Fig. 2.28).

2.1.7.2 Illicit Drugs

Cocaine Use Disorder (CUD): Chronic cocaine use can lead to a wide range of health issues, including cardiovascular, neurologic, or infectious complications—particularly in cases of intravenous or smoking use—but it can also result in psychiatric, cognitive, or social problems. Because cocaine is a highly addictive sub-

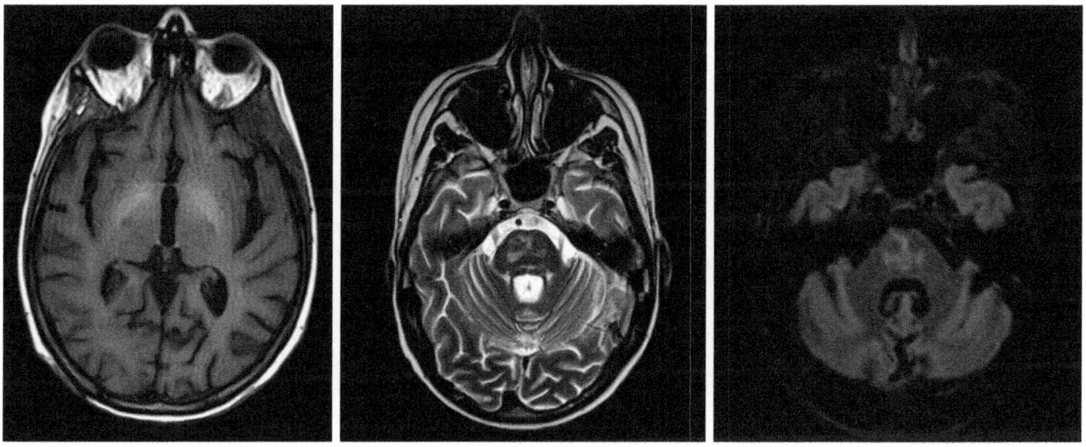

Fig. 2.28 38 y.o male patient with chronic alcoholism. On the left, T1-w image shows pallidal hyperintensity. The **Trident sign** is present in the pons (middle and right images), also visible in other metabolic conditions such as pontine myelinolysis

stance, repeated use can lead to the development of a Cocaine Use Disorder (CUD).

Chronic cocaine dependence is associated with both structural and functional changes in the brain. White matter volume has been found to be reduced in cocaine users, with a lack of normal age-related changes, and reduced gray matter density in the prefrontal cortex. Reductions in cortex thickness or alterations in white matter trophism can be appreciated on qualitative evaluation of brain MRI but they can also be more precisely characterized using advanced sequences such as DWI and DTI (Diffusion Tensor Imagin) in specific studies.

Furthermore, cocaine has been associated with cerebrovascular events, including cerebral infarction, intracerebral, and subarachnoid hemorrhage, and transient ischemic attacks, often due to a toxic related form of vasculitis, drug-induced vasculitis has been well described in the literature, with several substances—including methamphetamine, phenylephrine, ephedrine, heroin, barbiturates, lysergic acid diethylamide (LSD), and cocaine-known to cause toxic vasculitis.

The polysubstance nature of drug abuse frequently complicates efforts to attribute disease to a single agent; however, methamphetamine and structurally related substances are particularly known to induce necrotizing vasculitis [58–73, 75, 76] (Figs. 2.29 and 2.30).

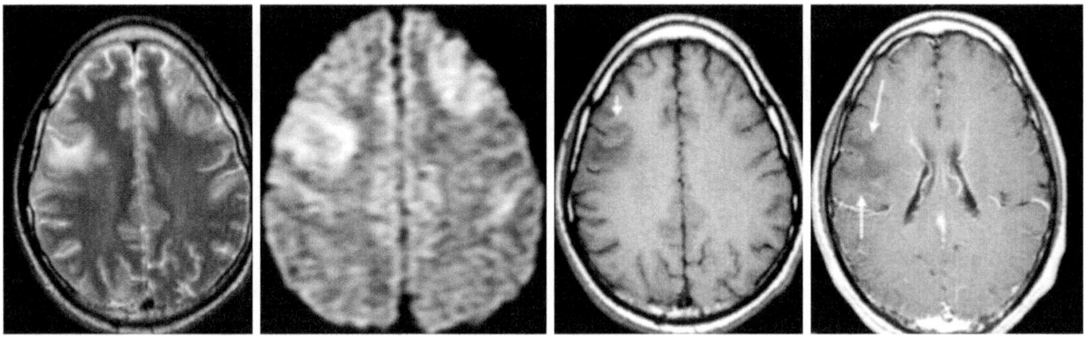

Fig. 2.29 Cocaine abuse, stroke-like symptoms—Toxic Vasculitis from Cocaine. Axial T2, DWI T1 pre and postgad shows: cortico-subcortical right frontal ischemic lesion (white arrows)

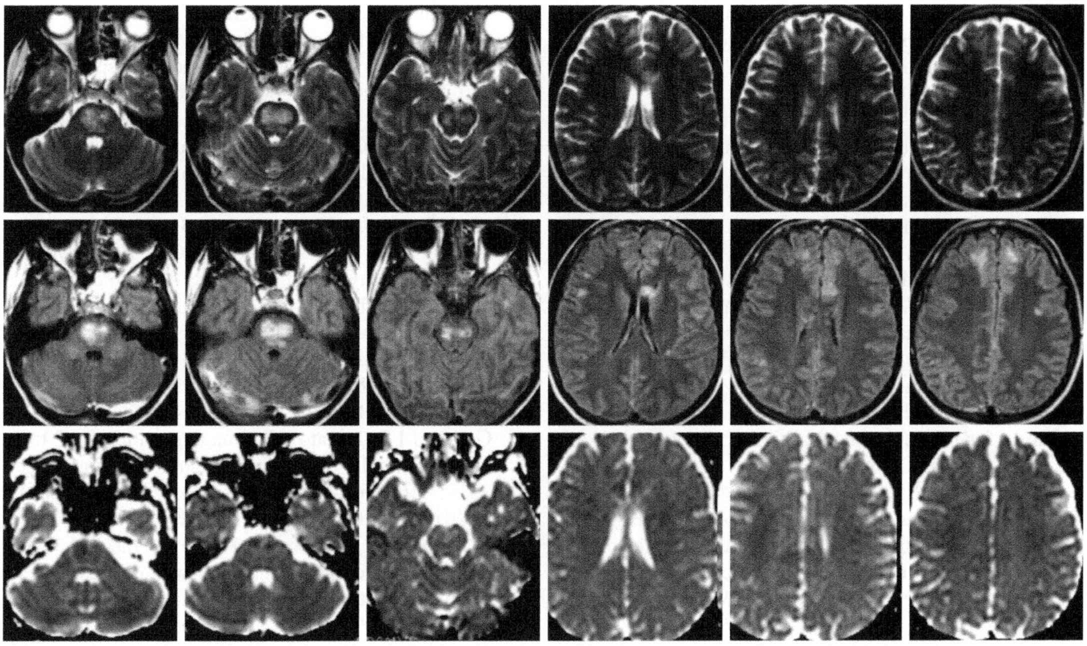

Fig. 2.30 18 y.o, female with cocaine abuse. Acute left hemisyndrome, dysarthria, then coma. Multiple hyperintense lesions with cortical and subcortical location in all the brain, with involvement of the pons, coherent with vascular lesions related to toxic vascular vessels modifications. Upper row: axial T2 images, middle row axial Flair images, lower row corrispondent ADC maps

References

1. Bathla G, Hegde AN. MRI and CT appearances in metabolic encephalopathies due to systemic diseases in adults. Clin Radiol. 2013;68(6):545–54. https://doi.org/10.1016/j.crad.2012.05.021.
2. Gavito-Higuera J MD, Mullins C MD, Gutierrez-Villalobos LI MD, Sandoval H PhD, Shewchuk J MD, Ramos-Duran L MD. MRI of toxic, metabolic, and autoimmune encephalopathies: a review. Appl Radiol. (www.appliedradiology.com January–February. 2020;
3. Chavhan G, Shroff M. Twenty classic signs in neuroradiology: A pictorial essay. Indian J Radiol Imaging. 2009;19(2):135–45. https://doi.org/10.4103/0971-3026.50835.
4. Rabinstein AA, Resnick SJ. Practical neuroimaging in stroke. Philadelphia: Saunders/Elsevier; 2009.
5. Singh D, Sharma A. White cerebellum sign: red flag in the emergency department. CJEM. 2014;16(05):413. https://doi.org/10.2310/8000.2013.131213.
6. Pereira C, De Carvalho A, Rabelo N, Kalkmann G, Crestani L, Santos L. White cerebellum sign: Case Series and Literature Review. Arch Pediat Neurosurg. 2020;2(3(September–December)):e512020. https://doi.org/10.46900/apn.v2i3(september-december).51.
7. Keijzer, H.M. • Hoedemaekers, C.W.E. • Meijer, F.J.A. Brain imaging in comatose survivors of cardiac arrest: pathophysiological correlates and prognostic properties Resuscitation 2018; 133:124–136. https://doi.org/10.1016/j.resuscitation.2018.09.012.
8. Gutierrez, L. • Rovira, À. • Portela, L. CT and MR in non-neonatal hypoxic-ischemic encephalopathy: radiological findings with pathophysiological correlations Neuroradiology 2010; 52:949–976. https://doi.org/10.1007/s00234-010-0728-z.
9. Simard JM, Kent TA, Chen M. Brain oedema in focal ischaemia: molecular pathophysiology and theoretical implications. Lancet Neurol. 2007;6:258–68. https://doi.org/10.1016/S1474-4422(07)70055-8.
10. Huang B, Castillo M. Hypoxic-ischemic brain injury: imaging findings from birth to adulthood. Radiographics. 2008;28(2):417–39.; quiz 617. https://doi.org/10.1148/rg.282075066.
11. Han BK, Towbin RB, De Courten-Myers G, McLaurin RL, Ball WS Jr. Reversal sign on CT: effect of anoxic/ischemic cerebral injury in children. AJNR Am J Neuroradiol. 1989 Nov-Dec;10(6):1191–8
12. Lim C, Hahm M, Lee H. Hepatic Encephalopathy on magnetic resonance imaging and its uncertain differential diagnoses: a narrative review. JYMS. 2023;40(2):136–45. https://doi.org/10.12701/jyms.2022.00689.

13. Geibprasert S, Gallucci M, Krings T. Alcohol-induced changes in the brain as assessed by MRI and CT. Eur Radiol. 2010;20(6):1492–501. https://doi.org/10.1007/s00330-009-1668-z.
14. McKinney AM, Lohman BD, Sarikaya B, et al. Acute hepatic encephalopathy: diffusion-weighted and fluid-attenuated inversion recovery findings, and correlation with plasma ammonia level and clinical outcome. AJNR Am J Neuroradiol. 2010;31(8):1471–9. https://doi.org/10.3174/ajnr.A2112.
15. U-King-Im JM, Yu E, Bartlett E, Soobrah R, Kucharczyk W. Acute hyperammonemic encephalopathy in adults: imaging findings. AJNR. Am J Neuroradiol. 2011;32(2):413–8. https://doi.org/10.3174/ajnr.A2290.
16. Hegde AN, Mohan S, Lath N, et al. Differential diagnosis for bilateral abnormalities of the basal ganglia and thalamus. Radiographics. 2011;31(1):5–30. https://doi.org/10.1148/rg.311105041.
17. Hathout L, Huang J, Zamani A, Morioka C, El-Saden S. White matter changes in chronic alcoholic liver disease: hypothesized association and putative biochemical mechanisms. Med Hypotheses. 2015;85(6):825–34. https://doi.org/10.1016/j.mehy.2015.10.002. Epub 2015 Oct 8.
18. Maffeo E, Montuschi A, Stura G, Giordana MT. Chronic acquired hepatocerebral degeneration, pallidal T1 MRI hyperintensity and manganese in a series of cirrhotic patients. Neurol Sci. 2014;35(4):523–30. https://doi.org/10.1007/s10072-013-1458-x. Epub 2013 May 28. PMID: 23712371 Free articles
19. Arora A, Mukund A, Rajesh S, Patidar Y, Sarin SK. The nervous liver: neurological complications associated with cirrhosis & liver transplantation. New Delhi. https://doi.org/10.1594/ecr2014/C-1397.
20. Long L-L, Li X-R, Huang Z-K, Jiang Y-M, Fu SX, Zheng W. Relationship between changes in brain MRI and 1H-MRS, severity of chronic liver damage, and recovery after liver transplantation. Exp Biol Med (Maywood). 2009;234(9):1075–85. https://doi.org/10.3181/0903-RM-118. Epub 2009 Jun 22.
21. da Rocha AJ, Maia ACM Jr, da Silva CJ, Sachetti SB. Lentiform fork sign in a child with dialysis disequilibrium syndrome: a transient MRI pattern which emphasizes neurologic consequence of metabolic acidosis. Clin Neurol Neurosurg. 2013;115(6):790–2. https://doi.org/10.1016/j.clineuro.2012.07.013. Epub 2012 Aug 14.
22. Vaysman T, Xu P, Vartanian T, Michalak P, Pike K, Liu A. "Highlighting" red nuclei by atypical posterior reversible encephalopathy syndrome in a patient with systemic lupus erythematosus. Clin Case Rep. 2019;7(7):1404–8. https://doi.org/10.1002/ccr3.2245. eCollection 2019 Jul.
23. Kim DM, Lee IH, Song CJ. Uremic encephalopathy: MR imaging findings and clinical correlation. AJNR Am J Neuroradiol. 2016;37(9):1604–9. https://doi.org/10.3174/ajnr.A4776. Epub 2016 Apr 28
24. Yanagawa Y, Isoi N, Tokumaru AM, Sakamoto T, Okada Y. Diffusion-weighted MRI predicts prognosis in severe hypoglycemic encephalopathy. J Clin Neurosci. 2006;13(6):696–9. https://doi.org/10.1016/j.jocn.2005.02.027. Epub 2006 Jul 11.
25. Fujioka M, Okuchi K, Hiramatsu KI, Sakaki T, Sakaguchi S, Ishii Y. Specific changes in human brain after hypoglycemic injury. Stroke. 1997;28(3):584–7. https://doi.org/10.1161/01.str.28.3.584.
26. Chuang KI, Hsieh KL, Chen CY. Hypoglycemic encephalopathy mimicking acute ischemic stroke in clinical presentation and magnetic resonance imaging: a case report. BMC Med Imaging. 2019;19(1):11. https://doi.org/10.1186/s12880-019-0310-z.
27. de Oliveira AM, Paulino MV, Vieira APF, McKinney AM, da Rocha AJ, Dos Santos GT, Leite CDC, Godoy LFS, Lucato LT. Imaging patterns of toxic and metabolic brain disorders. Radiographics. 2019;39(6):1672–95. https://doi.org/10.1148/rg.2019190016.
28. O'Donnell P, Buxton PJ, Pitkin A, Jarvis LJ. The magnetic resonance imaging appearances of the brain in acute carbon monoxide poisoning. Clin Radiol. 2000;55:273–80. https://doi.org/10.1053/crad.1999.0369.
29. Sener RN. Acute carbon monoxide poisoning: diffusion MR imaging findings. AJNR Am J Neuroradiol. 2003;24:1475–7.
30. Kim JH, Chang KH, Song IC, et al. Delayed encephalopathy of acute carbon monoxide intoxication: diffusivity of cerebral white matter lesions. AJNR. 2003;24:1592–7.
31. Lo CP, Chen SY, Lee KW, et al. Brain injury after acute carbon monoxide poisoning: early and late complications. AJR. 2007;189:W205–11. https://doi.org/10.2214/AJR.07.2425.
32. de Cerqueira ACR, dos Reis MC, Novis FD, Bezerra JMF, de Magalhães GC, Rozenthal M, Nardi AE. Cerebellar degeneration secondary to acute lithium carbonate intoxication. Case Reports Arq Neuropsiquiatr. 2008;66(3A):578–80. https://doi.org/10.1590/s0004-282x2008000400032.
33. Ono R, Nishiguchi S, Kitagawa I. Lithium intoxication-associated mild encephalitis/encephalopathy with a reversible splenial lesion: a case report. Case Reports Bipolar Disord. 2022;24(5):551–2. https://doi.org/10.1111/bdi.13242. Epub 2022 Jul 7.
34. Zhao C, Zhang Q, Zhang M, Zhang J, Bao X. Case Report: Metronidazole-induced encephalopathy in a patient with acute myeloid leukemia type 2 and a literature review of the pediatric case reports. Front Pediatr. 2025 Sep 29;13:1656227. https://doi.org/10.3389/fped.2025.1656227.
35. Bhattacharyya S, Darby RR, Raibagkar P, Gonzalez Castro LN, Berkowitz AL. Antibiotic-associated encephalopathy. Neurology. 2016;86:1–9. https://doi.org/10.1212/WNL.0000000000002455.
36. Isaac MFG, et al. MRI characteristics of chemotherapy-related central neurotoxicity: a picto-

rial review. Insights Imaging. 2024;15:56. https://doi.org/10.1186/s13244-023-01602-7.
37. Parasher A, Jhamb R. Posterior reversible encephalopathy syndrome (PRES): presentation, diagnosis and treatment. 2020;96(1140):623–8. https://doi.org/10.1136/postgradmedj-2020-137706. Epub 2020 May 28.
38. Hinchey J, Chaves C, Appignani B, et al. A reversible posterior leukoencephalopathy syndrome. N Engl J Med. 1996;334:494–500. https://doi.org/10.1056/NEJM199602223340803.
39. Onder AM LR, Teomete U, et al. Posterior reversible encephalopathy syndrome in the pediatric renal population. Pediatr Nephrol. 2007;22:1921–9. https://doi.org/10.1007/s00467-007-0578-z.
40. Bartynski WS. Posterior reversible encephalopathy syndrome, part 1: fundamental imaging and clinical features. AJNR Am J Neuroradiol. 2008;29:1036–42. https://doi.org/10.3174/ajnr.A0928.
41. Fugate JE, Rabinstein AA. Posterior reversible encephalopathy syndrome: clinical and radiological manifestations, pathophysiology, and outstanding questions. Lancet Neurol. 2015;14:914–25. https://doi.org/10.1016/S1474-4422(15)00111-8.
42. Mueller Mang C, Mang T, Pirker A, et al. Posterior reversible encephalopathy syndrome: do predisposing risk factors make a difference in MRI appearance? Neuroradiology. 2009;51:373–83. https://doi.org/10.1007/s00234-009-0504-0.
43. Doelken M, Lanz S, Rennert J, et al. Differentiation of cytotoxic and vasogenic edema in a patient with reversible posterior leukoencephalopathy syndrome using diffusion-weighted MRI. Diagn Interv Radiol. 2007;13:125–8.
44. Jennane S, Mahtat EM, Ababou M, El Maaroufi H, Doghmi K. Posterior reversible encephalopathy syndrome secondary to R-CHOP chemotherapy regimen. Cureus. 2022;14(5):e24988. https://doi.org/10.7759/cureus.24988. eCollection 2022 May
45. Aradillas E, Arora R, Gasperino J. Methotrexate-induced posterior reversible encephalopathy syndrome. 2011;36(4):529–36. https://doi.org/10.1111/j.1365-2710.2010.01207. Epub 2010 Sep 30.
46. Newey CR, Chandrasekaran PN, Mohebbi MR. Posterior reversible encephalopathy syndrome after high dose cytarabine in acute myelogenous leukemia. Neurol India. 2017 Jan;65(1):220. https://doi.org/10.4103/0028-3886.198171.
47. Sharma PK, Balachandar S, Vikram MA, Sukumar PD. Rituximab (monoclonal anti-CD20 antibody) induced posterior reversible encephalopathy syndrome (PRES): a case report and literature review. Radiol Case Rep. 2024;20(3):1538–47. https://doi.org/10.1016/jradcr202411070. eCollection 2025 Mar
48. Kazacheuskaya L, Brzezny J, De Alba L, Fowler MR, Traylor JG. Posterior reversible encephalopathy syndrome: a case report with contemporary literature review and neuropathological evidence from autopsy. Cureus. 2025;17(7):e87832. https://doi.org/10.7759/cureus.87832. eCollection 2025 Jul
49. Sheline GE, Wara WM, Smith V. Therapeutic irradiation and brain injury. Int J Radiat Oncol Biol Phys. 1980 Sep;6(9):1215–28. https://doi.org/10.1016/0360-3016(80)90175-3.
50. Jain RS, Gupta PK, Gupta ID, Agrawal R, Kumar S, Tejwani S. Reversible magnetic resonance imaging changes in a case of neuroleptic malignant syndrome. Am J Emerg Med. 2015;33(8):1113-e1. https://doi.org/10.1016/j.ajem.2015.01.029.
51. Zappella N, Perier F, Pico F, Palette C, Muret A, Merceron S, Girbovan A, Marquion F, Legriel S. Duloxetine-related posterior reversible encephalopathy syndrome A case report. Medicine. 2016;95(33):e4556. https://doi.org/10.1097/MD.0000000000004556.
52. Chopra S, Fornito A, Francey SM, O'Donoghue B, Cropley V, Nelson B, Graham J, Baldwin L, Tahtalian S, Yuen HP, Allott K, Alvarez-Jimenez M, Harrigan S, Sabaroedin K, Pantelis C, Wood SJ, McGorry P. Differentiating the effect of antipsychotic medication and illness on brain volume reductions in first-episode psychosis: a longitudinal, randomised, triple-blind, placebo-controlled MRI study. Neuropsychopharmacology. 2021;46:1494–501. https://doi.org/10.1038/s41386-021-00980-0.
53. Haggiag S, Alessandro LP, Carmela S, Carla G, Gasperini TC. Ozone-induced encephalopathy: a novel iatrogenic entity. Eur J Neurol. 28(8):2471–8. https://doi.org/10.1111/ene.14793.
54. Khosravi S, et al. Cerebral gas embolism and multifocal ischemic stroke during oxygen-ozone therapy (full text PMC). BMJ Neurol Open. 2024;6(2):e000885. https://doi.org/10.1136/bmjno-2024-000885.
55. Wu B, Zeng L, Peng K, Shao X, Liu L, Man R, Tang X, Zhong Y. Radiological findings of contrast-induced encephalopathy following cerebral angiography: a case report. Medicine (Baltimore). 2023;102(20):e33855. https://doi.org/10.1097/MD.0000000000033855.
56. Maclean MA, Rogers PS, Muradov JH, Pickett GE, Friedman A, Weeks A, Greene R, Volders D. Contrast-induced encephalopathy and the blood-brain barrier. Can J Neurol Sci. 2025;52(1):85–94. https://doi.org/10.1017/cjn.2024.38. Epub 2024 Mar 8
57. Diamandis E, Swiatek VM, Behme D. Fully reversible contrast-induced encephalopathy mimicking stroke after flow diverter treatment of carotid cave aneurysm. Neurointervention. 2023;18(1):58–62. https://doi.org/10.5469/neuroint.2022.00353.
58. Fowler JS, Volkow ND, Kassed CA, Chang L. Imaging the addicted human brain. Sci Pract Perspect. 2007 Apr;3(2):4–16. https://doi.org/10.1151/spp07324.
59. Eiden C, Vincent M, Serrand C, Serre A, Richard N, Picot MC, et al. Health consequences of cocaine use in France: data from the French Addictovigilance network. Fundam Clin Pharmacol. 2021;35(2):455–65. https://doi.org/10.1111/fcp.12603.

60. Bartzokis G. Age-related brain volume reductions in amphetamine and cocaine addicts and normal controls: implications for addiction research. Psychiatry Res Neuroimaging. 2000;98(2):93–102. https://doi.org/10.1016/s0925-4927(99)00052-9.
61. Beck AT, Steer RA, Brown G. Beck Depression Inventory–II (BDI-II) [Database record]. APA PsycTests. 1996. https://doi.org/10.1037/t00742-000.
62. Beheshti I. Cocaine destroys gray matter brain cells and accelerates brain aging. Biology (Basel). 2023;12(5):752. https://doi.org/10.3390/biology12050752.
63. Ersche KD, Barnes A, Jones PS, Morein-Zamir S, Robbins TW, Bullmore ET. Abnormal structure of frontostriatal brain systems is associated with aspects of impulsivity and compulsivity in cocaine dependence. Brain. 2011 Jul;134(Pt 7):2013–24. https://doi.org/10.1093/brain/awr138.
64. Xu H, Xu C, Guo C. Cocaine use disorder is associated with widespread surface- based alterations of the basal ganglia. J Psychiatr Res. 2023;158:95–103. https://doi.org/10.1016/j.jpsychires.2022.12.006.
65. Xu J, Kober H, Wang X, DeVito EE, Carroll KM, Potenza MN. Hippocampal volume mediates the relationship between measures of pre-treatment cocaine use and within-treatment cocaine abstinence. Drug Alcohol Depend. 2014;143:74–80. https://doi.org/10.1016/j.drugalcdep.2014.07.007.
66. Merkel PA, Koroshetz WJ, Irizarry MC, Cudkowicz ME. Cocaine-associated cerebral vaseulitis. Semin Arthritis Rheum. 1995;125(3):172–83. https://doi.org/10.1016/s0049-0172(95)80029-8.
67. Citron BP, Halpern M, McCarron M, et al. Necrotizing angiitis associated with drug abuse. N Engl J Med. 1970;283:1003–11. https://doi.org/10.1056/NEJM197011052831901.
68. Halpern M, Citron BP. Necrotizing angiitis associated with drug abuse. Am J Roentgenol Radium Therapy, Nucl Med. 1971;111:663–71. https://doi.org/10.2214/ajr.111.4.663.
69. Rumbaugh CL, Bergeron RT, Fang HCH, et al. Cerebral angiographic changes in the drug abuse patient. Radiology. 1971;101:335–44. https://doi.org/10.1148/101.2.335.
70. Glick R, Hoying J, Cerullo L, et al. Phenylpropanolamine: an over-the-counter drug causing central nervous system vasculitis and intracerebral hemorrhage. Neurosurgery. 1987;20:969–74. https://doi.org/10.1227/00006123-198706000-00027.
71. Forman HP, Levin S, Stewart B, et al. Cerebral tomography. Br J Psych. 1988;152:641–8.
72. Tumeh SS, Nagel JS, English RJ, et al. Cerebral abnormalities in cocaine abusers: demonstration by SPECT perfusion brain scintigraphy. Radiology. 1990;176:821–4. https://doi.org/10.1148/radiology.176.3.2389042.
73. Volpe JJ. Effect of cocaine use on the fetus. N Engl J Med. 1992;327:399–407. https://doi.org/10.1056/NEJM199208063270607.
74. Devenyi P, Schneiderman JF, Devenyi RG, et al. Cocaine-induced central retinal artery occlusion. CMAJ. 1988;138:129–30.
75. Rumbaugh CL, Fang HCH, Higgins RE, et al. Cerebral microvascular injury in experimental drug abuse. Investig Radiol. 1976;11:282–94. https://doi.org/10.1097/00004424-197607000-00005.
76. Leeds NE, Malhotra V, Zimmerman RD. The radiology of drug addiction affecting the brain. Semin Roentgenol. 1983;3:227–33. https://doi.org/10.1016/0037-198x(83)90027-5.

Long-Term Post-radiation Injury of the Central Nervous System: Neuroradiological Clues for Diagnosis

3

Marialuisa Zedde and Rosario Pascarella

3.1 Introduction

Radiation therapy is used to address a broad spectrum of malignant and benign conditions affecting the brain, skull base, and nearby structures, with both curative and palliative objectives. The most commonly employed administration modality is external beam radiation using photon therapy, in the form of X-rays or gamma rays. X-ray photon treatments can easily penetrate tissues and are typically prescribed in daily sessions (fractions) using a linear accelerator, with the total radiation dose delivered over several weeks. The exact dose fractionation depends on the type of target and clinical indication. Some smaller tumors, such as vestibular schwannomas and meningiomas, can be treated with a single session of radiation therapy (stereotactic radiosurgery) or a limited number of sessions (stereotactic radiotherapy), whereas larger tumors like gliomas require multiple fractions, usually over 3–6 weeks. Alternative delivery platforms include Gamma Knife (Elekta, Stockholm, Sweden) or CyberKnife (Accuray, California), which can provide more conformal radiation dose distributions to smaller targets. However, techniques for performing stereotactic treatments on standard linear accelerator platforms have also been developed and continue to evolve [1].

Proton beam therapy utilizes the specific physical properties associated with the dose deposition of a particle beam in tissue, notably that most of the energy is delivered at the end of its range, just before the particle comes to rest—known as the Bragg peak. When planned correctly, this can increase the dose delivered to the clinical target while minimizing the dose to normal tissues beyond the Bragg peak. There are two main indications for proton beam therapy in clinical practice: for dose escalation to radioresistant tumors such as skull base chordoma or chondrosarcoma, at sites where standard photon radiotherapy cannot deliver the necessary dose due to the proximity of critical structures; and to reduce radiation therapy toxicities to the brain and surrounding soft tissues, particularly in children, teenagers, and young adults, for whom the adverse effects of irradiating the developing brain are more significant.

M. Zedde (✉)
Neurology Unit, Stroke Unit, Azienda Unità Sanitaria Locale-IRCCS di Reggio Emilia, Reggio Emilia, Italy
e-mail: zedde.marialuisa@ausl.re.it

R. Pascarella
Neuroradiology Unit, Ospedale Santa Maria della Misericordia, AULSS 5 Polesana, Rovigo, Italy
e-mail: rosario.pascarella@aulss5.veneto.it

M. Zedde, R. Pascarella (eds.), *Neuroimaging of Treatment-Related Conditions in the Brain*,
https://doi.org/10.1007/978-3-032-23618-0_3

3.2 Mechanisms of Radiation Injury

Irradiation of tissue generates various types of DNA damage through the production of highly reactive free radicals, including single-strand breaks, double-strand breaks (the primary lethal lesion), base damage, and DNA crosslinks. Numerous DNA damage repair mechanisms are in place to help maintain genomic stability. However, some lesions are not adequately repaired, and the accumulation of these unrepaired lesions can eventually result in cell death. This can occur through programmed mechanisms such as apoptosis or autophagy, or via mitotic catastrophe during a future cell division. If the damage does not result in cell death, it may lead to late-onset radiation effects via highly reactive free radicals, including single-strand breaks, double-strand breaks (the primary lethal lesion), base damage, and DNA crosslinks. Multiple DNA damage repair mechanisms function to maintain genomic stability. However, some lesions fail to repair properly, leading to their accumulation, which can eventually cause cell death through programmed mechanisms such as apoptosis or autophagy, or via mitotic catastrophe during future cell divisions. If the damage does not result in cell death, it may lead to long-term effects of radiation exposure, such as the development of secondary tumors, sometimes manifesting several years or decades later.

The exact mechanisms responsible for radiation toxicity in the nervous system are not fully understood. Various hypotheses have been proposed to explain radiation-induced neurocognitive decline, supported by a range of preclinical and clinical data. Evidence suggests that radiation reduces neurogenesis in the hippocampus, with preclinical models indicating a depletion of neural progenitor cells over multiple cell divisions. Changes in the cellular microenvironment also play a crucial role in determining cell fate and reducing neurogenesis. Radiation-induced oxidative stress leads to the upregulation of proinflammatory pathways and an increase in the number of activated microglia, which serve as potent inhibitors of neurogenesis. Additionally, radiation can induce endothelial cell death, causing thrombus formation on the exposed matrix and small vessel occlusion. Accelerated atherosclerosis and microangiopathy following radiation can result in vascular encephalopathy and infarction [1].

In the central nervous system (CNS), radiation effects can be broadly categorized into those affecting vascular endothelial cells and direct effects on neuroglial cells, particularly oligodendroglial cells [2]. Vascular endothelial damage can lead to altered permeability, resulting in vasogenic edema and disruption of the blood–brain barrier (BBB) or blood–spinal cord barrier. Preclinical studies suggest that endothelial damage may occur within the first 24 h after irradiation [3]. Subsequent late vascular effects may include telangiectasia, thrombosis, occlusion of small vessels, fibrinoid deposits, and hyaline thickening of vessel walls [2], potentially leading to ischemic stroke or hemorrhage months to years after radiation therapy [4]. Oligodendrocytes are notably sensitive to radiation, with cell death occurring relatively early even at low doses of irradiation [2]. Radiation not only reduces the number of mature oligodendrocytes but also induces loss of their precursors, the oligodendrocyte type 2 astrocyte. This failure to replace normally turned over oligodendrocytes ultimately leads to demyelination [2].

Moreover, radiation induces changes in cellular composition such as increased numbers of reactive astrocytes (gliosis) and microglia [2]. These reactive cells have been reported to produce reactive oxygen species, proinflammatory cytokines, and growth factors (e.g., vascular endothelial growth factor [VEGF]), leading to a cycle of further cellular toxic effects and tissue damage [2]. Experimental studies [5] increasingly indicate that radiation is cytotoxic to proliferating neuroglial progenitor cells, including neural stem cells, neuronal precursor cells, and glial precursor cells. Chronic damage to these progenitor cell populations responsible for hippocampal neurogenesis and white matter integrity may play a significant role in late delayed radiation-induced neurotoxic effects, including cognitive impairment and white matter disease [5].

3.3 Late Complications

In the CNS too, radiation-induced injury can be categorized into three phases based on the time of expression: acute, early delayed, and late delayed. Acute and early delayed injuries are typically transient and reversible, while late delayed injuries tend to be irreversible. Neuroradiologists play a crucial role in correctly interpreting imaging studies following RT by being familiar with the expected imaging appearances and distinguishing them from tumor recurrence. Key factors in recognizing radiation-induced changes on follow-up imaging include:

1. Time Elapsed Since RT: The duration since radiation therapy is vital in understanding the expected changes. Acute effects may manifest within days to weeks after treatment, while early delayed effects can occur within a few months. Late delayed effects often emerge several months to years after RT.
2. Location of the Target Lesion: Understanding the location of the target lesion helps in assessing the specific areas that may exhibit radiation-induced changes. Different regions of the body may respond differently to radiation therapy, and recognizing these patterns is essential for accurate interpretation.
3. Inclusion of Normal Structures: The extent to which normal structures are included in the radiation field influences the potential for radiation-induced changes. Structures within the radiation field may exhibit alterations over time, while those outside the field typically remain unaffected.

Neuroradiologists rely on their expertise and knowledge of these factors to differentiate between expected postradiation changes and signs of tumor recurrence, ensuring appropriate patient management and care.

Late-onset complications from radiation therapy typically emerge 6–12 months post-treatment, though they can be delayed for several years or even decades. The most significant issues are radionecrosis and late-delayed radiation encephalopathy, but several other complications might be considered, as given in Table 3.1.

3.4 Brain

3.4.1 Leukoencephalopathy

For many years, it has been established that radiotherapy can lead to delayed cognitive impairments, ranging from mild memory loss to severe dementia [6]. This complication is more commonly seen in adult survivors of childhood brain tumors and in patients with low-grade gliomas where the tumor remains in remission for extended periods [7]. The MRI hallmarks of these patients are typically varying degrees of high T2-weighted signal changes in the subcortical white matter and brain atrophy (Figs. 3.1 and 3.2). While some patients experience a gradual decline, most remain stable. In some cases, cerebral atrophy can be strikingly focal, affecting specific lobes of the brain that have been

Table 3.1 Delayed CNS complications following radiation therapy

Brain	Spine
Parenchymal injury	*Secondary neoplasms*
Leukoencephalopathy	Osteoradionecrosis
Radiation-induced secondary normal pressure hydrocephalus	Spinal cord myelopathy
Radiation necrosis	Secondary neoplasms
Stroke-like migraine attacks after RT (SMART syndrome)[a]	
Radiation-induced vasculopathy	
Steno-occlusive and moyamoya-like vasculopathy	
Intracranial aneurysm	
Cavernous malformation (hemorrhagic vasculopathy)	
Mineralizing microangiopathy (dystrophic calcification)	
Chronic expanding encapsulated hematoma	
Other structures	
Cranial nerve injury	
Endocrine complications	

[a]It will be discussed in a separate chapter

irradiated. Unfortunately, there is no recognized treatment for this syndrome, although some authors suggest using anticholinesterases for symptomatic relief [8].

Its pathophysiological mechanisms involve damage to oligodendrocytes, resulting in axonal demyelination and disruption of vascular endothelial cells. This disruption leads to coagulative necrosis, vessel thickening, and focal mineralization [9, 10].

Radiation-induced leukoencephalopathy may initially be subclinical but can progress to cognitive deficits, including impairments in learning, memory, executive function, attention, and concentration. In some cases, these deficits may advance to dementia and gait disturbance [5, 9]. Cognitive impairments are frequently observed following whole-brain RT [9]. It has been suggested that cognitive dysfunction is correlated with the volume and amount of irradiated tissue in the hippocampus dentate gyrus due to the presence of neural stem cells [5, 9]. Consequently, sparing the hippocampus has become a crucial consideration in the treatment planning process [9, 11].

The long-term cognitive effects of radiotherapy in patients with low-grade gliomas were highlighted in a study [12] that compared 195 patients with low-grade gliomas (104 of whom had undergone radiotherapy) with a matched group of patients with low-grade hematological malignancies and healthy controls, all followed for at least 6 years. This study found that patients with low-grade gliomas faced significant challenges in various health-related quality of life domains, including neurocognitive deficits, primarily associated with tumor changes. Notably, only high-dose per fraction radiotherapy (>2 Gy) resulted in significant additional cognitive decline. Follow-up findings after 12 years indicated that even doses less than 2 Gy/fraction led to progressive declines in attentional and executive functions and information processing speed. 53% of patients who received radiotherapy developed cognitive deficits in at least five out of 18 neuropsychological test areas, compared to 27% of patients who had not undergone radiation therapy [13].

Until the last decade, whole brain radiotherapy was the standard treatment for brain metastases but caused cognitive decline in over 60% of patients within 2–6 months post-treatment [14]. This approach has now been largely replaced by stereotactic radiosurgery for fit patients with stable or controlled extracranial disease and a reasonable prognosis of at least 6 months. Hippocampal-sparing techniques are becoming more popular for patients unsuitable for stereotactic radiosurgery, although these methods have not yet consistently demonstrated cognitive benefits.

In patients with primary CNS lymphoma traditionally treated with combined high-dose intravenous methotrexate chemotherapy followed by whole brain radiotherapy, the incidence of severe cognitive impairment increases with age, reaching 83% in patients over 60 years old [15]. Based on the findings of a randomized phase 2 study by a European consortium (IELSG-32 study), the standard care for fit patients under 70 years with primary CNS lymphoma in Europe now involves a chemotherapy regimen known as Methotrexate, Ara-C, Thiotepa, and Rituximab (MATRIX), followed by autologous stem cell transplantation. This strategy avoids the use of whole brain radiotherapy, thereby reducing the risk of potentially fatal neurotoxicity [16].

The incidence of radiation-induced leukoencephalopathy varies among previous reports but tends to increase with longer follow-up periods. For instance, in patients who underwent whole-brain RT for brain metastases, the incidence of radiation-induced leukoencephalopathy was approximately 30% at 6-months post-treatment, rising to 100% by 3 years [9]. Risk factors associated with radiation-induced leukoencephalopathy include higher total radiation dose, higher dose per fraction, and a larger volume of tissue irradiated. Additionally, the use of concurrent or sequential chemotherapy, particularly methotrexate, may significantly heighten the incidence and severity of radiation-induced leukoencephalopathy [5].

Radiation-induced leukoencephalopathy typically presents specific imaging characteristics [17]. On T2-weighted or fluid-attenuated

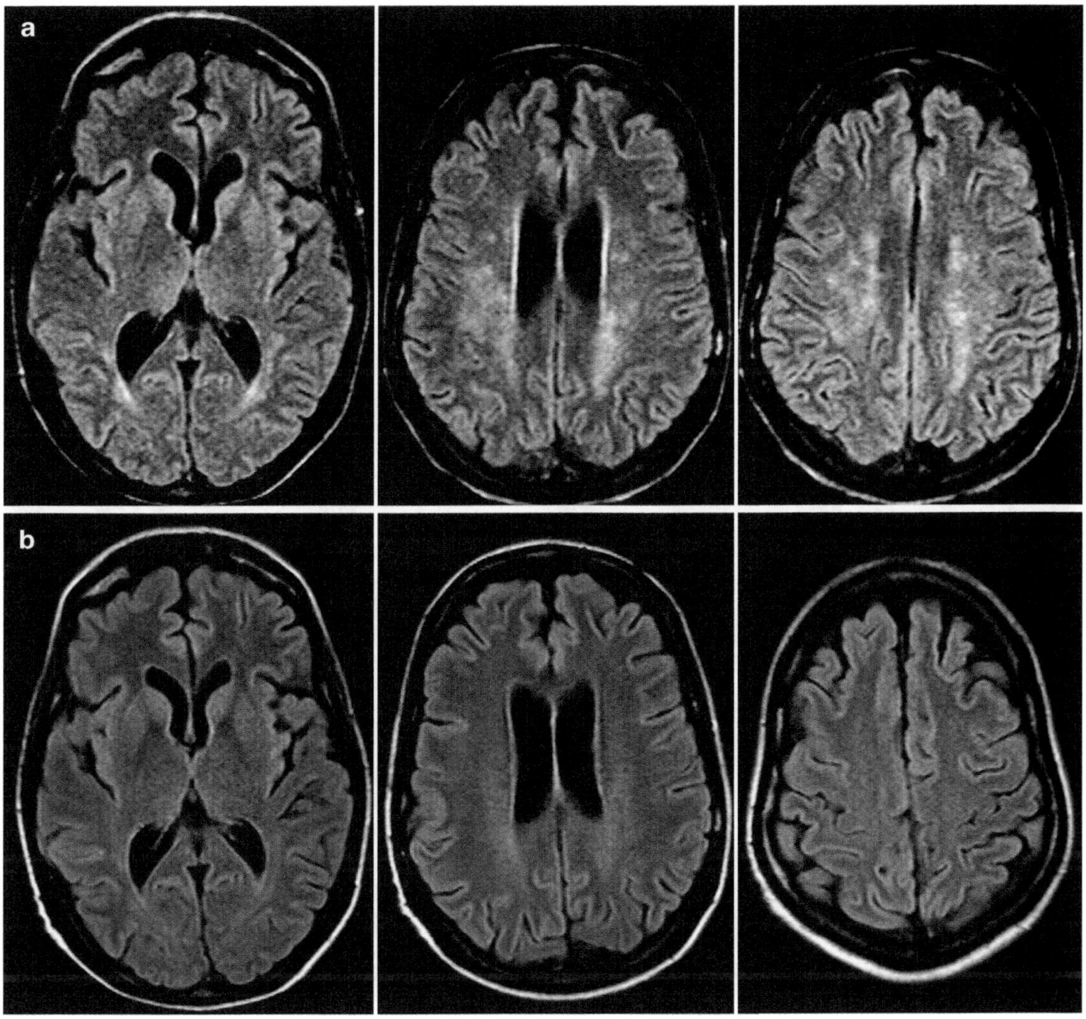

Fig. 3.1 Brain MRI (axial FLAIR) of the same patient in this figure and Fig. 3.2 year after radiation therapy (panel **a**) and before radiation therapy (panel **b**)

inversion-recovery (FLAIR) images, cerebral white matter appears with high signal intensity. Notably, there is usually an absence of enhancement or significant mass effect [5, 9, 10]. In cases following whole-brain RT, radiation-induced leukoencephalopathy typically demonstrates diffuse and symmetric involvement. Notably, certain areas like the subcortical U-fiber, corpus callosum, and gray matter may show relative sparing [9]. The progression of white matter lesions typically initiates around the periventricular white matter and advances to diffuse white matter changes over time, often accompanied by varying degrees of cerebral atrophy. This progression can unfold gradually over months to years [5, 9].

3.4.2 Radiation-Induced Secondary Normal Pressure Hydrocephalus

Radiation-induced dementia is characterized by a pattern of "subcortical dementia" associated with diffuse white matter injury, typically emerging within 2 years post-treatment. Patients may exhibit symptoms similar to normal pressure hydrocephalus, including progressive memory loss, decreased

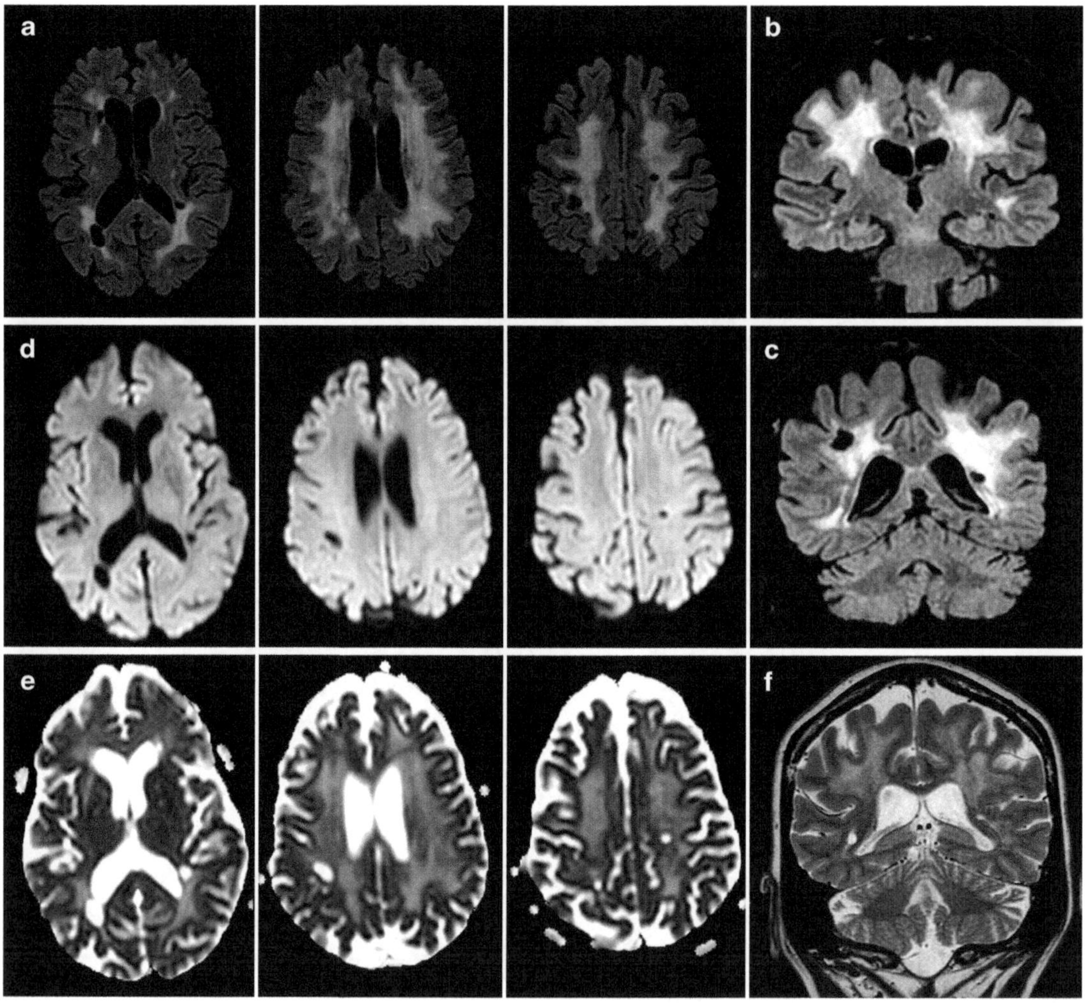

Fig. 3.2 Brain MRI with severe postradiation leukoencephalopathy found 15 years after radiation therapy. Panel **a** shows axial FLAIR sequences with severe, extensive, confluent supratentorial white matter hyperintensity neat to the cortical–subcortical junction and some cavitated lesion within it. Panel **b** shows the corresponding coronal FLAIR, highlighting both features, i.e. the involvement of the cortical-subcortical junction from leukoencephalopathy and the presence of multiple cavitated lesions. Panels **c** and **d** show the corresponding axial DWI and ADC map, where the leukoencephalopathy appears hypointense and slightly hyperintense, respectively. Panel **f** shows the coronal T2W sequence with the same features as in panel **b**

attention, gait difficulties, urinary incontinence, and fatigue. Emotional lability and apathy are common and can be challenging to distinguish from depression. While antidepressants are frequently used, they do not improve cognitive function. Over time, patients may develop akinetic mutism. MRI scans reveal ventricular enlargement, diffuse confluent subcortical white matter changes, and cortical and subcortical atrophy.

Currently, there is no specific treatment for radiation-induced dementia. Ventriculoperitoneal shunting [18] is occasionally attempted, offering incomplete and short-lived improvement. Unfortunately, deterioration occurs in about 80% of cases, and death generally follows within 4 years after the onset of the disorder.

3.4.3 Radiation Necrosis

Radionecrosis is the most common late complication of radiation therapy, first described pathologically in 1948 [19] in patients with conditions such as recurrent "rodent ulcer of the scalp" and a normal brain. It can be challenging to differentiate from tumor recurrence both clinically and radiologically. Today, radionecrosis most often follows focal radiation therapy for brain metastases, but it can also occur in patients treated for extracranial and extra-axial tumors, where normal brain tissue was included within the radiation field, such as in head and neck cancer, skull osteosarcoma, pituitary adenoma, and clival chordoma. A typical example is bilateral medial temporal lobe necrosis following radiation therapy for pituitary tumors or nasopharyngeal cancer.

Cerebral radiation necrosis represents a severe late delayed complication that typically appears after a latency period of several months, though cases have been reported even more than 10 years after irradiation [10, 20–22]. Histopathological examination of radiation necrosis reveals fibrinoid changes in blood vessels, coagulative necrosis, demyelination, and gliosis [10, 20]. The disruption of the BBB, visualized on gadolinium-enhanced images, may be partly mediated through VEGF released in response to hypoxia [2].

The reported incidence of radiation necrosis following RT for brain tumors varies from 3% to 24% [20, 23, 24]. Radiation necrosis is more likely to occur with the administration of high doses per fraction, and the combined use of chemotherapy with RT may also contribute to its development [24]. Additionally, targeted therapy and immunotherapy may increase the risk of treatment-related necrosis [25].

This complication is now less common due to reductions in dose per fraction and advancements in radiation therapy delivery. It is recognized that administering a "safe dose" of 55–60 Gy to a focal field with daily fractions of 1.8–2 Gy carries less than a 5% risk of radionecrosis. Patients with vascular risk factors, such as hypertension, diabetes, and advanced age, are at higher risk, as are those undergoing concomitant chemotherapy [26–30]. Some patients without specific risk factors may develop radionecrosis due to increased sensitivity to radiation at conventional dose fractionation [31].

Currently, radionecrosis most frequently occurs after stereotactic radiosurgery, such as Gamma Knife treatment for brain metastases (affecting 5–25% of cases) and non-neoplastic conditions like arteriovenous malformations (up to 20% of cases). The symptoms of radionecrosis are indistinguishable from those of tumor recurrence or progression, and brain imaging shows similar patterns. Recently, an MRI sequence with delayed contrast known as TRAMS (treatment response assessment maps) or contrast clearance analysis has become routine in clinical practice due to its sensitivity and specificity [32]. This involves acquiring two standard 3D T1-weighted MRI brain scans—one five minutes after gadolinium injection and another an hour later. The first series is digitally subtracted from the second, resulting in high-resolution, volumetric maps that distinguish regions of contrast clearance (blue) from contrast accumulation (red). Radionecrosis appears red due to poor contrast clearance in non-viable tissue with irradiated vessels, while tumor recurrence appears blue due to rapid clearance through tumor vasculature (Fig. 3.3).

Radiation necrosis typically arises at or near the original tumor site, which received the highest radiation dose [33]. However, it can also occur in parts of the normal brain parenchyma encompassed within the treatment field of a tumor located outside the brain. For example, some patients treated for nasopharyngeal cancer may develop temporal lobe necrosis. Symptoms resulting from localized brain necrosis depend on the lesion's location and may include focal neurologic deficits or more generalized signs and symptoms of increased intracranial pressure.

In many instances, radiation necrosis resolves spontaneously and can be managed conservatively without intervention. However, symptomatic relief may be necessary for some patients, often achieved through the administration of steroids and resection of necrotic tissue. Corticosteroid dependence can occur. Other treatments, such as hyperbaric oxygen or drugs like pentoxifylline, alpha-tocopherol, and pentobarbital, have been tried without clear evidence of efficacy. A recent systematic review concluded that bevacizumab [34, 35] appears to be more effective and just as safe as corticosteroids.

Conventional MRI typically reveals an enhancing mass lesion with central necrosis and reactive edema [20, 22, 36]. The enhancement pattern is often described as a "spreading wavefront," where the margins of enhancement are ill-defined, or as "soap bubble-like" or "Swiss cheese-like," indicating that the enhancing lesion includes central nonenhancing necrotic components of varying size [20]. Multiple lesions may be present, and some lesions may develop distant from the original tumor site if the distant site was within the radiation field [20, 22]. As radiation necrosis progresses with tumor-like growth, it can lead to marked shrinkage of the white matter and cortex, resulting in focal brain atrophy [20]. The periventricular white matter is among the areas most susceptible to radiation necrosis [20]. This vulnerability may be explained by the relatively poor blood supply from long medullary arteries lacking collateral vessels, making it susceptible to ischemic effects produced by postirradiation vasculopathy [20].

Imaging findings of radiation necrosis are not always irreversible and progressive but can be static, decrease, or even resolve at follow-up. For instance, Wang et al. [33] retrospectively analyzed the MRI features of the temporal lobes in patients previously treated with radiation for nasopharyngeal cancer. They found that T2-hyperintense white matter lesions were the earliest and most common manifestation after RT, followed by enhancing lesions, which often became necrotic with increasing size. Both white matter lesions and enhancing lesions were more likely than cysts to regress and could show complete resolution. Cysts were the least frequent pattern of radiation-induced injury and typically developed from enhancing lesions that exhibited necrosis.

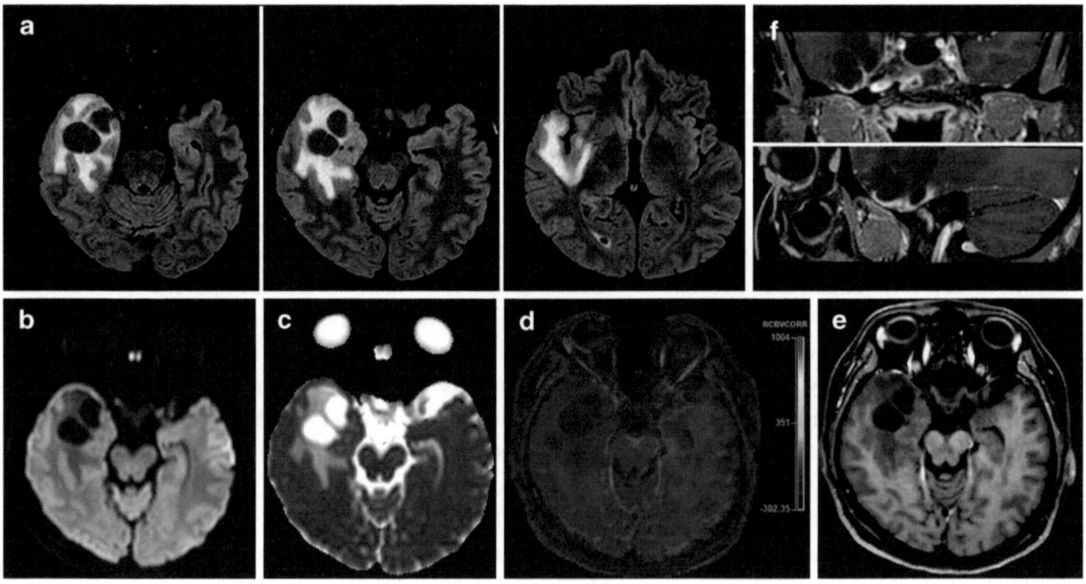

Fig. 3.3 Radionecrosis in a patient treated by surgery and radiation therapy because of a right temporal bone chondrosarcoma, showing the confluent white matter hyperintensity surrounding the surgical cavity and extending to the insular region (panel **a**, axial FLAIR) with corresponding hypointense signal in DWI (panel **b**) and slightly hyperintense signal on ADC maps (panel **c**), low CBV on MR perfusion (panel **d**) and absence of lesional contrast enhancement on postcontrast T1W (axial panel **e**, coronal and sagittal in panel **f**). In panels **e** and **f**, there is a focal contrast enhancement in the pachymeningeal layer of the right anterior fossa

Radiologic features of radiation necrosis at conventional imaging can overlap with those of recurrent tumors, including high-grade primary brain tumors and brain metastases, making image interpretation challenging. This issue is the topic of Chap. 5 of this book.

3.4.4 Radiation-Induced Vasculopathy

Radiation can damage intracranial vasculature, leading to ischemic stroke or hemorrhage. The carotid artery can become stenotic after cervical radiotherapy for lymphomas or head and neck cancers and may occasionally rupture a few weeks post-treatment, causing death. However, late-delayed complications are more frequent and generally occur many years after treatment, with a median onset of about 20 years for extracranial arteries and 7 years for intracranial arteries. Radiation-induced vasculopathy is an accelerated form of atherosclerosis and often occurs in unusual locations, such as the distal internal carotid artery (ICA). It has been observed within 2 years of proton beam therapy for childhood brain tumors [27–31].

The lesions typically consist of one or more arterial stenoses or occlusions of the carotid or cerebral arteries within the radiation portal. Pathological findings include the destruction of the internal elastic lamina and the replacement of the normal intima and media with fibrous tissue. Treatment involves managing vascular risk factors and, where appropriate, performing carotid endarterectomy. However, surgery can be more challenging due to vascular fibrosis and poor wound healing. If a patient with a history of radiation therapy develops a stroke, it should not be assumed to be due to radiation vasculopathy unless it is within the radiation portal, and other risk factors should be considered (Fig. 3.4).

3.4.4.1 Moyamoya-Like Arteriopathy

Steno-occlusive vasculopathy of the large cerebral arteries may evolve slowly after irradiation and predominantly affects patients younger than 18 years at the time of RT [37]. In a retrospective study [38] of 75 consecutive pediatric patients with primary brain tumors treated with proton RT, the crude incidence of radiation-induced steno-occlusive vasculopathy was approximately 6.7%. The terminal internal carotid artery (ICA) and the major branches of the circle of Willis are especially vulnerable [37, 39]. Patients with suprasellar or chiasmatic lesions have a high risk for this complication because these tumors often require intense RT near the circle of Willis [37, 39].

Clinical manifestations of radiation-induced steno-occlusive vasculopathy include transient ischemic attacks, infarcts, and seizures [37, 39]. Histologic studies have revealed subintimal collections of foam cells with myointimal proliferation, broadly characterized as premature or accelerated arteriosclerosis. At imaging, there is wall thickening and enhancement of the large cerebral arteries, resulting in a stenotic or occlusive state. The terminal parts of the ICA and its branches, such as the middle cerebral artery, are most frequently involved, and multivessel involvement is common [40]. Furthermore, moyamoya-like collateral circulation and transdural anastomoses may be observed [37, 39, 40].

Risk factors for developing radiation-induced moyamoya-like vasculopathy include young age at the time of RT, high radiation dose, combined chemotherapy, and comorbid neurofibromatosis type 1 (NF1) [37]. In a review of 345 children treated with RT for a primary brain tumor, 12 patients (3.5%) developed evidence of moyamoya-like vasculopathy [38]. The onset of moyamoya-like vasculopathy was more rapid in patients with NF1 and those who received more than 50 Gy of radiation to the optic chiasm. Children with NF1 treated for optic pathway glioma have a high risk for radiation-induced moyamoya-like vasculopathy and may develop this vasculopathy earlier than non-neurofibromatosis patients or after lower radiation exposure. The risk of infarction is higher in patients with radiation-induced moyamoya-like vasculopathy than in those with idiopathic moyamoya disease [38].

The strong association between neurofibromatosis type 1 and moyamoya disease is one reason

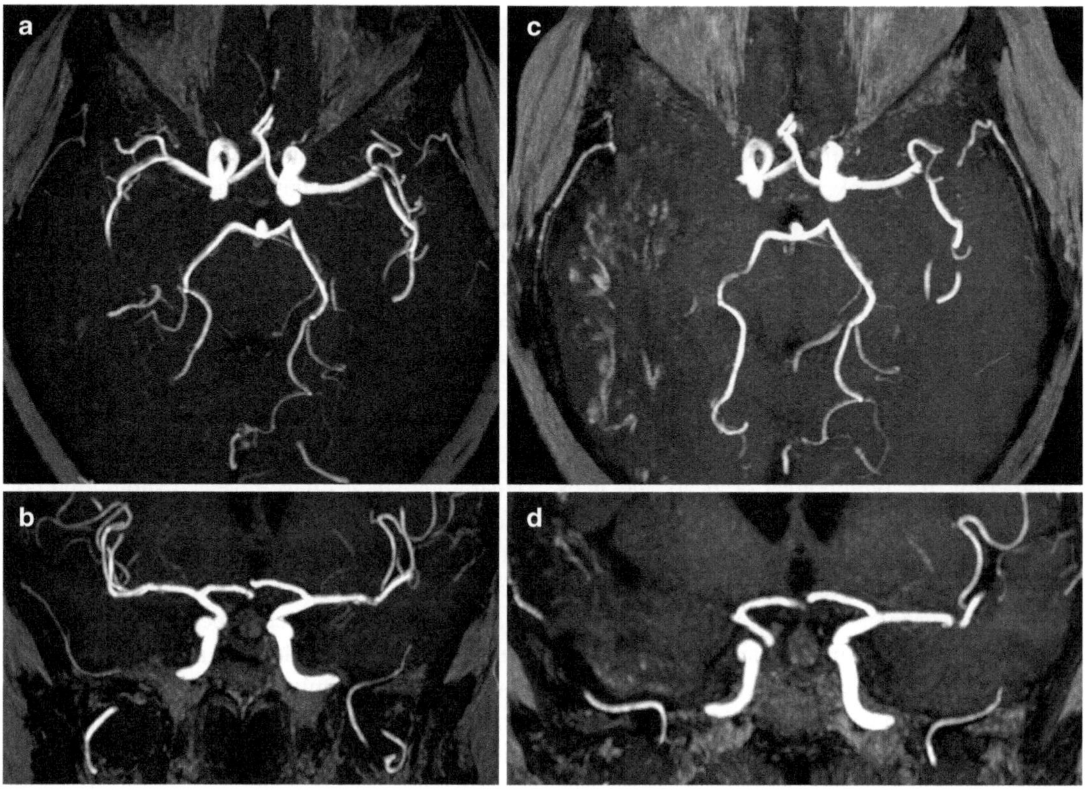

Fig. 3.4 MRA of the same patient in Fig. 3.5 reconstructed in MIP/MPR in axial (**a** and **c**) and coronal (**b** and **d**) plane, showing the evolution of radiation-induces arteriopathy from 10 years after radiation (**a** and **b**) with focal left M2 stenosis and 16 years after radiation (**c** and **d**) with right MCA steno-occlusion

why radiation therapy has been largely replaced by chemotherapy in young children with optic pathway gliomas. Treatment focuses on preventing further strokes through surgical revascularization procedures.

3.4.4.2 Radiation-Induced Intracranial Aneurysms

Radiation-induced intracranial aneurysms are rare but potentially fatal complications of RT that may develop across a wide age group [41]. They can be discovered during routine radiologic follow-up or incidentally during workup for other symptoms. A review [41] of patients irradiated for various tumors found that 46 patients developed 69 intracranial aneurysms within the irradiated fields over a median period of 12 years. The lag time between RT and diagnosis may be shorter in patients older than 40 years, potentially due to increased follow-up diagnostic procedures. Stereotactic radiosurgery may also shorten the lag time due to the high-energy focused radiation received by a vessel during the procedure.

The pathogenesis of radiation-induced aneurysms is speculative, but injuries to endothelial cells, elastic lamina, and smooth muscle cells of the involved vessels have been proposed as primary mechanisms. Accelerated atherosclerosis secondary to irradiation may also contribute to aneurysm formation. Radiation-induced intracranial aneurysms are more likely to be saccular, with a higher incidence in the anterior circulation and a high likelihood of multiple aneurysms in a single patient. These aneurysms may originate directly from the arterial wall rather than from a branching site like ordinary saccular aneurysms, possibly due to vessel wall degradation caused by radiation. Combined with weaken-

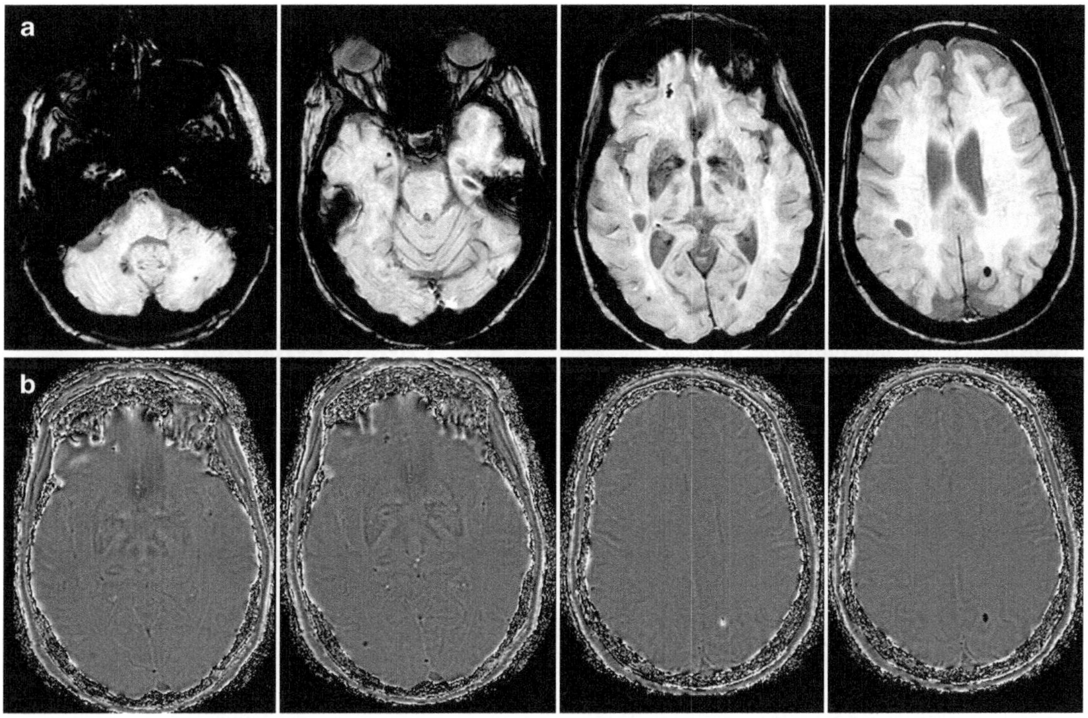

Fig. 3.5 Brain MRI (axial SWI images in panel **a** and phase images in panel **b**) showing the coexistence of SWI focal hypointensities with a different signal in the phase images, referring to both de novo telangiectasias and calcification (as for mineralizing angiopathy)

ing of the vessel wall, constant shear pressure may precipitate changes leading to formation of saccular and fusiform aneurysms, pseudoaneurysms, and eventual rupture. The reported frequency of rupture is greater than expected for non–radiation-induced aneurysms, although selection bias may influence reporting tendencies [41].

3.4.4.3 Radiation-Induced Cavernous Malformations

RT is associated with the development of cavernous malformations in the CNS [42]. The cumulative incidence of cerebral cavernous malformations following RT is approximately 3–4% at 10 years, 7–14% at 20 years, and potentially as high as 60% at 25 years [43]. These radiation-induced cavernous malformations are more common in pediatric patients than in adults [42, 44]. Children aged 10 years or younger at the time of RT have a shorter latency period and an increased incidence of cavernous malformations [44]. Studies have shown a correlation between radiation doses greater than 30 Gy and shorter latency periods for the development of these malformations. While spinal cord cavernous malformations after irradiation are rare, they have been reported. When present, their main risk is intracranial hemorrhage, but this is rare [45].

The mechanism underlying the development of radiation-induced cavernous malformations likely involves vascular injury. Radiation causes endothelial proliferation with hyalinization and fibrinoid necrosis of the vessel walls, leading to ischemia and infarction due to narrowing of the vascular lumen [44]. Ischemia activates hypoxia-inducible factor 1 (HIF-1), which induces vascular endothelial growth factor (VEGF), promoting reactive angiogenesis. The expression of these factors decreases with age, indicating that the origin of acquired cavernous malformations is more frequent at younger ages.

MRI typically shows a reticulated core of heterogeneous signal intensity on T2-weighted images with a dark peripheral rim of hemosiderin [42]. Cavernous malformations can be detected as multiple hypointense lesions on T2*-weighted images and are better identified with susceptibility-weighted imaging [46]. Some lesions may increase in size over time [42]. Compared with non-radiation-induced cavernous malformations, radiation-induced cavernous malformations are more likely to present as multiple lesions, manifest at a younger age, and are at least as likely to cause symptomatic hemorrhage [42].

3.4.5 Mineralizing Microangiopathy (Dystrophic Calcification)

Mineralizing microangiopathy with dystrophic calcification is a distinctive histopathologic process affecting the microvasculature of the CNS [47]. It typically develops after combined CNS irradiation and chemotherapy in childhood, though it can also occur following RT alone [10, 47]. An autopsy study of children with leukemia treated with cranial irradiation found mineralizing microangiopathy in 28 (17%) of 163 patients, with detection as early as 10 months post-RT [48].

Histologically, calcification in mineralizing microangiopathy occurs in the walls of precapillary arterioles, capillaries, venules, and smaller arteries such as the lenticulostriate artery. Dystrophic calcification also develops in the perivascular neural tissue due to mineralization of plasma fluids leaking from damaged vessels and regional ischemia from circulatory impairment. The patient's age at the time of CNS irradiation significantly impacts the development of mineralizing microangiopathy, with a higher risk in children under 10 years old who have undergone RT [47].

CT scans typically show multiple punctate foci of calcification, mainly involving the basal ganglia and subcortical white matter. Calcification may also be present in the cerebellar structures and brainstem. On MRI, calcified areas may exhibit paradoxical hyperintensity on T1-weighted images and hypointensity on T2-weighted images, likely due to a surface-relaxation mechanism associated with particulate calcium. It remains unclear whether these lesions correlate with clinical symptoms. In most cases, mineralizing microangiopathy is asymptomatic and is an incidental finding on follow-up CT scans (Fig. 3.5).

3.4.6 Chronic Expanding Encapsulated Hematoma

Cysts and chronic expanding encapsulated hematomas [49, 50] can emerge as late delayed complications following stereotactic radiosurgery for arteriovenous malformations. These conditions are thought to result from increased permeability of the blood vessels within the nidus, breakdown of the BBB, and liquefaction of coagulation necrosis. Shuto et al. [49] documented that these complications are caused by repeated minor hemorrhages from a nodular angiomatous lesion developing within the brain parenchyma adjacent to the irradiated nidus. If the hemorrhage primarily spreads into the brain parenchyma, a cyst develops and enlarges. Conversely, if the hemorrhage occurs mainly within the angiomatous lesion, a chronic expanding encapsulated hematoma forms. These cysts and chronic expanding encapsulated hematomas typically develop more than 2 years after stereotactic radiosurgery. Hasegawa et al. [50] reported actuarial incidences of cyst formation or chronic expanding encapsulated hematoma of 1.2%, 5.2%, and 6.3% at 5, 10, and 15 years, respectively, with a median interval to progression of 9.4 years. A large nidus volume is the most significant risk factor for developing these complications.

The typical imaging pattern [49, 50] of a chronic expanding encapsulated hematoma is a nodule with low or mixed signal intensity on T2-weighted images, with or without a cyst. Enhancement occurs due to BBB disruption. The cysts can be multilobulated and are often accompanied by perilesional edema. A fluid—fluid level with different signal intensities within the cyst may be observed due to multiple hemorrhages at different stages. These cysts and hematomas may increase in size over time and become symptomatic due to mass effect, potentially necessitating surgical intervention. Symptomatic cysts may require the insertion of an Ommaya reservoir for repeated aspiration of contents or a cystoperitoneal shunt.

3.4.7 Radiation-Induced Brain Tumors

Patients who have undergone radiation therapy are more susceptible than the general population to developing secondary brain and spine tumors. The most common types of these tumors are meningiomas (70%), gliomas (20%), and sarcomas (10%), which typically appear many years, or even decades, after treatment, with an average onset of 12 years. A study involving over 10,000 patients treated for tinea capitis with low-dose radiation (1.5 Gy) found the relative risk for all tumors to be 6.9 and for gliomas to be 2.6 [51]. This increased risk has been corroborated by several other studies. In patients treated for childhood acute lymphoblastic leukemia, the relative risk is exceptionally high [52], justifying the use of screening MRI brain imaging for adult survivors.

To diagnose a radiation-induced tumor, several criteria must be met: a long interval must exist between the initial radiation treatment and the development of the second tumor (with some cases appearing over 60 years later), the tumor must grow within or at the margins of the radiation field, and it must be of a different histological subtype than the primary tumor. These secondary tumors generally have a poor prognosis, as the patients typically have limited capacity for additional radiotherapy. However, the longer the interval between the original treatment and the development of the secondary tumor, the greater the potential for normal tissue recovery, which may offer some treatment options.

3.4.8 Cranial Nerves

Late-delayed complications of radiation therapy in the cranial nerves are rare, occurring in fewer than 1% of cases after conventional radiotherapy. However, patients previously exposed to more than 50 Gy to the posterior fossa have a higher risk of hearing impairment. Current radiotherapy planning techniques aim to minimize this risk.

The optic nerve stands out as the most clinically significant cranial nerve affected by delayed radiation toxicity, often occurring years after treatment for orbital, pituitary, or suprasellar tumors. Considered a major organ at risk during treatment planning for nearby targets, radiation-induced optic neuropathy typically manifests as subacute painless visual loss, progressing to monocular or binocular blindness with optic atrophy. Anterior lesions may present with papilloedema and peripapillary hemorrhage, occasionally accompanied by radiation-induced retinal lesions, whereas funduscopy usually appears normal in posterior lesions. MR imaging of the anterior visual pathways, employing fat saturation, can aid diagnosis by revealing optic nerve and chiasm enlargement and signal changes, along with contrast enhancement. Like in late-delayed radiation myelopathy, steroids prove beneficial in the acute phase of optic neuropathy, yet there are no established treatments for its progressive form. Optic nerve sheath fenestration has shown promise in some cases [53].

Eye movement disorders may transiently manifest as sixth nerve palsy following radiation to the pituitary gland, cavernous sinus, or nasopharynx. Neuromyotonia, characterized by spontaneous eye muscle spasms and intermittent diplopia lasting seconds and recurring frequently, may respond to phenytoin or carbamazepine.

Trigeminal neuropathy may result in facial numbness, notably observed after radiosurgery for trigeminal neuralgia, trigeminal, and vestibular schwannomas.

In patients treated for head and neck cancer, ageusia is commonly reported, while facial motor neuropathy is rare after fractionated radiation therapy and should prompt suspicion of perineural invasion. Facial palsy occurs in less than 5% of cases following stereotactic radiosurgery for vestibular schwannoma.

Early-delayed hearing loss is often attributed to otitis media, stemming from eustachian tube edema, rather than direct vestibulocochlear nerve damage.

Late-onset hearing loss due to cochlear damage presents with high-frequency hearing loss and tinnitus. Damage to the glossopharyngeal, vagus, spinal accessory, and hypoglossal nerves can occur months to years after high radiation doses for head and neck cancer. Symptoms include tongue atrophy, dysarthria, dysphagia, and shoulder drop. Dropped head syndrome may occur years after cervical region irradiation, resembling myasthenia gravis or motor neuron disease.

Radiation-induced cranial nerve injury, as observed in histopathological studies, is attributed to several mechanisms including the breakdown of the nerve-blood barrier, demyelination, ischemia, coagulation necrosis, and fibrosis [54]. For the lower cranial nerves, this type of injury is primarily due to tissue fibrosis, which entraps the nerve trunks, particularly those running through the neck muscles. Factors such as the total radiation dose, fraction size, and concurrent chemotherapy significantly influence the likelihood of these injuries. The onset of clinical symptoms typically occurs years after radiation therapy, necessitating long-term monitoring to fully understand the treatment's complications [55].

Imaging studies on radiation-induced cranial neuropathy are generally limited to single-case or small-series reports, with radiation-induced optic neuropathy being the most documented. The incidence of this condition varies from 0.5% to 9.0%, depending on the primary tumor's size and location [56]. MRI findings of radiation-induced optic neuropathy include smooth thickening and enhancement of the affected nerves, which may precede symptoms and persist for months [54, 56]. Although intraorbital enhancement is rare, it has been reported, and nerve atrophy may become apparent over time [56].

In clinical settings, balanced steady-state free-precession sequences, such as FIESTA (Fast Imaging Employing Steady-State Acquisition) from General Electric and CISS (Constructive Interference Steady-State) imaging from Siemens Healthineers, are crucial for detailing the anatomy of cranial nerves. It is essential to rule out tumor infiltration, including local recurrence, leptomeningeal dissemination, neoplastic meningitis, and perineural spread of malignancy, in patients presenting with symptoms indicative of cranial nerve issues [54, 57].

3.4.9 Radiation-Induced Endocrinopathy

Radiation-induced neuroendocrine dysfunction, particularly anterior hypopituitarism, is a late-onset consequence of cranial irradiation [58]. This condition often arises due to the inclusion of the hypothalamopituitary axis in radiation fields used for treating various tumors, including primary brain, nasopharyngeal, and skull base tumors, as well as during CNS prophylaxis for acute lymphoblastic leukemia and total body irradiation before bone marrow transplantation. A systematic review found that 66% of adults who underwent cranial irradiation for primary nonpituitary tumors developed some degree of hypopituitarism [58, 59].

The severity and onset of neuroendocrine dysfunction are influenced by the total radiation dose, fraction size, younger age at irradiation, and prior pituitary compromise from the tumor and surgery. Endocrine dysfunction can appear as early as 1 year post-therapy and increases over time. Consequently, patients should have baseline endocrine evaluations within a year of completing irradiation, followed by regular testing for timely diagnosis and treatment.

The exact mechanism of radiation-induced damage to the hypothalamopituitary axis is not fully understood, but it is believed to involve direct neuronal damage rather than vascular injury [53]. The growth hormone axis is most vulnerable, followed by the gonadotropin, adrenocorticotropic hormone, and thyroid-stimulating hormone axes. Growth hormone deficiency is common after radiation doses below 40 Gy, while higher doses (≥60 Gy), particularly used for nasopharyngeal carcinoma or skull base tumors, can lead to panhypopituitarism. Imaging may reveal pituitary gland atrophy and radiation-induced changes in surrounding structures, such as leukoencephalopathy and ICA stenosis.

3.5 Spine

3.5.1 Late-Delayed Radiation Myelopathy

Late-delayed radiation myelopathy typically emerges 1–10 years following exposure to radiation therapy. Similar to brain neurotoxicity, risk factors for this condition include older age, total radiation dose exceeding 60 Gy, higher dose per fraction, and the volume of irradiated cord. Symptoms manifest as slowly progressive sensorimotor deficits, often presenting as a hemicord (Brown-Séquard) syndrome with eventual bladder involvement leading to paraparesis or tetraparesis. While MR imaging may initially appear normal, the cord usually becomes swollen, with gadolinium enhancement observed in about half of cases. Eventually, cord atrophy with occasional cystic cavitation occurs. Diagnosis relies on identifying cord signal changes within the radiation-exposed area and ruling out other potential causes of myelopathy (Fig. 3.6). The natural history varies, with symptoms stabilizing in some patients while progressing to complete deficit in others.

Neuropathological findings typically include demyelination, focal necrosis, axonal loss, fibrinoid necrosis of vessel walls, perivascular fibro-

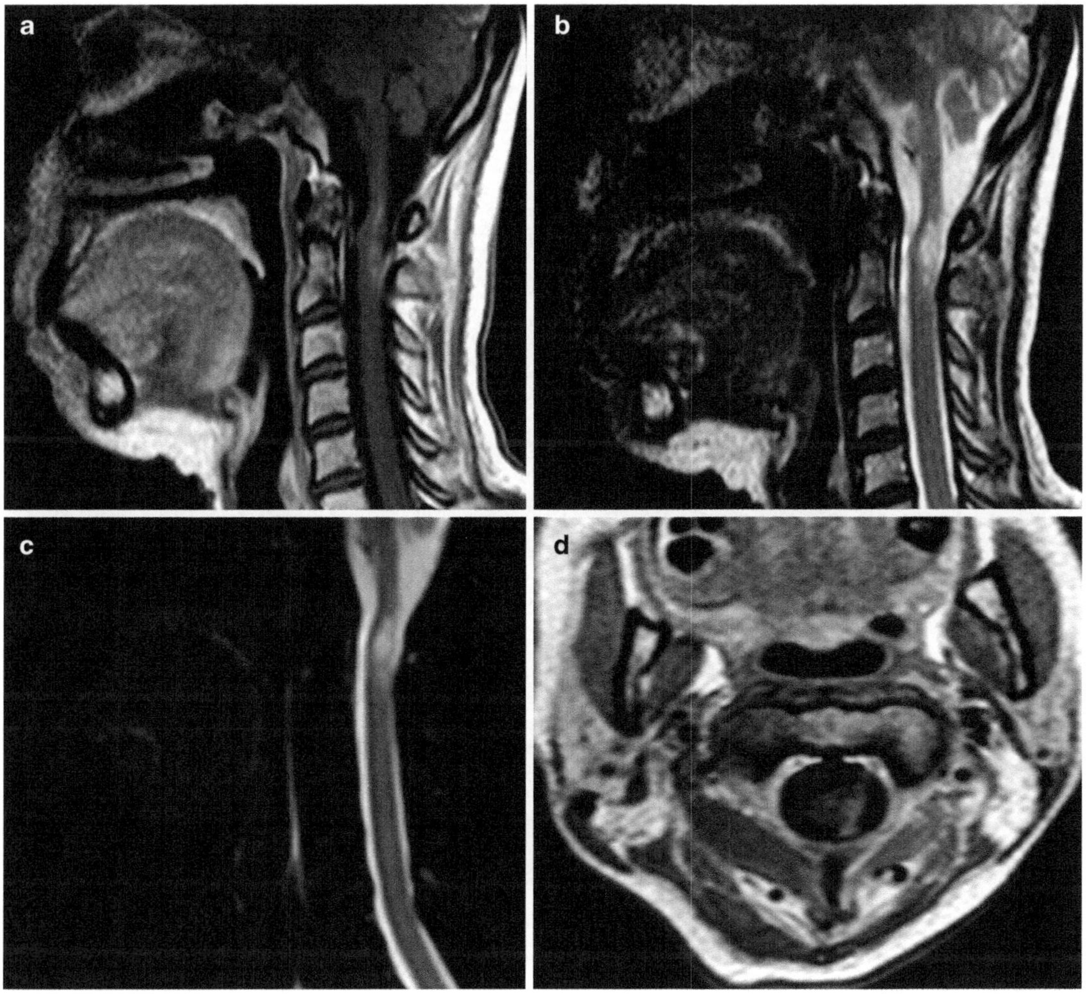

Fig. 3.6 Spine MRI (sagittal plane on T1W—panel **a**, T2W—panel **b**—and STIR sequences—panel **c**; axial T1W at C1 level), showing a focal signal change in the left posterior hemiportion of the spinal cord

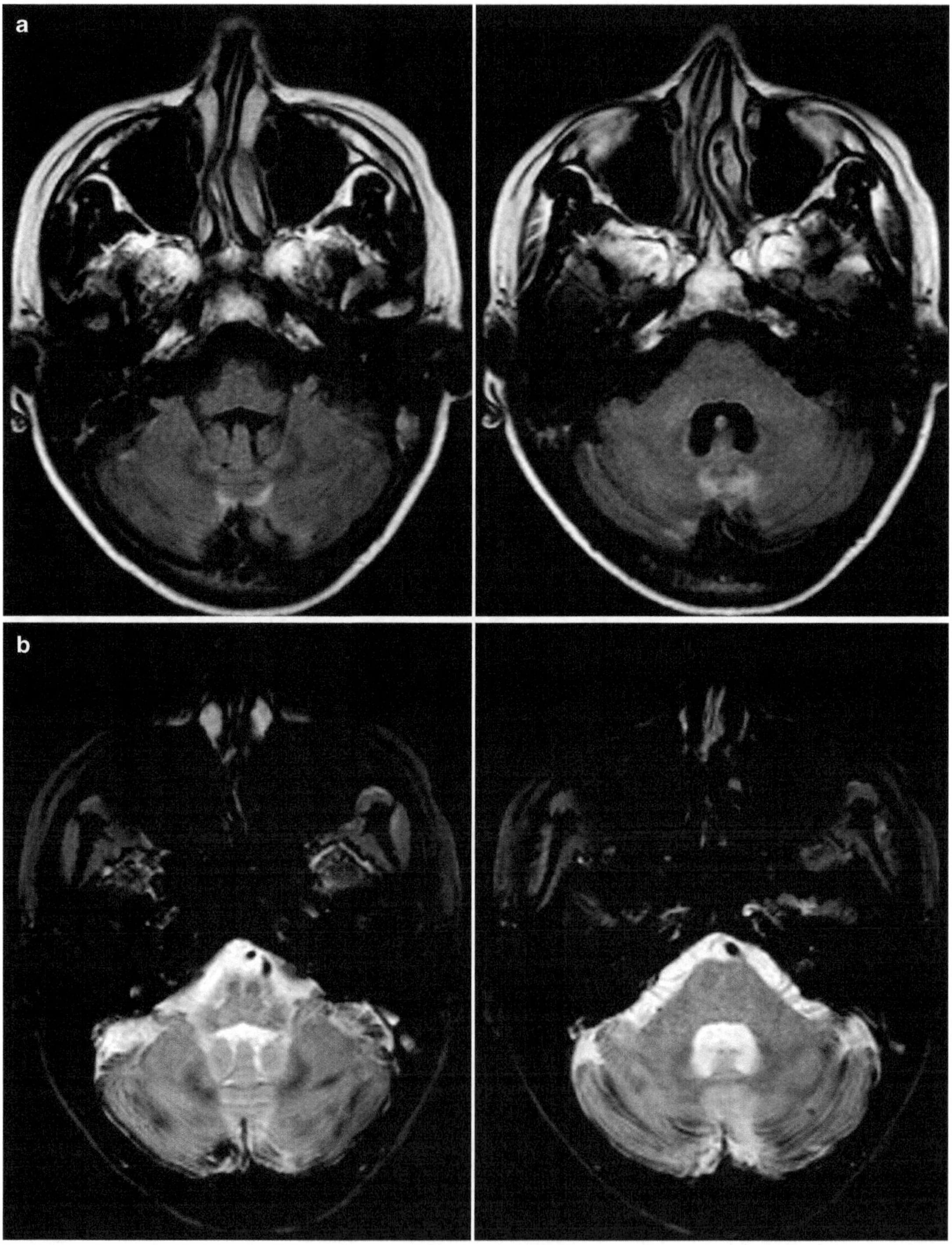

Fig. 3.7: Brain MRI (axial FLAIR in panel **a** and T2* in panel **b**) of the posterior fossa in a patient several years after radiation therapy because an aggressive hematological malignancy, showing both leukoencephalopathy and superficial siderosis in the cerebellar folia

sis, and sometimes vasculitis. Corticosteroids may help reduce inflammation in the subacute stages, but patients often become steroid-dependent with few experiencing long-term improvement. Currently, there is no proven treatment, although hyperbaric oxygen and anticoagulation have been explored in small series (Fig. 3.7).

3.5.2 Lower Motor Neuron Syndrome

A lower motor neuron syndrome resembling motor neuron disease has been reported following radiation therapy to the distal spinal cord and cauda equina, particularly in the treatment of testicular cancer and lymphoma. This syndrome presents with progressive proximal and/or distal symmetrical leg weakness, muscle fasciculation, and wasting, but with preserved sensation initially [53]. Sphincter disturbance and sensory loss may develop later. MR imaging is usually normal, but contrast enhancement of cauda equina roots may occur. Electromyography typically shows denervation with preserved sural action potentials. This condition is best understood as a motor neuronopathy rather than a radiculopathy based on neurophysiological evidence.

References

1. Kosmin M, Rees J. Radiation and the nervous system. Pract Neurol. 2022;22(6):450–60. https://doi.org/10.1136/pn-2022-003343.
2. Tofilon PJ, Fike JR. The radioresponse of the central nervous system: a dynamic process. Radiat Res. 2000;153(4):357–70.
3. Nordal RA, Wong CS. Molecular targets in radiation-induced blood-brain barrier disruption. Int J Radiat Oncol Biol Phys. 2005;62(1):279–87.
4. Roongpiboonsopit D, Kuijf HJ, Charidimou A, et al. Evolution of cerebral microbleeds after cranial irradiation in medulloblastoma patients. Neurology. 2017;88(8):789–96.
5. Dietrich J, Monje M, Wefel J, Meyers C. Clinical patterns and biological correlates of cognitive dysfunction associated with cancer therapy. Oncologist. 2008;13(12):1285–95.
6. Crossen JR, Garwood D, Glatstein E, et al. Neurobehavioral sequelae of cranial irradiation in adults: a review of radiation-induced encephalopathy. J Clin Oncol. 1994;12:627–42.
7. Lawrie TA, Gillespie D, Dowswell T, et al. Long-term neurocognitive and other side effects of radiotherapy, with or without chemotherapy, for glioma. Cochrane Database Syst Rev. 2019;8:CD013047.
8. Cramer CK, Cummings TL, Andrews RN, et al. Treatment of radiation-induced cognitive decline in adult brain tumor patients. Curr Treat Options in Oncol. 2019;20:42.
9. Zhong X, Huang B, Feng J, Yang W, Liu H. Delayed leukoencephalopathy of non-small cell lung cancer patients with brain metastases underwent whole brain radiation therapy. J Neuro-Oncol. 2015;125(1):177–81.
10. Valk PE, Dillon WP. Radiation injury of the brain. AJNR Am J Neuroradiol. 1991;12(1):45–62.
11. Brown PD, Gondi V, Pugh S, et al. Hippocampal avoidance during whole-brain radiotherapy plus Memantine for patients with brain metastases: phase III trial NRG oncology CC001. J Clin Oncol. 2020;38(10):1019–29.
12. Klein M, Heimans JJ, Aaronson NK, et al. Effect of radiotherapy and other treatment-related factors on mid-key term to long-term cognitive sequelae in low-grade gliomas: a comparative study. Lancet. 2002;360:1361–8.
13. Douw L, Klein M, Fagel SS, et al. Cognitive and radiological effects of radiotherapy in patients with low-grade glioma: long-term follow-up. Lancet Neurol. 2009;8:810–8.
14. van Grinsven EE, Nagtegaal SHJ, Verhoeff JJC, et al. The impact of stereotactic or whole brain radiotherapy on neurocognitive functioning in adult patients with brain metastases: a systematic review and meta-analysis. Oncol Res Treat. 2021;44:622–36.
15. Abrey LE, Yahalom J, DeAngelis LM. Treatment for primary CNS lymphoma: the next step. J Clin Oncol. 2000;18:3144–50.
16. Ferreri AJM, Cwynarski K, Pulczynski E, et al. Whole-brain radiotherapy or autologous stem-cell transplantation as consolidation strategies after high-dose methotrexate-based chemoimmunotherapy in patients with primary CNS lymphoma: results of the second randomisation of the international extranodal lymphoma study Group-32 phase 2 trial. Lancet Haematol. 2017;4:e510–23.
17. Katsura M, Sato J, Akahane M, Furuta T, Mori H, Abe O. Recognizing radiation-induced changes in the central nervous system: where to look and what to look for. Radiographics. 2021;41(1):224–48. https://doi.org/10.1148/rg.2021200064.
18. Perrini P, Scollato A, Cioffi F, et al. Radiation leukoencephalopathy associated with moderate hydrocephalus: intracranial pressure monitoring and results of ventriculoperitoneal shunting. Neurol Sci. 2002;23:237–41.

19. Pennybacker J, Russell DS. Necrosis of the brain due to radiation therapy; clinical and pathological observations. J Neurol Neurosurg Psychiatry. 1948;11:183–98.
20. Kumar AJ, Leeds NE, Fuller GN, et al. Malignant gliomas: MR imaging spectrum of radiation therapy- and chemotherapy-induced necrosis of the brain after treatment. Radiology. 2000;217(2):377–84.
21. Wang YX, King AD, Zhou H, et al. Evolution of radiation-induced brain injury: MR imaging-based study. Radiology. 2010;254(1):210–8.
22. Shah R, Vattoth S, Jacob R, et al. Radiation necrosis in the brain: imaging features and differentiation from tumor recurrence. Radiographics. 2012;32(5):1343–59.
23. Brandsma D, Stalpers L, Taal W, Sminia P, van den Bent MJ. Clinical features, mechanisms, and management of pseudoprogression in malignant gliomas. Lancet Oncol. 2008;9(5):453–61.
24. Ruben JD, Dally M, Bailey M, Smith R, McLean CA, Fedele P. Cerebral radiation necrosis: incidence, outcomes, and risk factors with emphasis on radiation parameters and chemotherapy. Int J Radiat Oncol Biol Phys. 2006;65(2):499–508.
25. Galldiks N, Kocher M, Ceccon G, et al. Imaging challenges of immunotherapy and targeted therapy in patients with brain metastases: response, progression, and pseudoprogression. Neuro-Oncology. 2020;22(1):17–30.
26. Kralik SF, Watson GA, Shih C-S, et al. Radiation-induced large vessel cerebral vasculopathy in pediatric patients with brain tumors treated with proton radiation therapy. Int J Radiat Oncol Biol Phys. 2017;99:817–24.
27. Hall MD, Bradley JA, Rotondo RL, Hanel R, Shah C, Morris CG, Aldana PR, Indelicato DJ. Risk of radiation vasculopathy and stroke in pediatric patients treated with proton therapy for brain and Skull Base tumors. Int J Radiat Oncol Biol Phys. 2018;101(4):854–9. https://doi.org/10.1016/j.ijrobp.2018.03.027.
28. Bavle A, Srinivasan A, Choudhry F, Anderson M, Confer M, Simpson H, Gavula T, Thompson JS, Clifton S, Gross NL, McNall-Knapp R. Systematic review of the incidence and risk factors for cerebral vasculopathy and stroke after cranial proton and photon radiation for childhood brain tumors. Neurooncol Pract. 2020;8(1):31–9. https://doi.org/10.1093/nop/npaa061.
29. Winter SF, Vaios EJ, Shih HA, Grassberger C, Parsons MW, Gardner MM, Ehret F, Kaul D, Boehmerle W, Endres M, Dietrich J. Mitigating radiotoxicity in the central nervous system: role of proton therapy. Curr Treat Options in Oncol. 2023;24(11):1524–49. https://doi.org/10.1007/s11864-023-01131-x.
30. Hess CB, Thompson HM, Benedict SH, Seibert JA, Wong K, Vaughan AT, Chen AM. Exposure risks among children undergoing radiation therapy: considerations in the era of image guided radiation therapy. Int J Radiat Oncol Biol Phys. 2016;94(5):978–92. https://doi.org/10.1016/j.ijrobp.2015.12.372.
31. Malone S, Raaphorst GP, Gray R, et al. Enhanced in vitro radiosensitivity of skin fibroblasts in two patients developing brain necrosis following AVM radiosurgery: a new risk factor with potential for a predictive assay. Int J Radiat Oncol Biol Phys. 2000;47:185–9.
32. Bodensohn R, Forbrig R, Quach S, et al. Mri-based contrast clearance analysis shows high differentiation accuracy between radiation-induced reactions and progressive disease after cranial radiotherapy. ESMO Open. 2022;7:100424.
33. Wang YX, King AD, Zhou H, et al. Evolution of radiationinduced brain injury: MR imaging–based study. Radiology. 2010;254(1):210–8.
34. Liao G, Khan M, Zhao Z, et al. Bevacizumab treatment of radiation-induced brain necrosis: a systematic review. Front Oncol. 2021;11:593449.
35. Deibert CP, Ahluwalia MS, Sheehan JP, et al. Bevacizumab for refractory adverse radiation effects after stereotactic radiosurgery. J Neuro-Oncol. 2013;115(2):217–23.
36. Mullins ME, Barest GD, Schaefer PW, Hochberg FH, Gonzalez RG, Lev MH. Radiation necrosis versus glioma recurrence: conventional MR imaging clues to diagnosis. AJNR Am J Neuroradiol. 2005;26(8):1967–72.
37. Bitzer M, Topka H. Progressive cerebral occlusive disease after radiation therapy. Stroke. 1995;26(1):131–6.
38. Kralik SF, Watson GA, Shih CS, Ho CY, Finke W, Buchsbaum J. Radiation-induced large vessel cerebral vasculopathy in pediatric patients with brain tumors treated with proton radiation therapy. Int J Radiat Oncol Biol Phys. 2017;99(4):817–24.
39. Ullrich NJ, Robertson R, Kinnamon DD, et al. Moyamoya following cranial irradiation for primary brain tumors in children. Neurology. 2007;68(12):932–8.
40. Aoki S, Hayashi N, Abe O, et al. Radiation-induced arteritis: thickened wall with prominent enhancement on cranial MR images—report of five cases and comparison with 18 cases of moyamoya disease. Radiology. 2002;223(3):683–8.
41. Nanney AD 3rd, El Tecle NE, El Ahmadieh TY, et al. Intracranial aneurysms in previously irradiated fields: literature review and case report. World Neurosurg. 2014;81(3–4):511–9.
42. Cutsforth-Gregory JK, Lanzino G, Link MJ, Brown RD Jr, Flemming KD. Characterization of radiation-induced cavernous malformations and comparison with a nonradiation cavernous malformation cohort. J Neurosurg. 2015;122(5):1214–22.
43. Nagy G, McCutcheon BA, Giannini C, Link MJ, Pollock BE. Radiation-induced cavernous malformations after single-fraction meningioma radiosurgery. Oper Neurosurg (Hagerstown). 2018;15(2):207–12.
44. Heckl S, Aschoff A, Kunze S. Radiation-induced cavernous hemangiomas of the brain: a late effect predominantly in children. Cancer. 2002;94(12):3285–91.
45. Koester SW, Scherschinski L, Srinivasan VM, Karahalios K, Rumalla K, Benner D, Catapano JS,

Spetzler RF, Lawton MT. Radiation-induced cavernous malformations in the spine: patient series. J Neurosurg Case Lessons. 2023;5(23):CASE22482. https://doi.org/10.3171/CASE22482.
46. Khasminsky V, Yalon M, Greenberg G, Tsarfaty G, Atar E, Hoffmann C. Detection of cavernous malformations after whole-brain radiotherapy in primitive neuroectodermal tumor patients: comparing susceptibility-weighted imaging and T2 gradient-echo sequences. Neuroradiology. 2018;60(9):913–9.
47. Shanley DJ. Mineralizing microangiopathy: CT and MRI. Neuroradiology. 1995;37(4):331–3.
48. Price RA, Birdwell DA. The central nervous system in childhood leukemia. III. Mineralizing microangiopathy and dystrophic calcification. Cancer. 1978;42(2):717–28.
49. Shuto T, Ohtake M, Matsunaga S. Proposed mechanism for cyst formation and enlargement following gamma knife surgery for arteriovenous malformations. J Neurosurg. 2012;117(Special_Suppl, Suppl):135–43.
50. Hasegawa T, Kato T, Naito T, et al. Long-term outcomes for pediatric patients with brain arteriovenous malformations treated with gamma knife radiosurgery. II. The incidence of cyst formation, encapsulated hematoma, and radiation-induced tumor. World Neurosurg. 2019;126:e1526–36.
51. Ron E, Modan B, Boice JD, et al. Tumors of the brain and nervous system after radiotherapy in childhood. N Engl J Med. 1988;319:1033–9.
52. Neglia JP, Meadows AT, Robison LL, et al. Second neoplasms after acute lymphoblastic leukemia in childhood. N Engl J Med. 1991;325:1330–6.
53. Abraham A, Drory VE. Postradiation lower motor neuron syndrome: case series and literature review. J Neurol. 2013;260:1802–6.
54. Saremi F, Helmy M, Farzin S, Zee CS, Go JL. MRI of cranial nerve enhancement. AJR Am J Roentgenol. 2005;185(6):1487–97.
55. Kong L, Lu JJ, Liss AL, et al. Radiation-induced cranial nerve palsy: a cross-sectional study of nasopharyngeal cancer patients after definitive radiotherapy. Int J Radiat Oncol Biol Phys. 2011;79(5):1421–7.
56. Archer EL, Liao EA, Trobe JD. Radiation-induced optic neuropathy: clinical and imaging profile of twelve patients. J Neuroophthalmol. 2019;39(2):170–80.
57. Crush AB, Howe BM, Spinner RJ, et al. Malignant involvement of the peripheral nervous system in patients with cancer: multimodality imaging and pathologic correlation. Radiographics. 2014;34(7):1987–2007.
58. Darzy KH, Shalet SM. Hypopituitarism as a consequence of brain tumours and radiotherapy. Pituitary. 2005;8(3–4):203–11.
59. Appelman-Dijkstra NM, Kokshoorn NE, Dekkers OM, et al. Pituitary dysfunction in adult patients after cranial radiotherapy: systematic review and meta-analysis. J Clin Endocrinol Metab. 2011;96(8):2330–40.

4 Smart Syndrome: Clinical and Neuroimaging Clues of a Underrecognized Iatrogenic Disease

Marialuisa Zedde and Rosario Pascarella

4.1 Introduction

SMART syndrome, acronym for "stroke-like migraine attacks after radiation therapy," is a rare condition that manifests in patients with a history of brain radiotherapy. These patients experience a unique set of clinical-radiological symptoms, including recurrent prolonged hemispheric neurological issues, headaches, and sometimes seizures. These symptoms are associated with transient cortical gadolinium enhancement and swelling [1]. Some patients have a prior history of migraines or seizures before their SMART episodes [2]. The exact minimum dose of brain irradiation required to predispose someone to SMART syndrome is unknown. However, most documented cases involve significantly higher radiation exposure (>50 Gy) [1].

SMART syndrome appears to be quite rare, first reported in 1995 [3], involving four children with "complicated migraine-like episodes after cranial irradiation." Since then, additional cases have been documented, typically showing a latent period between irradiation and symptom onset ranging from 14 months to 30 years. Neurological impairments from SMART syndrome may not be fully reversible [2, 4].

MRI findings in SMART syndrome usually show cortical T2 and fluid-attenuated inversion recovery hyperintensity in one hemisphere, with gyral enhancement. These abnormalities are most prominent in the temporal, parietal, and occipital regions, with minimal or absent diffusion-weighted abnormalities [2]. MRI changes can occur without clinical or EEG evidence of epileptic seizures and may not be present in every attack [1, 2]. These changes can also be delayed by 2–7 days after onset and typically resolve within 2–5 weeks. SMART syndrome can be complicated by cerebral infarction, and some scans show permanent damage due to cortical laminar necrosis [2].

4.2 Definition and Diagnostic Criteria

Stroke-like migraine attacks after radiation therapy (SMART) syndrome is recognized as a delayed complication of cranial irradiation. It manifests as migraine-like headaches and the sudden onset of stroke-like symptoms, affecting both adult and pediatric patients who have previously undergone treatment for brain tumors [1, 2, 5–10].

M. Zedde (✉)
Neurology Unit, Stroke Unit, Azienda Unità Sanitaria Locale-IRCCS di Reggio Emilia, Reggio Emilia, Italy
e-mail: zedde.marialuisa@ausl.re.it

R. Pascarella
Neuroradiology Unit, Ospedale Santa Maria della Misericordia, AULSS 5 Polesana, Rovigo, Italy

M. Zedde, R. Pascarella (eds.), *Neuroimaging of Treatment-Related Conditions in the Brain*,
https://doi.org/10.1007/978-3-032-23618-0_4

In 2006, Black et al. [1] proposed diagnostic criteria for SMART syndrome, which include (Table 4.1): (I) a remote history of external beam cranial irradiation; (II) prolonged, reversible signs and symptoms referable to a unilateral cortical region beginning years after cranial irradiation, such as seizures, migraines with or without aura, and stroke-like symptoms; (III) transient, diffuse, unilateral gyriform enhancement sparing the white matter within a previous radiation field; (IV) symptoms not attributable to another disorder (Table 4.1).

Since these initial diagnostic criteria were proposed, subsequent cases of SMART syndrome have revealed additional clinical and imaging manifestations that do not strictly fit these criteria, despite matching the overall features of SMART syndrome. Updates regarding clinical and imaging prognostic factors have been made, and a spectrum of SMART syndrome variants, including peri-ictal pseudoprogression (PIPG) and acute late-onset encephalopathy after radiation therapy (ALERT), have been proposed [11, 12].

After Black et al. [1] proposed diagnostic criteria for SMART syndrome encompassing both clinical and imaging features. However, clinical manifestations are known to vary, sometimes persisting, recurring, or leading to infarction. Notably, while migraines are a hallmark feature, they may not always manifest despite the syndrome's name. Regarding imaging features, besides classic cortical changes, involvement of the brainstem has been suggested, and T2-weighted imaging (T2WI) and FLAIR sequences may reveal prolonged hyperintensity in cortical and underlying white matter regions. Diffusion-weighted imaging (DWI), susceptibility-weighted imaging (SWI), and T2*-weighted imaging (T2*WI), routinely included in brain MRI protocols, can detect acute alterations in affected areas and serve as prognostic indicators for clinical recovery [1, 8, 10]. Because of these clinical and imaging characteristics, modifications to the 2006 diagnostic criteria have been proposed (Table 4.2), incorporating updates such as the potential persistence of clinical symptoms and the presence of T2WI and FLAIR hyperintensity in irradiated cortical and white matter areas.

Table 4.1 Diagnostic criteria for stroke-like migraine attack after cranial radiation therapy syndrome [1]

CRITERIA	
A	Remote history of external beam cranial irradiation without evidence of residual or recurrent neoplasm
B	Prolonged, reversible signs and symptoms referable to a unilateral cortical region beginning years after irradiation Manifestations may include confusion seizures headache with the attacks visuospatial deficits hemisensory deficits hemiparesis aphasia antecedent migraine with or without aura starting after irradiation.
C	Transient, diffuse, unilateral cortical gadolinium enhancement of the cerebral gyri sparing the white matter within a previous radiation field
D	Not attributable to another disorder

Table 4.2 Revised diagnostic criteria of SMART

Criteria	
A	Remote history of external beam cranial irradiation
B	Prolonged signs and symptoms, which may be reversible or persistent, attributable to a unilateral cortical region. Clinical manifestations may include migraine-type headache with or without an aura, seizures, confusion, and stroke-like symptoms, including visuospatial deficits, hemisensory deficits, hemiparesis, and aphasia
C	Reversible or sustained unilateral gyriform enhancement with or without T2WI/FLAIR hyperintensity involving the cortex and subjacent cerebral white matter in the irradiated area
D	No definitive evidence of residual or recurrent brain tumor, and not attributable to other disorders

4.3 Epidemiological Notes

SMART syndrome can affect both adult and pediatric populations, with a higher incidence in males [6, 7]. Due to its rarity, the overall incidence is not well-established. The age of onset ranges from 3.5 to 88 years, with an average onset at approximately 45 years, typically occurring around 14 years postbrain irradiation [9].

Radiation therapy associated with SMART syndrome can be administered through whole-brain radiation or focal irradiation techniques such as stereotactic radiosurgery, intensity-modulated radiation therapy, or 3D conformal radiation therapy. The condition is often linked to radiation doses of 50 Gy or higher. Most patients recover within 1.5–2.5 months [6]; however, some experience incomplete recovery or recurrent episodes [2, 6].

Recent reports indicate that older patients are more likely to experience incomplete recovery and prolonged symptoms, while female patients tend to have higher recurrence rates [10].

4.4 Pathomechanisms

The pathophysiology of SMART syndrome is not fully understood but is believed to be multifactorial. It involves delayed brain irradiation injury leading to white matter necrosis, vascular endothelial damage, demyelination, and gliosis, though histological evidence is sparse. Radiation-induced mitochondrial dysfunction has also been implicated [5, 13, 14]. Three main pathomechanisms have been postulated.

(I) Radiation-Induced Mitochondrial Dysfunction.

Ionizing radiation damages DNA in both tumor and normal brain cells, primarily through free radicals and reactive oxygen species (ROS) produced in the mitochondria. This damage causes persistent mitochondrial ROS production, impairing neuron and endothelial cell function by disrupting the electron transport chain and reducing available ATP. This impairment leads to neuronal and blood-brain barrier (BBB) endothelial dysfunction, affecting ion homeostasis and resulting in neuronal hyperexcitability [5, 13–15]. Similar mitochondrial dysfunction is observed in MELAS syndrome.

(II) Neuronal Dysfunction.

Radiation-induced mitochondrial dysfunction in neurons leads to Na, K-ATPase dysfunction due to ATP depletion. This dysfunction causes an extracellular shift of K+ ions and glutamate, which binds to NMDA and AMPA receptors, leading to an influx of Na + and Ca2+ into neurons. While Na + influx causes reversible swelling, elevated Ca2+ levels lead to neuronal hyperexcitability [16–18].

(III) BBB Endothelial Dysfunction.

BBB endothelial cells maintain extracellular ion homeostasis. Reduced Na, K-ATPase function due to ATP shortage increases K+ concentration in cerebrospinal fluid (CSF), causing neuronal hyperexcitability. This hyperexcitability can trigger cortical spreading depression, a wave of transient regional depolarization seen in acute MELAS, hemiplegic migraine, and status epilepticus. Nuclear and perfusion imaging shows hypermetabolism/hyperperfusion during neuronal excitability and hypometabolism/hypoperfusion during spreading depression [17–20], distinguishing it from other conditions like tumor recurrence.

Delayed radiation brain injury may cause vascular dysregulation, BBB disruption, and cerebral edema, similar to posterior reversible encephalopathy syndrome (PRES) [21–23]. However, unlike PRES, which affects the bilateral posterior circulation, SMART syndrome usually occurs unilaterally and does not follow vascular boundaries. The commonality between the pathophysiology of these conditions remains uncertain due to different mechanisms and patterns of vascular injury.

4.5 Clinical Presentation

Patients with SMART syndrome often experience severe, unilateral migraine-type headaches (35%–72%), frequently accompanied by nausea, vomiting, and photophobia, with or without an aura. Seizures, which can be focal or generalized, are also common (35–83%) [6, 7, 12] and can be life-threatening, necessitating prompt treatment with antiseizure medications. Stroke-like neurological deficits are reported in 33%–87% of patients, including visuospatial deficits, hemisensory deficits, hemiparesis, and speech impairment. Subsequent infarctions occur in 14–18% [10, 11] of cases, and the recurrence rate of SMART syndrome is 55–62%. A recent study indicates that hemiparesis, speech impairment, and visual impairment are likely to have incomplete recovery [8].

4.6 Neuroradiological Features

Neuroimaging is a key component of SMART diagnosis and it has been recently updated and reviewed [8]. Brain MR imaging [2, 6, 7] being the primary modality of choice. In the acute phase of SMART syndrome, typical MR imaging features [2, 6–8] include (Fig. 4.1):

- reversible, unilateral gyriform enhancement with T2 and FLAIR hyperintense cortical swelling,
- distribution pattern not consistent with vascular territories,
- predominantly unilateral, reflecting the distribution of the high-dose radiation treatment field [11] (bilateral [2, 10, 11] cerebral involvement has been reported in rare cases),
- temporal and parietal lobes more frequently affected than occipital and frontal lobes [12].

In the delayed phase, conventional MRI typically shows resolution or mitigation of the previously described features along with symptom improvement. Gyriform enhancement typically resolves within 14–35 days but may persist for up to 84 days in some cases [2] (Figs. 4.2 and 4.3).

Additional imaging features beyond the standard criteria for SMART syndrome include findings from advanced neuroimaging and nuclear medicine studies, which are important for

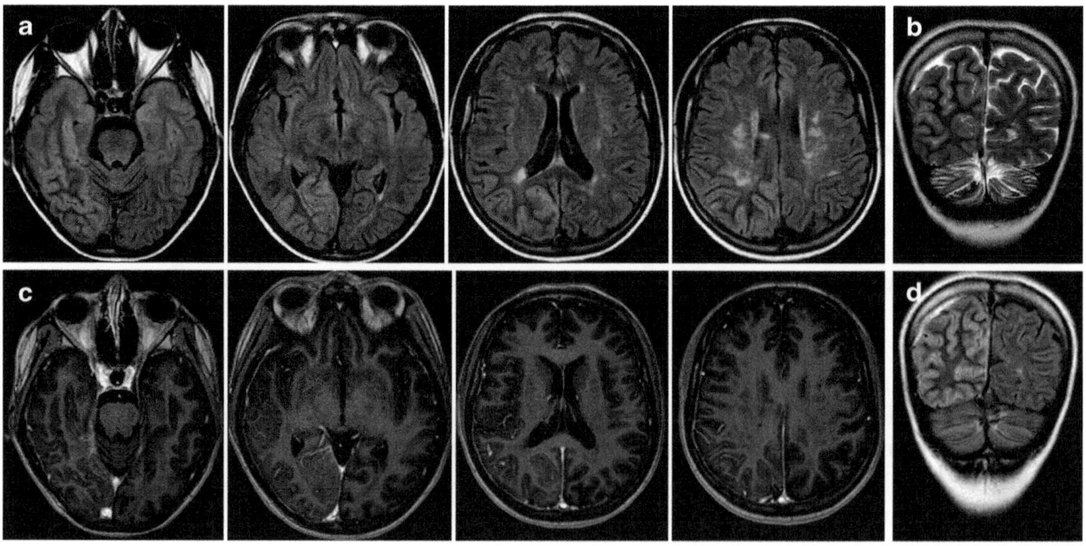

Fig. 4.1 Brain MRI of a patient presenting with left hemianopsia, headache, and seizures, showing left temporal, occipital, and parietal cortical swelling and hyperintensity in FLAIR sequence (axial view in panel a and coronal view in panel b) with corresponding contrast enhancement on postcontrast T1W sequence (axial view in panel c and coronal view in panel d). This pattern is suggestive for SMART syndrome in a patient who underwent whole brain and spine radiation therapy 15 years before

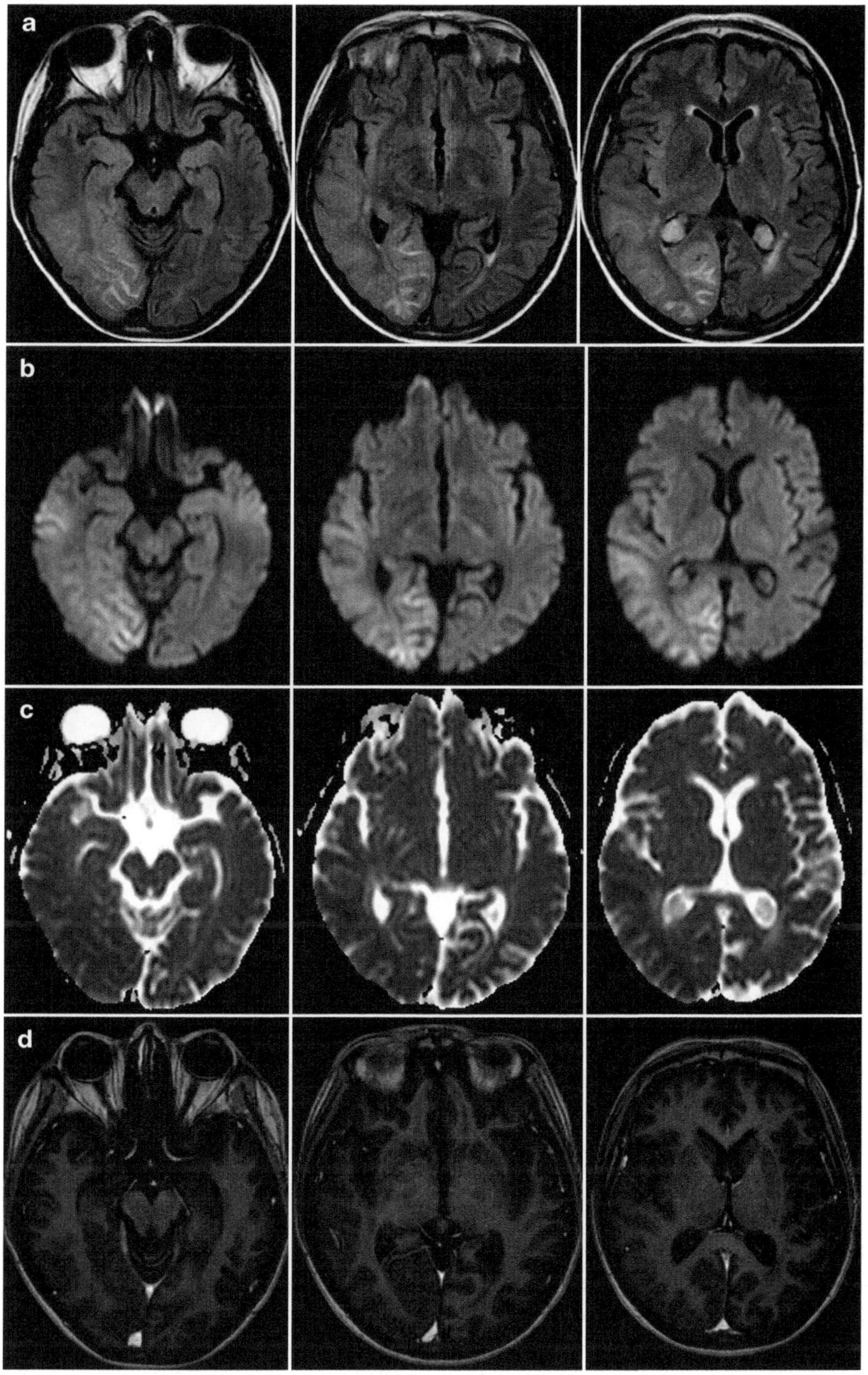

Fig. 4.2 Brain MRI after one month of steroid therapy in the same patient of Fig. 4.1, showing brain swelling, sulcal effacement and subcortical hyperintensities on FLAIR (panel a) as for vasogenic edema (DWI in panel b and ADC map in panel c) wit resolution of contrast enhancement on postcontrast T1W (panel d)

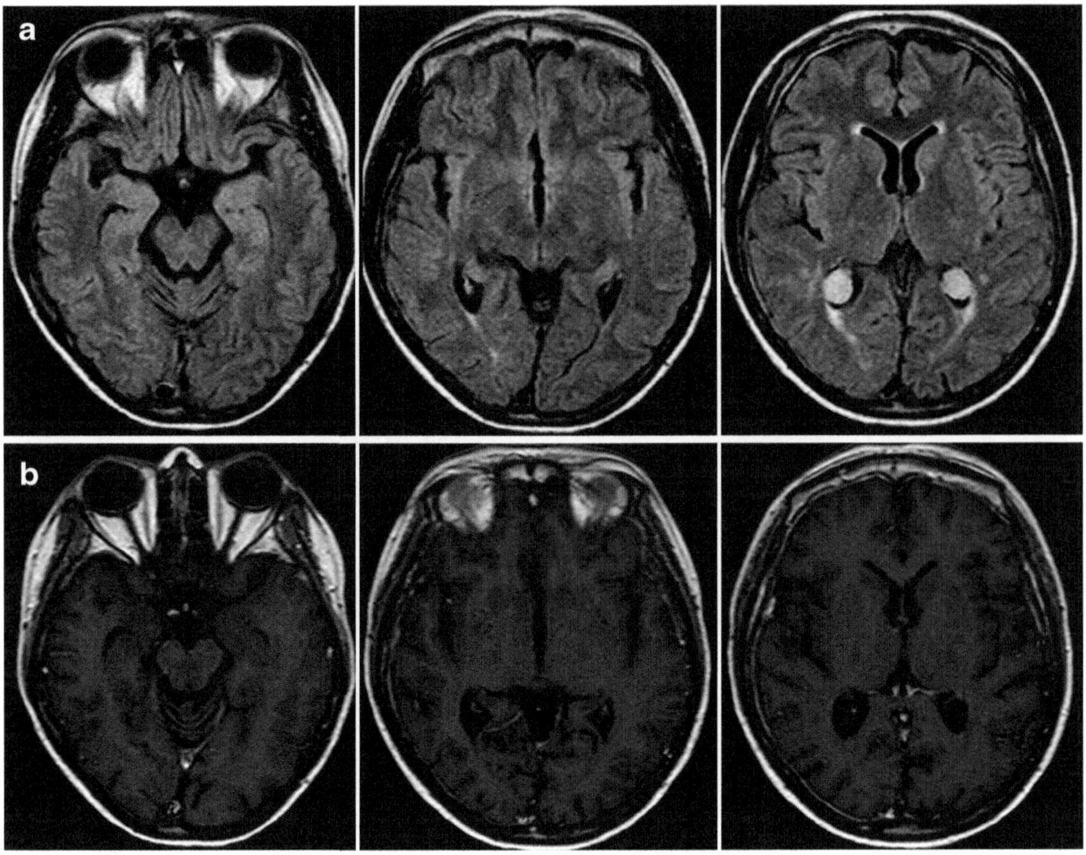

Fig. 4.3 Complete resolution of SMART pattern after 3 months in the same patient of Figs. 4.1 and 4.2. Panel a shows FLAIR MRI and panel b post contrast T1W MRI

comprehensive assessment and prognosis. Variants of SMART syndrome such as PIPG and ALERT also exhibit distinct imaging characteristics, warranting specific attention in clinical evaluation and management [8].

4.6.1 Conventional MRI and White Matter Involvement

In addition to the typical MR imaging features described in the diagnostic criteria, some cases of SMART syndrome also exhibit involvement of the white matter adjacent to the gyriform enhancement and cortical swelling. This white matter involvement is believed to indicate edema, particularly in severe cases of SMART syndrome. The presence of white matter abnormalities is associated with poorer recovery outcomes in SMART syndrome [8].

4.6.2 DWI

Diffusion-weighted imaging (DWI) detects differences in the Brownian motion of water molecules, where abnormalities in diffusion signal are believed to indicate changes in the random movement of water molecules within tissues. These changes typically reflect alterations in the internal microarchitecture of tissues and are observed in various neurological conditions. In the context of SMART syndrome, DWI can also characterize neuronal hyperexcitability and cortical spreading phenomena. This phenomenon arises from transient impairment of neuronal cell Na, K-ATPase pumps due to abnormal ion homeostasis at synapses, leading to restricted diffusion in affected areas [24, 25]. In some cases of acute SMART syndrome attacks, regions involving the underlying white matter may show restricted diffusion on DWI. The presence of restricted diffusion in SMART syndrome is associated with delayed or incomplete recovery, suggesting its potential utility as a prognostic indicator in assessing the severity and outcome of the condition [8, 10] (Figs. 4.1 and 4.3).

4.6.3 SWI and GRE

Susceptibility-weighted imaging (SWI) and T2*-weighted imaging (T2*WI) [26] are sensitive to detect susceptibility effects related to iron, particularly within hemosiderin deposits. These imaging modalities are capable of identifying microhemorrhages and radiation-induced intracranial cavernomas, which are common delayed complications of intracranial radiation therapy. SWI, in particular, is more sensitive than T2*WI for detecting these iron-related effects [27–29]. In the context of SMART syndrome, SWI and T2*WI demonstrate linear hypointensity in the subcortical white matter of regions affected during acute SMART attacks (Fig. 4.4). While there is no pathological confirmation of this SWI finding, it is hypothesized to reflect hemorrhagic transformation acutely influenced by SMART syndrome [6]. Patients with SMART syndrome showing this SWI feature are reported to experience incomplete recovery more frequently than those without it. Therefore, the inclusion of susceptibility imaging in routine brain protocols is crucial across medical institutions. Reporting findings from SWI or T2*WI, whether positive or negative, is essential for radiologists and clinicians to ensure appropriate clinical management and prognostic assessment [6].

4.6.4 Perfusion Imaging

CT perfusion and dynamic susceptibility contrast (DSC) MR imaging findings have been documented in cases of SMART syndrome. CT perfusion assesses the passage of iodinated contrast from intravascular to extravascular spaces within the region of interest (ROI) [30]. On the other hand, DSC MR imaging tracks the initial passage of a paramagnetic contrast agent through the ROI using a dynamic series of T2- or T2*-weighted images [31]. Both techniques provide insights into local perfusion dynamics through first-pass contrast bolus analysis, including cerebral blood volume (CBV) and cerebral blood flow (CBF). During the acute phase of a SMART syndrome attack, both CBV and CBF typically show increased values, indicating heightened perfusion in the affected region. In contrast, during the postictal phase, CBV and CBF are expected to decrease or return to normal levels. This distinct perfusion pattern can aid in distinguishing SMART syndrome from other conditions such as local tumor recurrence or carcinomatosis, which typically exhibit persistent elevated perfusion in the absence of targeted treatments [32–35]. Therefore, sequential perfusion imaging is recommended to monitor changes over time and guide appropriate clinical management.

4.6.5 Spectroscopy

MR spectroscopy is a noninvasive imaging technique used to evaluate the concentration of biomolecules within a region of interest (ROI). In the context of SMART syndrome, its role remains under investigation with mixed findings reported in the literature. One study showed a decrease in N-acetylaspartate (NAA) levels and an increase in creatine (Cr) and choline (Cho) peaks in affected regions [36, 37]. However, conflicting results have been reported in another study that did not observe significant differences in these biomarkers. Currently, there is insufficient data

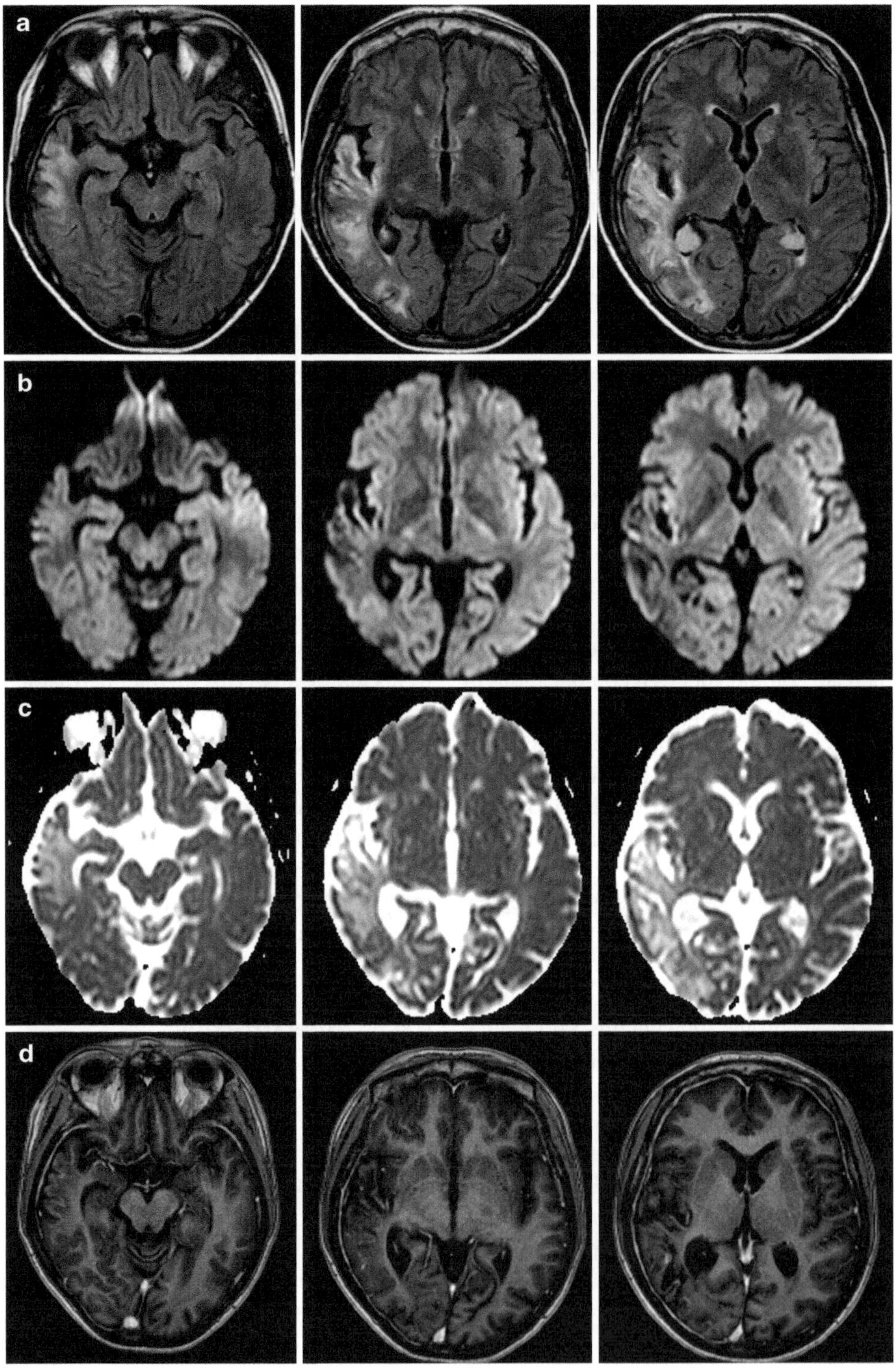

Fig. 4.4 In the same patient of the Figs. 4.1, 4.2 and 4.3 the recurrency of symptoms 1 year later was associated to right temporal and occipital cortical hyperintensities with more prominent leptomeningeal space in the dame side (FLAIR on panel a) without DWI (panel b) and ADC (panel c) signal changes and with minimal cortical contrast enhancement on postcontrast T1W-MRI (panel d)

to conclusively establish the role of MR spectroscopy in diagnosing or monitoring SMART syndrome. Further research is needed to clarify its potential utility and to standardize its application in clinical practice.

4.6.6 Widening the Neuroimaging Patterns: SMART Syndrome Spectrum

Other delayed complications of radiation therapy that fall within the spectrum akin to SMART syndrome include Postirradiation Perilesional Glioma (PIPG) and Acute Late Encephalopathy of Radiation Therapy (ALERT) [11, 12]. PIPG was first proposed in 2011, characterized by clinical features such as the absence of acute headache, stroke-like deficits, and MR imaging

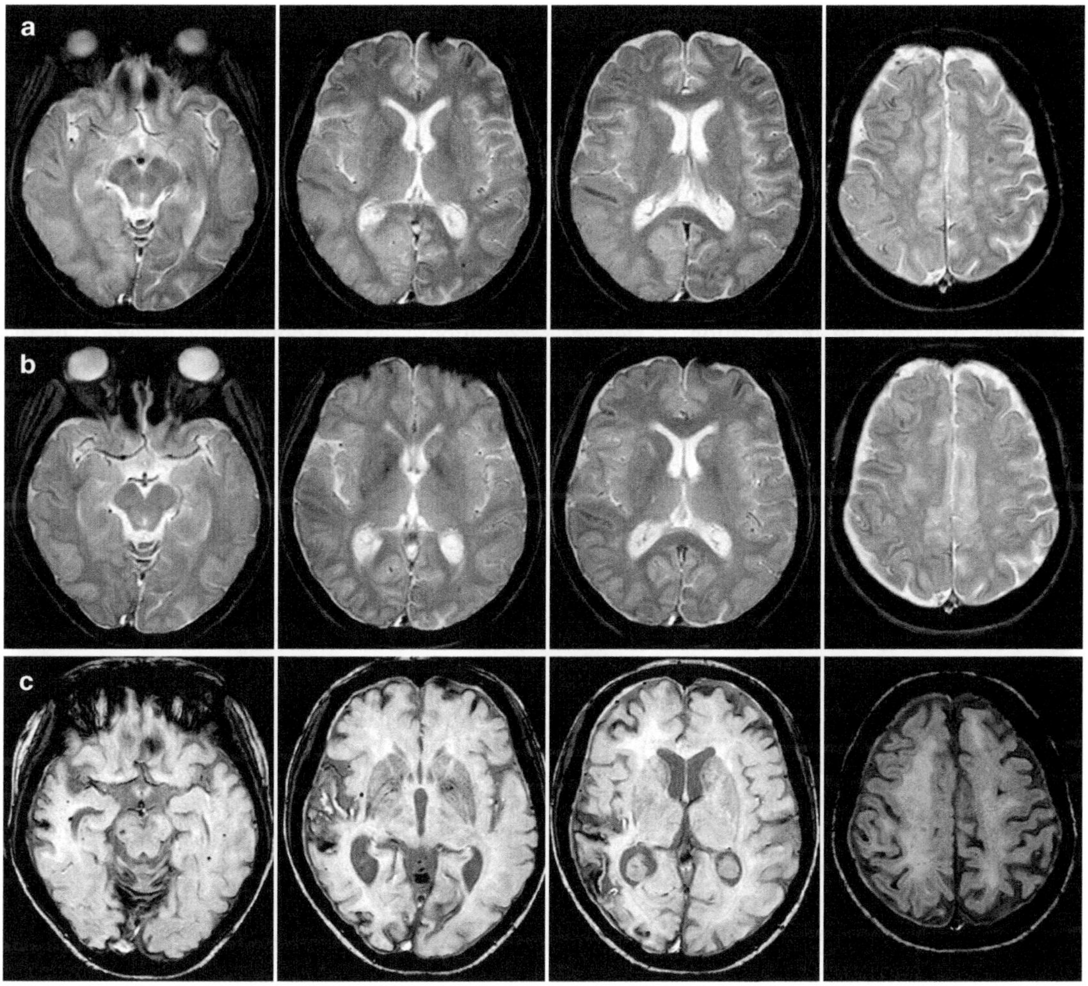

Fig. 4.5 GRE and SWI cortical and leptomeningeal hypointense signal developing over years in the same patients of Figs. 4.1, 4.2, 4.3, and 4.4 (baseline in panel a corresponding to the time of Figs. 4.1, 4.3-months control in panel b as in Fig. 4.3 and 1 year control as in Fig. 4.4)

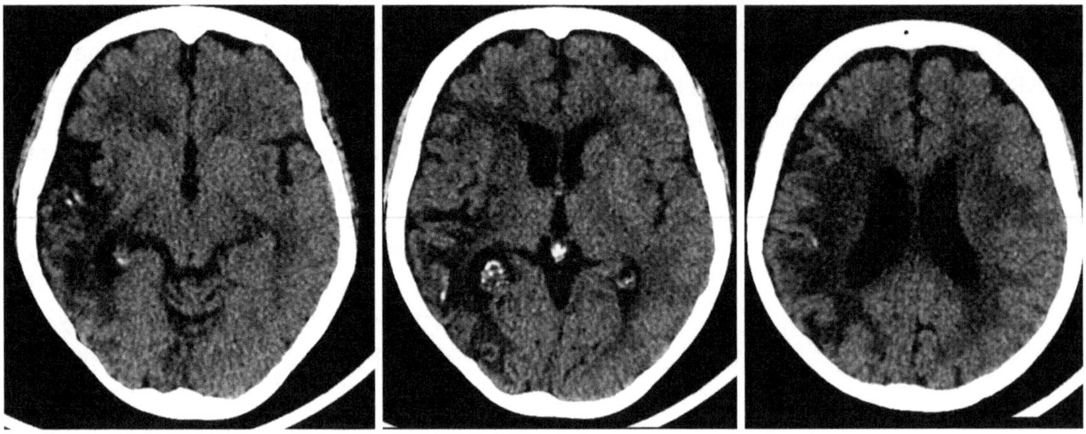

Fig. 4.6 Some hypointensities in T2* and SWI sequences showed in Fig. 4.5 correspond to hyperintense mineralized foci on brain CT

showing focal cortical or leptomeningeal enhancement over an ictal region, without involvement of adjacent white matter [12] (Figs. 4.5 and 4.6). Unlike SMART syndrome, PIPG can affect all cortical regions, while SMART syndrome typically manifests with a predilection for the temporal, parietal, and occipital lobes. Notably, the introduction of steroids did not show a consistent correlation with clinical improvement in PIPG, unlike in SMART syndrome or ALERT syndrome [11].

ALERT syndrome, established in 2013, is marked by clinical features including prolonged impaired consciousness, seizures, and stroke-like symptoms. Its MR imaging characteristics reveal multifocal patchy enhancement or focal leptomeningeal enhancement associated with abnormal T2/FLAIR signal intensity in corresponding areas [11]. Unlike PIPG, patients with ALERT syndrome typically show rapid symptom improvement within days following steroid administration, highlighting the efficacy of steroids in managing this condition. These syndromes, while sharing some clinical and imaging features with SMART syndrome, demonstrate distinct characteristics that aid in their differentiation and management strategies.

4.6.7 Differential Diagnoses

The assessment of SMART syndrome relies significantly on MR imaging for diagnosis. However, CSF testing and electroencephalography (EEG) are also vital to rule out infectious or neoplastic conditions and are commonly included in the diagnostic evaluation [2, 8]. CSF analysis typically reveals nonspecific results, showing no evidence of neoplastic growth, inflammation, or infectious processes [38, 39]. EEG, particularly with long-term video monitoring, can detect electrographic activities associated with both nonconvulsive and convulsive status epilepticus in many cases. This capability enables clinicians to initiate appropriate treatment with antiseizure medications when necessary.

Pathological examinations of four cases [2] have shown only nonspecific gliosis. Proposed mechanisms include an impaired trigemino--vascular system, cerebral hyperexcitability, post-radiation neuronal dysfunction, mitochondrial damage, and vascular endothelial injury [1–3]. The unilateral MRI abnormalities in SMART syndrome resemble familial hemiplegic migraine, which can sometimes be associated with cortical edema and enhancement opposite the hemiplegic side [2] (Table 4.3).

Table 4.3 Neuroradiological differential diagnosis of SMART [40]

Acute infarction (arterial or venous)
Posterior reversible encephalopathy syndrome
Viral encephalitis
Mitochondrial disorders, for example, mitochondrial encephalomyopathy, lactic acidosis, and stroke-like episodes (MELAS), and other metabolic conditions, for example, urea cycle disorders
Postseizure cortical swelling
Hemiplegic migraine

Patients with SMART syndrome typically have a history of central nervous system (CNS) tumors treated with cranial irradiation. When diagnosing SMART syndrome, it is crucial to differentiate it from potential differential diagnoses such as tumor recurrence and leptomeningeal carcinomatosis. These conditions require distinct clinical management strategies. Tumor recurrence may present with similar imaging features to SMART syndrome, such as leptomeningeal or gyriform enhancement on MR imaging, particularly if the initial tumors were aggressive or metastatic [41]. Differentiating between these involves reviewing preirradiation images and confirming the original tumor site. Follow-up MR imaging shortly after therapy initiation is advisable, as SMART syndrome's gyriform enhancement often resolves quickly [2] compared to persistent findings in tumor recurrence [32, 35, 42].

Leptomeningeal carcinomatosis, which involves persistent gyriform or leptomeningeal enhancement, can be ruled out with CSF analysis despite its low sensitivity but high specificity [43]. Contrastingly, SMART syndrome does not show persistent enhancement without treatment.

Subacute brain infarction [44], presenting with T2 and FLAIR hyperintensity along vascular territories, can mimic SMART syndrome's MR findings but typically respects vascular boundaries, unlike SMART syndrome. MR venography can exclude cortical vein thrombosis if vascular concerns arise [45]. Posterior reversible encephalopathy syndrome (PRES) [46] may resemble SMART syndrome clinically but usually exhibits bilateral imaging features, making it distinguishable from the unilateral nature of SMART syndrome.

Infectious processes like cerebritis and meningoencephalitis can be ruled out through CSF analysis and clinical history.

Conditions like hemiplegic migraine or status epilepticus [47, 48] may mimic SMART syndrome's clinical and imaging features but are typically differentiated by personal or family history and absence of prior intracranial irradiation.

Mitochondrial encephalomyopathy, lactic acidosis, and stroke-like episodes (MELAS) [49, 50] may present similarly to SMART syndrome with migraine-like headaches and imaging findings but can be distinguished by characteristic MR spectroscopy and genetic testing demonstrating mitochondrial mutations.

Each of these differential diagnoses requires careful consideration and thorough clinical and imaging evaluation to accurately diagnose and treat SMART syndrome.

4.7 Treatment and Natural History

There is no established treatment for SMART syndrome. Various treatments, including corticosteroids, antiplatelet agents, propranolol, and verapamil, have been used with uncertain benefits. Early symptomatic treatment of seizures is crucial. SMART syndrome is a diagnosis of exclusion, requiring ongoing surveillance for other potential causes. Awareness of SMART syndrome can help avoid unnecessary investigations.

Treatment for SMART syndrome typically involves specific medications to manage migraines, seizures, and prevent recurrence of symptoms. Antimigraine medications are used for migraine-type headaches, while antiseizure medications are essential for controlling seizures, which can be focal or generalized and potentially life-threatening. Aspirin and verapamil [2, 6] are considered to help reduce the severity and frequency of SMART syndrome episodes. Antiplatelet therapy and blood pressure medications are also utilized, especially in cases where acute infarction is suspected following an attack. In instances of severe headache and neurological deficits, corticosteroids (steroids) are often prescribed to alleviate focal cerebral edema. However, their use in the acute phase has been associated with incomplete symptom recovery, necessitating careful evaluation of risks versus benefits before administration [7, 8, 51].

L-arginine, known for improving endothelial function and used in stroke-like episodes of MELAS syndrome [52], has emerged as a potential treatment option for SMART syndrome due to similarities in clinical and imaging features, as well as shared pathophysiology.

Treatment decisions should be tailored to individual patient needs, considering the specific symptoms and their severity, as well as potential risks associated with each therapeutic approach.

4.8 Conclusion

SMART is a rare and incompletely understood late manifestation after radiation therapy in the CNS. It is important to be aware of its presence and of its clinical and neuroimaging features in order to properly diagnose and treat it.

References

1. Black DF, Bartleson JD, Bell ML, et al. SMART: stroke-like migraine attacks after radiation therapy. Cephalalgia. 2006;26:1137–42.
2. Black DF, Morris JM, Lindell EP, et al. Stroke-like migraine attacks after radiation therapy (SMART) syndrome is not always completely reversible: a case series. AJNR Am J Neuroradiol. 2013;34:2298–303.
3. Shuper A, Packer RJ, Vezina LG, et al. 'Complicated migraine-like episodes' in children following cranial irradiation and chemotherapy. Neurology. 1995;45:1837–40.
4. Partap S, Walker M, Longstreth WT, et al. Prolonged but reversible migraine-like episodes long after cranial irradiation. Neurology. 2006;66:1105–7.
5. Turnquist C, Harris BT, Harris CC. Radiation-induced brain injury: current concepts and therapeutic strategies targeting neuroinflammation. Neurooncol Adv. 2020;2:vdaa057.
6. Zheng Q, Yang L, Tan LM, et al. Stroke-like migraine attacks after radiation therapy syndrome. Chin Med J. 2015;128:2097–101.
7. Dominguez M, Malani R. Stroke-like migraine attacks after radiation therapy (SMART) syndrome: a comprehensive review. Curr Pain Headache Rep. 2021;25:33.
8. Ota Y, Leung D, Lin E, et al. Prognostic factors of stroke-like migraine attacks after radiation therapy (SMART) syndrome. AJNR Am J Neuroradiol. 2022;43:396–401.
9. Rigamonti A, Lauria G, Mantero V, et al. SMART (stroke-like migraine attack after radiation therapy) syndrome: a case report with review of the literature. Neurol Sci. 2016;37:157–61.
10. Singh TD, Hajeb M, Rabinstein AA, et al. SMART syndrome: retrospective review of a rare delayed complication of radiation. Eur J Neurol. 2021;28:1316–23.
11. Rheims S, Ricard D, van den Bent M, et al. Peri--ictal pseudoprogression in patients with brain tumor. Neuro-Oncology. 2011;13:775–82.
12. Di Stefano AL, Berzero G, Vitali P, et al. Acute late-onset encephalopathy after radiotherapy: an unusual life-threatening complication. Neurology. 2013;81:1014–7.
13. Kam WW, Banati RB. Effects of ionizing radiation on mitochondria. Free Radic Biol Med. 2013;65:607–19.
14. Averbeck D, Rodriguez-Lafrasse C. Role of mitochondria in radiation responses: epigenetic, metabolic, and signaling impacts. Int J Mol Sci. 2021;22:11047.
15. Iizuka T, Sakai F, Suzuki N, et al. Neuronal hyperexcitability in stroke-like episodes of MELAS syndrome. Neurology. 2002;59:816–24.
16. Verma M, Lizama BN, Chu CT. Excitotoxicity, calcium and mitochondria: a triad in synaptic neurodegeneration. Transl Neurodegener. 2022;11:3.
17. Ayata C, Lauritzen M. Spreading depression, spreading depolarizations, and the cerebral vasculature. Physiol Rev. 2015;95:953–93.
18. Auffenberg E, Hedrich UB, Barbieri R, et al. Hyperexcitable interneurons trigger cortical spreading depression in an Scn1a migraine model. J Clin Invest. 2021;131:e142202.
19. Vinogradova LV. Initiation of spreading depression by synaptic and network hyperactivity: insights into trigger mechanisms of migraine aura. Cephalalgia. 2018;38:1177–87.

20. Dreier JP, Major S, Pannek HW, COSBID Study Group, et al. Spreading convulsions, spreading depolarization and epileptogenesis in human cerebral cortex. Brain. 2012;135:259–75.
21. Greene-Schloesser D, Robbins ME, Peiffer AM, et al. Radiation-induced brain injury: a review. Front Oncologia. 2012;2:73.
22. Kessler AT, Bhatt AA. Brain tumour post-treatment imaging and treatment-related complications. Insights Imaging. 2018;9:1057–75.
23. Anderson RC, Patel V, Sheikh-Bahaei N, et al. Posterior reversible encephalopathy syndrome (PRES): pathophysiology and neuroimaging. Front Neurol. 2020;11:463.
24. Pai V, Sitoh YY, Purohit B. Gyriform restricted diffusion in adults: looking beyond thrombo-occlusions. Insights Imaging. 2020;11:20.
25. Moritani T, Smoker WR, Sato Y, et al. Diffusion--weighted imaging of acute excitotoxic brain injury. AJNR Am J Neuroradiol. 2005;26:216–28.
26. Greenberg SM, Vernooij MW, Cordonnier C, Microbleed Study Group, et al. Cerebral microbleeds: a guide to detection and interpretation. Lancet Neurol. 2009;8:165–74.
27. Khanipour Roshan S, Salmela MB, McKinney AM. Susceptibility weighted imaging in stroke-like migraine attacks after radiation therapy syndrome. Neuroradiology. 2015;57:1103–9.
28. Goos JD, van der Flier WM, Knol DL, et al. Clinical relevance of improved microbleed detection by susceptibility-weighted magnetic resonance imaging. Stroke. 2011;42:1894–900.
29. Cheng AL, Batool S, McCreary CR, et al. Susceptibility-weighted imaging is more reliable than T2*-weighted gradient-recalled echo MRI for detecting microbleeds. Stroke. 2013;44:2782–6.
30. Hoeffner EG, Case I, Jain R, et al. Cerebral perfusion CT: technique and clinical applications. Radiology. 2004;231:632–44.
31. Welker K, Boxerman J, Kalnin A, et al. American Society of Functional Neuroradiology MR perfusion standards and practice subcommittee of the ASFNR clinical practice committee. ASFNR recommendations for clinical performance of MR dynamic susceptibility contrast perfusion imaging of the brain. AJNR Am J Neuroradiol. 2015;36:E41–51.
32. Nar Senol P, Gocmen R, Karli Oguz K, et al. Perfusion imaging insights into SMART syndrome: a case report. Acta Neurol Belg. 2015;115:807–10.
33. Teske N, Albert NL, Forbrig R, et al. Advanced imaging findings in stroke-like migraine attacks after radiation therapy (SMART) syndrome. Eur J Nucl Med Mol Imaging. 2023;50:1264–5.
34. Biju RD, Dower A, Moon BG, et al. SMART (stroke--like migraine attacks after radiation therapy) syndrome: a case study with imaging supporting the theory of vascular dysfunction. Am J Case Rep. 2020;21:e921795.
35. Gelfand JM, Wintermark M, Josephson SA. Cerebral perfusion-CT patterns following seizure. Eur J Neurol. 2010;17:594–601.
36. Gomez-Cibeira E, Calleja-Castano P, Gonzalez de la Aleja J, et al. Brain magnetic resonance spectroscopy findings in the stroke-like migraine attacks after radiation therapy (SMART) syndrome. J Neuroimaging. 2015;25:1056–8.
37. Farid K, Meissner WG, Samier-Foubert A, et al. Normal cerebrovascular reactivity in stroke-like migraine attacks after radiation therapy syndrome. Clin Nucl Med. 2010;35:583–5.
38. Fan EP, Heiber G, Gerard EE, et al. Stroke-like migraine attacks after radiation therapy: a misnomer? Epilepsia. 2018;59:259–68.
39. Winter SF, Klein JP, Vaios EJ, Karschnia P, Lee EQ, Shih HA, Loebel F, Dietrich J. Clinical presentation and management of SMART syndrome. Neurology. 2021;97(3):118–20. https://doi.org/10.1212/WNL.0000000000012150.
40. Patel UK, Patel K, Malik P, Elkady A, Patel N, Lunagariya A. Stroke-like migraine attacks after radiation therapy (SMART) syndrome-a case series and review. Neurol Sci. 2020;41(11):3123–34.
41. Andersen BM, Miranda C, Hatzoglou V, et al. Leptomeningeal metastases in glioma: the memorial Sloan Kettering cancer center experience. Neurology. 2019;92:e2483–91.
42. BundC, Fahrer P, GebusO, et al. Sequential FDG PET andMRI findings in a case of SMART syndrome. Seizure. 2017;51:50–1.
43. Chamberlain MC, Glantz M, Groves MD, et al. Diagnostic tools for neoplastic meningitis: detecting disease, identifying patient risk, and determining benefit of treatment. Semin Oncol. 2009;36:S35–45.
44. Karonen JO, Partanen PL, Vanninen RL, et al. Evolution of MR contrast enhancement patterns during the first week after acute ischemic stroke. AJNR Am J Neuroradiol. 2001;22:103–11.
45. Idiculla PS, Gurala D, Palanisamy M, et al. Cerebral venous thrombosis: a comprehensive review. Eur Neurol. 2020;83:369–79.
46. Fugate JE, Rabinstein AA. Posterior reversible encephalopathy syndrome: clinical and radiological manifestations, pathophysiology, and outstanding questions. Lancet Neurol. 2015;14:914–25.
47. Guerriero RM, Gaillard WD. Imaging modalities to diagnose and localize status epilepticus. Seizure. 2019;68:46–51.
48. Pellerin A, Marois C, Mezouar N, et al. Neuronal injuries evidenced by transient cortical magnetic resonance enhancement in hemiplegic migraine: a case report. Cephalalgia. 2019;39:323–5.
49. Bhatia KD, Krishnan P, Kortman H, et al. Acute cortical lesions in MELAS syndrome: anatomic distribution, symmetry, and evolution. AJNR Am J Neuroradiol. 2020;41:167–73.
50. Cheng W, Zhang Y, He L. MRI features of stroke-like episodes in mitochondrial encephalomyopathy with

lactic acidosis and strokelike episodes. Front Neurol. 2022;13:843386.
51. Jia W, Saito R, Kanamori M, et al. SMART (stroke--like migraine attacks after radiation therapy) syndrome responded to steroid pulse therapy: report of a case and review of the literature. eNeurologicalSci. 2018;12:1–4.
52. Wai K, Balabanski A, Chia N, et al. Reversible hemispheric hypoperfusion in two cases of SMART syndrome. J Clin Neurosci. 2017;43:146–8.

5 Dilemmas in Neuroimaging of Brain Tumors: Distinguishing Pseudoprogression from True Progression

Nicoletta Anzalone, Maurizio Barbera, and Edoardo Masiello

5.1 Introduction

Radiotherapy (RT) continues to be a fundamental treatment for brain tumors, significantly aiding in disease control and extending patient survival, especially when combined with chemotherapy and immunotherapy. However, this implementation may lead to an increase in treatment-related changes (TRC) from combined chemoradiotherapy (CRT), especially after completion of the Stupp protocol based on temozolomide (TMZ). One of the most difficult tasks for neuroradiologists in monitoring brain tumors is distinguishing between disease progression and treatment effects that can be clinically classified based on timing into early ones such as pseudoprogression (PsP) and late ones such as radiation necrosis (RN). PsP typically arises within 6 months after CRT for gliomas specifically described in the Stupp protocol and is characterized by self-limiting enhancing lesions that spontaneously stabilize and resolve without additional treatment related to an excessive inflammatory response that mimics disease progression. Conversely, RN generally manifests 12–18 months post-RT, featuring progressively enhancing lesions linked to increased morbidity. Although PsP and RN are considered to result from different clinical and pathophysiological processes, they share numerous histologic features such as inflammatory infiltrates and necrosis, leading to similar imaging appearances, pushing conventional gadolinium-enhanced Magnetic Resonance Imaging (MRI) to its diagnostic limits, often resulting in inconclusive findings. This chapter will focus on the current knowledge in accurate interpretation of post-treatment imaging with a particular attention on differentiating PsP from TP. We will explore the definitions, incidence, and clinical aspects of PsP, as well as the limitations of conventional imaging techniques in distinguishing these entities. Advanced imaging modalities such as MR spectroscopy (MRS), perfusion MRI (PWI), diffusion-weighted imaging (DWI), and positron emission tomography (PET) will be discussed for their roles in improving diagnostic accuracy.

5.2 Definition

The criteria that define PsP have not been well-established and most articles on PsP vary in the criteria they use to define it. This phenomenon is thought to result from an inflammatory response and increased vascular permeability within the tumor and surrounding brain tissue, leading to

N. Anzalone (✉)
Neuroradiology Unit, IRCCS San Raffaele Scientific Institute, Milan, Italy

Vita-Salute San Raffaele University, Milan, Italy
e-mail: anzalone.nicoletta@hsr.it

M. Barbera · E. Masiello
Neuroradiology Unit, IRCCS San Raffaele Scientific Institute, Milan, Italy

M. Zedde, R. Pascarella (eds.), *Neuroimaging of Treatment-Related Conditions in the Brain*,
https://doi.org/10.1007/978-3-032-23618-0_5

edema and enhancement that resemble disease progression on imaging. In general, PsP refers to a phenomenon observed in the neuroimaging of brain tumors, particularly following treatment with radiotherapy and chemotherapy, where there is an apparent increase in tumor size and/or enhancement that mimics true tumor progression (TP). This change typically occurs within the first three to 6 months after the completion of neuro-oncological therapy, especially CRT, but it can also happen outside the commonly described period following the start of treatment. This phenomenon has become a major challenge in brain tumor follow-up, as failure to recognize it may lead to inappropriate management decisions for patients with TP.

5.3 Epidemiology

The occurrence of PsP varies widely depending on the type of primary tumor, treatment regimen, and imaging criteria used for diagnosis. A recent meta-analysis reports that the incidence of PsP reaches approximately 36% following CRT for adult high-grade glioma [1]. PsP is not unique to high-grade gliomas and may also occur after radiotherapy in lower-grade gliomas [2]. Similarly, nearly 30% of metastases treated with stereotactic radiosurgery (SRS) exhibit a temporary, moderate increase in volume approximately 6 weeks post-treatment, and this can occasionally persist for over 15 months [3]. Higher doses of RT approaching 60 Gy and above have been associated with the development of PsP, with whole-brain radiation therapy (WBRT) also contributing to this in metastatic disease [4–6]. Moreover, proton therapy in gliomas might be associated with an increased risk of PsP [7]. Particularly, PsP is reported up to 90% of patients affected from gliomas with hypermethylation of the O-6-methylguanine-DNA methyltransferase (MGMT) gene promoter, which is present in up to 45% of glioblastoma (GBM) with proposed mechanism of increased tumor sensitivity to the alkylating effects of TMZ and radiotherapy in the Stupp protocol [8]. The incidence may be higher with the use of novel systemic therapies, such as immune checkpoint inhibitors, which can potentiate inflammatory responses within the brain [9]. Neither age nor size of the irradiated tumors volume were noted to be related to the occurrence of PsP [10].

5.4 Clinical Aspects

Patients may or may not experience clinical deterioration or worsening symptoms during PsP. Clinicians may notice worsening neurological symptoms similar to those seen with TP, including headaches, seizures, and focal neurological deficits. These symptoms are often a result of increased edema and mass effect from the inflammatory response.

Patients with PsP, despite having a worsening radiological picture, are less often symptomatic compared to those with early TP. (34% vs. 57%) [10]. A correlation between PsP and favorable MGMT promoter status has been reported, and when present, it is associated with improved survival rates [11].

5.5 Pathophysiology

The pathophysiology of PsP involves various mechanisms, including treatment-induced inflammation, vascular changes, tissue injury, and immune-mediated effects (Fig. 5.1). Following radiotherapy and chemotherapy, the release of cytokines and chemokines triggers an inflammatory response in the tumor microenvironment, leading to increased permeability of the blood–brain barrier and accumulation of immune cells and further inflammatory mediators. One key mechanism is radiation-induced endothelial cell apoptosis. Radiation causes membrane damage, leading to the activation of acid sphingomyelinase and the production of ceramide. Ceramide then activates multiple apoptotic pathways, including the mitogen-activated protein kinase (MAPK) pathway, the mitochondrial pathway, and the death receptor pathway. These processes contribute to endothelial cell death, which in turn affects vascular permeability and tissue

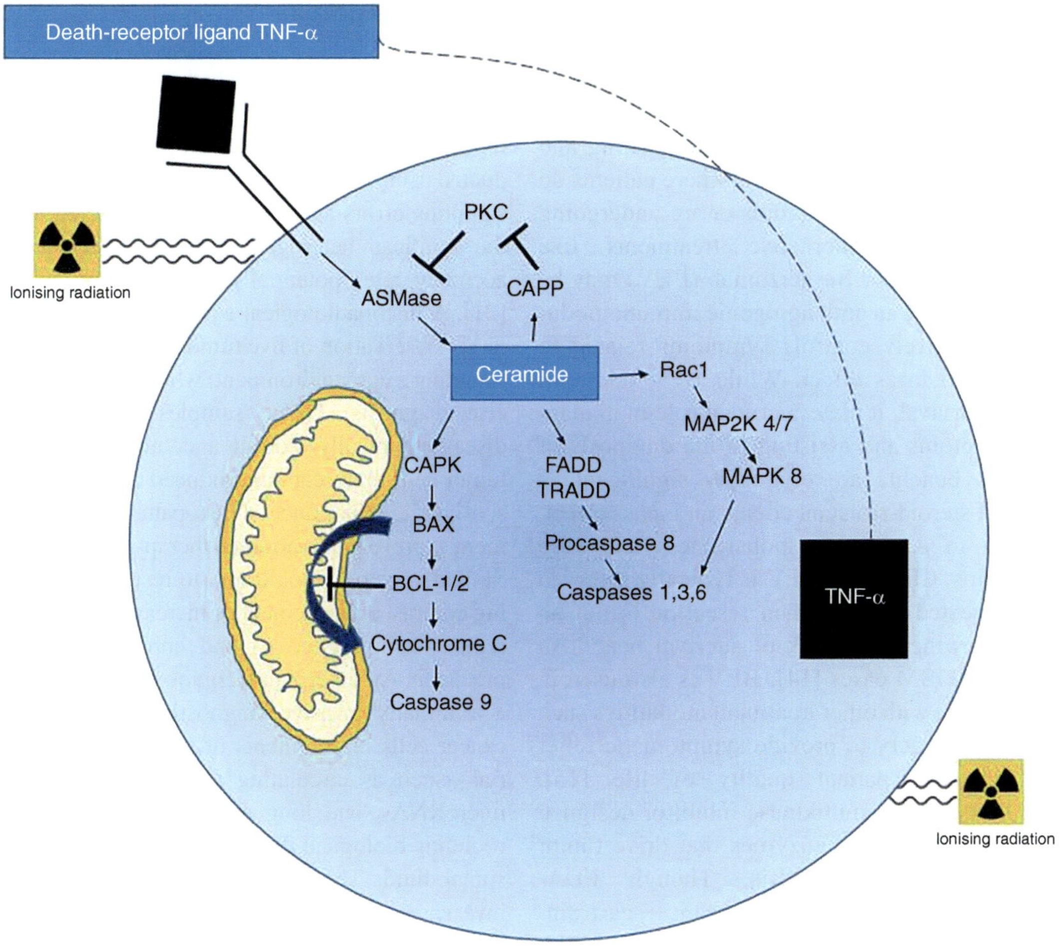

Fig. 5.1 Pathophysiology of Pseudoprogression: Radiotherapy leads to cytokine and chemokine release, which triggers an inflammatory response. Radiation causes endothelial cell apoptosis via acid sphingomyelinase activation and ceramide production, engaging apoptotic pathways (MAPK, mitochondrial, and death receptor) that heighten vascular permeability, oxygenation disruption, and necrosis. (Modified by Brandsma et al. [6])

oxygenation. The combined impact of radiation-induced membrane and DNA damage and temozolomide-induced DNA damage results in heightened endothelial cell apoptosis, increased vascular permeability, and subsequent hypoxia and necrosis. This creates a scenario where the treated area shows features such as reactive gliosis, microvascular changes, and inflammatory infiltrates [6]. The most radiation-sensitive glial cell type in the central nervous system, oligodendrocytes, is assumed to be the cause of early delayed (or subacute) damage. White matter injury is caused by damage to oligodendrocytes and their progenitors. This damage can limit myelin synthesis, which may culminate in temporary, diffuse demyelination [12].

5.6 Treatment

The treatment of PsP is complex and requires careful consideration to avoid mistaking it for TP, which could lead to unnecessary changes in therapy. Treatment strategies often involve continued monitoring and supportive care, as PsP can resolve spontaneously over time. In some cases, adjusting the current treatment regimen may be necessary if clinical symptoms become severe or if there is significant uncertainty in the diagnosis. Corticosteroids are regarded as the primary treatment for symptomatic PsP, mainly because their anti-inflammatory effects help reduce symptoms associated with swelling and mass impact [13]. In situations where patients do not respond to corticosteroids or are undergoing immunotherapy, alternative treatments like repeat resection or Bevacizumab (BEV) may be required. BEV, an antiangiogenic immunomodulator, effectively controls symptoms related to edema and mass effect. While BEV does not extend survival, it plays a crucial role in managing symptoms and assisting in the diagnosis of PsP. Its benefits are especially significant in cases of steroid-resistant edema and mass effect, helping to establish responsiveness and ease symptoms. Clinically, BEV is typically reserved for suspected PsP or when resection is not an option, owing to its lack of survival benefit in recurrent GBM cases [14]. BEV is also used in conjunction with other treatment modalities such as repeat surgery to provide symptomatic relief and improve patient quality of life [15]. Regorafenib is a multikinase inhibitor designed to target several key enzymes that drive tumor growth and angiogenesis. Though FDA-approved for treating colorectal cancer, gastrointestinal stromal tumors, and hepatocellular carcinoma, Regorafenib is also being investigated for its potential in treating brain tumors, especially GBM. Clinical trials, including the REGOMA study, have shown promising results, suggesting that Regorafenib may improve overall survival in patients with recurrent glioblastoma [16, 17]. Laser Interstitial Thermal Therapy (LITT) is presented as a minimally invasive surgical option that can help distinguish between true TP and PsP through simultaneous biopsy [18]. This technique is beneficial in directly treating post-treatment changes if present [19]. Although no survival benefit has been established compared to medical management, LITT has been associated with earlier weaning from steroids and reductions in contrast-enhancing volume, which suggests potential utility in managing PsP [20]. However, further investigation is needed to validate the efficacy of LITT in this context.

5.7 Diagnosis

To definitively determine whether imaging changes are TP or PsP, tissue must be obtained via biopsy or repeat resection. Although biopsies can be conducted using either open or stereotactic techniques, sampling errors are frequently encountered due to the significant heterogeneity of GBMs, resulting in accuracy rates potentially being as low as 76% [21]. A histopathological examination enables the direct observation of live tumor cells and their surrounding microenvironment, which is vital for precise diagnosis. Tissue samples from recurrent diseases typically exhibit a combination of live tumor cells and treatment-induced changes, underscoring the importance of histopathological assessment to prevent unwarranted therapy modifications. Skilled surgeons should aim to resect areas showing contrast enhancement or increased perfusion to reduce sampling errors and enhance diagnostic precision. An emerging technique, liquid biopsy is a minimally invasive diagnostic test that detects cancer cells or fragments of tumor-derived material—such as circulating tumor DNA (ctDNA), microRNAs, and long noncoding RNA—in surrounding biological fluids like plasma and cerebrospinal fluid. These biomarkers allow for a less invasive assessment of tumor activity [22].

Research indicates that in 83% of glioma patients, cf-tDNA concentrations decrease following radiation treatment, often before observable changes are detected on MRI [23]. High plasma cf-tDNA levels have been associated with poorer outcomes in cases of TP, while lower levels are linked to irradiation changes and PsP, with a sensitivity and specificity of 90% and 100%, respectively [24]. Moreover, microRNAs have shown a similar capability to distinguish between PsP and TP, though the evidence is limited [25]. The main limitation of liquid biopsy in the context of GBM management is its current technological and methodological constraints, which affect its reliability and generalizability. This often necessitates the use of large blood samples to obtain sufficient material for analysis, posing practical challenges in clinical settings. Additionally, the ability of circulating nucleic acids to cross the BBB can be inconsistent, potentially leading to variable detection rates. Therefore, the diagnosis of PsP relies heavily on imaging techniques where both MRI with advanced sequence and PET play a central role.

5.8 Response Assessment

The evaluation of tumor response to treatments is crucial in neuro-oncology, particularly for assessing the effectiveness of therapies and making informed decisions on patient management. Over time, various response assessment criteria have been developed to address the evolving needs of clinical practice, ensuring that imaging accurately reflects the changes in tumor behavior and response to treatment. The first version of the Response Assessment in Neuro-Oncology (RANO) criteria was created to improve upon the limitations of McDonald criteria [26]. The McDonald criteria, although widely used, were primarily based on changes in tumor size and enhancement on MRI, which did not fully account for the effects of newer treatments such as antiangiogenic therapies, which can alter contrast enhancement without necessarily reflecting a true reduction in tumor burden [27]. The modified RANO (mRANO) classification was developed to address specific challenges and limitations of the original RANO criteria [28]. One significant advancement in mRANO is the adoption of the postradiotherapy scan as the baseline for all subsequent comparisons, which helps to standardize assessments and reduce variability caused by postoperative changes and timing differences. The mRANO criteria focus primarily on measurable enhancing disease, excluding nonenhancing T2/FLAIR changes to reduce interrater variability. Table 5.1 captures the main differences between RANO and mRANO criteria.

Table 5.1 Comparison of RANO and mRANO criteria for assessing tumor response and progression in gliomas

Criteria	RANO	mRANO
Baseline for assessment	Postsurgical scan	Postradiotherapy scan
Measurable disease	Enhancing lesion on T1 postcontrast, both diameters ≥10 mm on a single slice and seen on ≥2 slices	
Nonmeasurable disease	Enhancing lesion on T1 postcontrast, at least one diameter <10 mm, seen on <2 slices, or with poorly defined margins, predominantly cystic/necrotic components, or non-enhancing T2/FLAIR lesions considered tumor but not reliably measurable.	
Complete response (CR)	Disappearance of all enhancing lesions (measurable/non measurable), stable/improved T2/FLAIR lesions, and no new lesions	Disappearance of all enhancing lesions (measurable/nonmeasurable) compared to postradiotherapy baseline
Partial response (PR)	≥50% decrease in sum of products of perpendicular diameters of measurable enhancing lesions, no progression of nonmeasurable disease, stable/improved T2/FLAIR lesions, and no new lesions	≥50% decrease in sum of products of perpendicular diameters of measurable enhancing lesions compared to postradiotherapy baseline
Stable disease (SD)	<50% decrease and < 25% increase in sum of products of perpendicular diameters of enhancing lesions, stable T2/FLAIR lesions, and no new lesions	<50% decrease and < 25% increase in sum of products of perpendicular diameters of enhancing lesions compared to postradiotherapy baseline
Progressive disease (PD)	≥25% increase in sum of products of perpendicular diameters of enhancing lesions, significant increase in T2/FLAIR lesions, or appearance of new lesions	≥25% increase in sum of products of perpendicular diameters of enhancing lesions compared to postradiotherapy baseline; confirmed on subsequent scans
Pseudoprogression definition	Suspected if progression observed within 12 weeks postradiotherapy and the new or increased enhancement remains within the radiation field; follow-up scan recommended	Suspected if at least a 25% increase in bidimensional area compared to postradiotherapy baseline; follow-up scan required to confirm; third scan may be needed

This table outlines the differences between the RANO and mRANO criteria for evaluating tumor response and progression in gliomas. It includes baseline requirements for assessment, definitions of measurable and nonmeasurable disease, and criteria for categorizing complete response (CR), partial response (PR), stable disease (SD), and progressive disease (PD). Notably, mRANO uses postradiotherapy scans as the baseline and adds specificity in pseudoprogression definition, requiring a follow-up or third scan to confirm suspected pseudoprogression based on increases in the bidimensional area postradiotherapy

The current version of RANO criteria v. 2.0 (Table 5.2) incorporate measurements of the target lesions, clinical status, and steroid use to provide a comprehensive assessment. RANO 2.0 specifies the use of the postradiotherapy scan as the baseline for all subsequent comparisons, avoiding the confounding effects of postoperative changes and providing a consistent reference point for evaluating treatment response, reducing the likelihood of misclassifying treatment effects as disease progression by providing clear timeframes for follow-up. However, in recurrent tumors or newly diagnosed gliomas that do not involve RT, a pretreatment scan is used instead [29]. In RANO 2.0 if TP is suspected within the first 3 months after completion of radiotherapy, additional follow-up scans are required to confirm whether the observed changes are due to TP or PsP. PsP is considered if the enhancing lesions observed on the initial post-treatment scan decrease or stabilize on the follow-up scan at 4–8 weeks, no new enhancing lesions appear outside the radiation field and the clinical status remains stable or improves without significant changes attributable to the tumor. If there is at least a 25% increase in the bidimensional area of the lesion on the initial post-treatment scan compared to the baseline, this increase is classified as preliminary progression (Figs. 5.2, 5.3 and 5.4). If the second scan shows a further 25% increase

Table 5.2 Summary of RANO 2.0 criteria for assessing treatment response in glioma

RANO 2.0 criteria	Description
Baseline for assessment	Newly diagnosed tumors: postradiotherapy scan as baseline (21–35 days post-RT) Recurrent tumors or newly diagnosed gliomas that do not involve RT: pretreatment (pre-Tx) scan
Tumor components	Contrast-enhancing (CE) tissue: evaluated in all tumors Noncontrast-enhancing (non-CE) tissue: evaluated in non-CE and mixed tumors
Measurable disease	≥10 mm in all dimensions (3D) or ≥10 mm in 2 perpendicular diameters (2D). Non-measurable disease includes lesions that are too small, poorly defined, or confluent, and are followed qualitatively or semi-quantitatively.
Complete response (CR)	Disappearance of all lesions sustained for ≥4 weeks, no new lesion, improved or stable clinical status and off corticosteroids (or on physiologic replacement dose)
Partial response (PR)	≥50% (2D) or ≥65% (3D) decrease in tumor burden (sum of products of perpendicular diameters or total volume of target lesions) compared to baseline, sustained for ≥4 weeks, no newly-measurable lesion, improved or stable clinical status and corticosteroid dose is stable compared to baseline (or on physiologic replacement dose)
Minor response (MR; only applicable to non-CE disease)	25–50% decrease in tumor burden with 2D measurements, or 40–65% with 3D measurements compared to baseline, sustained for ≥4 weeks, no newly-measurable lesion, improved or stable clinical status and corticosteroid dose is stable compared to baseline (or on physiologic replacement dose)
Progressive disease (PD)	≥25% increase in tumor burden (2D) or ≥40% increase (3D) compared to the appropriate reference scan (baseline or nadir), or the appearance of new measurable lesions, or clinical deterioration not attributable to other causes
Stable disease (SD)	Does not meet criteria for CR, PR, MR, or PD
Confirmation scan	required for CR, PR, and MR, sustained ≥4 weeks for PD: Mandatory ≤12 weeks post-RT for CE tumors; optional >12 weeks or for non-CE tumors
Pseudoprogression (PsP)	A follow-up scan after ≥4 weeks after the initial scan is required to distinguish true progression from PsP, especially for CE tumors ≤12 weeks post-RT. if the follow-up scan shows stability or improvement without further increase in tumor burden, the initial finding is classified as PsP, and treatment continues
Clinical and steroid use	Clinical deterioration unrelated to steroid use may define PD Steroid increase during response (CR/PR/MR) downgrades response to SD

Modified by Ellingson et al. [29]

RANO 2.0 criteria for radiographic response assessment in adult gliomas. Key assessment points include baseline scans, criteria for measurable and nonmeasurable disease, and definitions for complete response (CR), partial response (PR), minor response (MR), stable disease (SD), and progressive disease (PD). pseudoprogression (PsP) is addressed within specific time frames—3 months postradiotherapy for RANO 2.0, with additional follow-up scans recommended to confirm findings if no clinical deterioration is observed

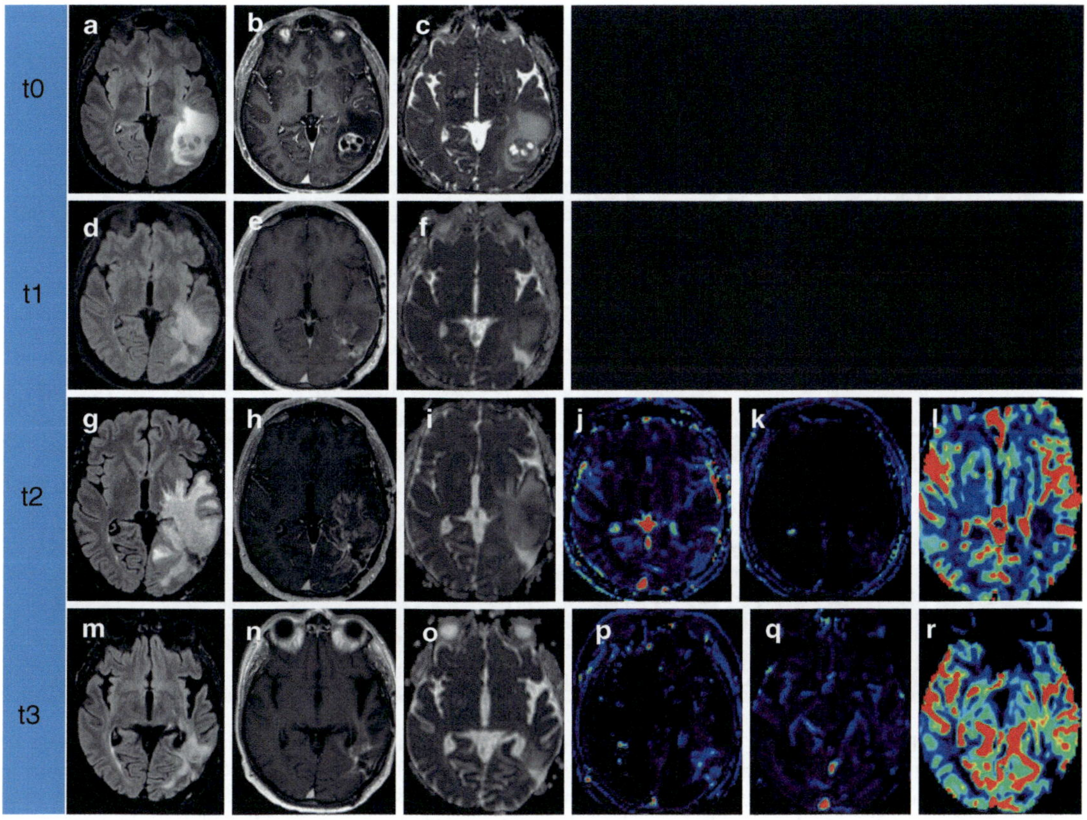

Fig. 5.2 Baseline (t0) FLAIR (**a**), post-contrast T1-weighted (**b**) and ADC maps (**c**) show an expansive cortico-subcortical lesion in the left temporo-occipital region, heterogeneous on FLAIR with necrotic-multicystic enhancement. Histology post-surgical resection confirmed IDH-wildtype grade IV glioblastoma [30], treated with radiotherapy (60 Gy in 30 sessions) and temozolomide. At the end of chemoradiotherapy (t1), FLAIR (**d**) and post-contrast T1-weighted (**e**) images revealed increased pericavitary enhancement and necrosis, predominantly in the peritrigonal cortico-subcortical area. Additionally, FLAIR hyperintensity extended into the temporo-occipital region, accompanied by mildly increased diffusivity (**f**). One month later (t2), FLAIR (**g**) and post-contrast T1-weighted (**h**) imaging showed an increase in pathological tissue with inhomogeneous reduction of diffusivity (**i**) and enhancement along the margins of the surgical cavity, extending into the white matter with a characteristic finger-like morphology. Post-gadolinium imaging revealed irregular and necrotic enhancement, accompanied by mild increases in Vp (**j**), Ktrans (**k**), and rCBV (**l**), favoring a diagnosis of pseudoprogression. Two months later, FLAIR (**m**), post-contrast T1-weighted (**n**), showed significant reduction in pathological tissue and enhancement, with decreased edema and normalized diffusivity (**o**). Perfusion imaging demonstrated a reduction in Vp (**p**), Ktrans (**q**), and rCBV values, with residual pericavitary foci consistent with post-radiation reactive changes

compared to the first post-treatment scan, the progression is confirmed [31].

Immunotherapy Response Assessment in Neuro-Oncology (iRANO) criteria were introduced in 2015 to evaluate treatment responses in patients receiving immunotherapy. These criteria address the challenge of distinguishing TP from PsP caused by immunotherapy. It recommends a repeat scan 3 months after the initial scan showing progression, particularly if the progression is detected within 6 months of starting immunotherapy and the patient is clinically stable. This is because PsP is more common and can be more prolonged with immunotherapy [32].

The Brain Metastases RANO (BM-RANO) criteria were published in 2015, considering up to five measurable lesions as targets based on size, measurement reliability, or active recurrence after local treatment. PsP in the context of BM-RANO is recognized but less common compared to primary brain tumors [33] (Table 5.3).

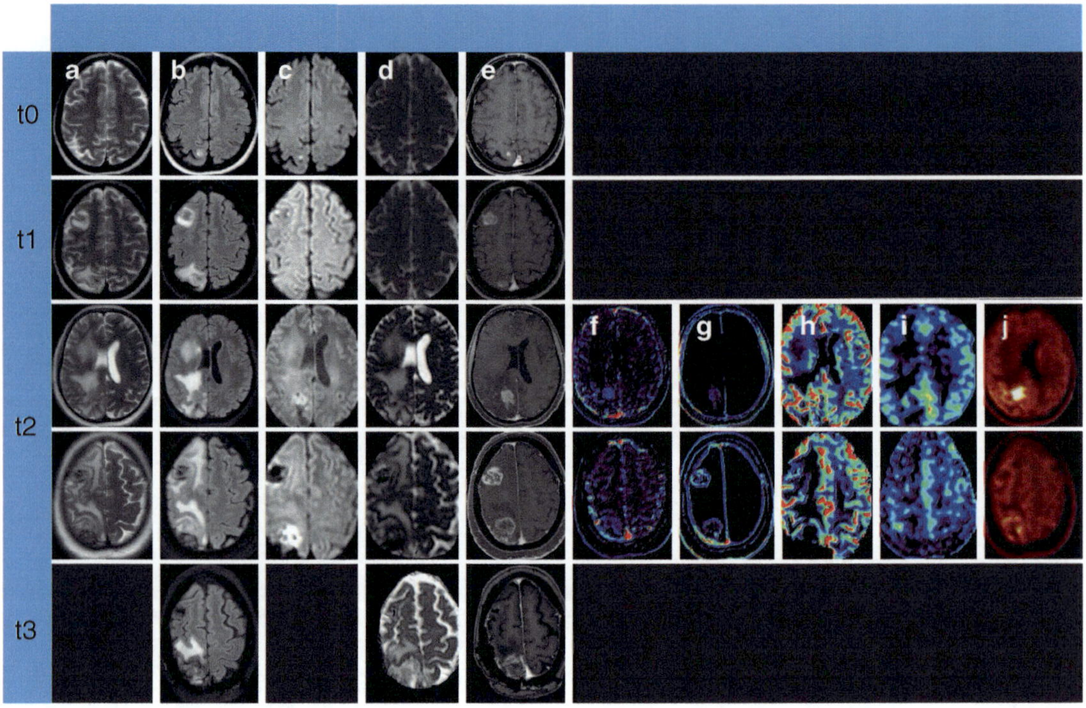

Fig. 5.3 T2-weighted (**a**), FLAIR (**b**), DWI b1000 (**c**), ADC (**d**), and post-contrast T1-weighted images (**e**) illustrate brain metastases from gestational choriocarcinoma. At baseline (t0), a small, non-edematous lesion in the right parietal region was treated with stereotactic radiosurgery. Six months later (t1), the lesion showed enlargement with perilesional edema, and a new edematous lesion appeared in the right frontal region, also treated with stereotactic radiosurgery. At the 12-month follow-up (t2), both lesions showed further enlargement and increased vasogenic edema. The frontal lesion lacked significant increases in Vp (**f**), Ktrans (**g**), rCBV (**h**), ASL (**i**) values, or elevated amino acid metabolism on MET-PET (**j**). In contrast, the parietal lesion, especially in its inferior portion, displayed hyperperfusion and hypermetabolism. Three months later (t3), follow-up imaging revealed regression of the frontal lesion. The parietal lesion underwent partial surgical resection, with histology confirming disease recurrence

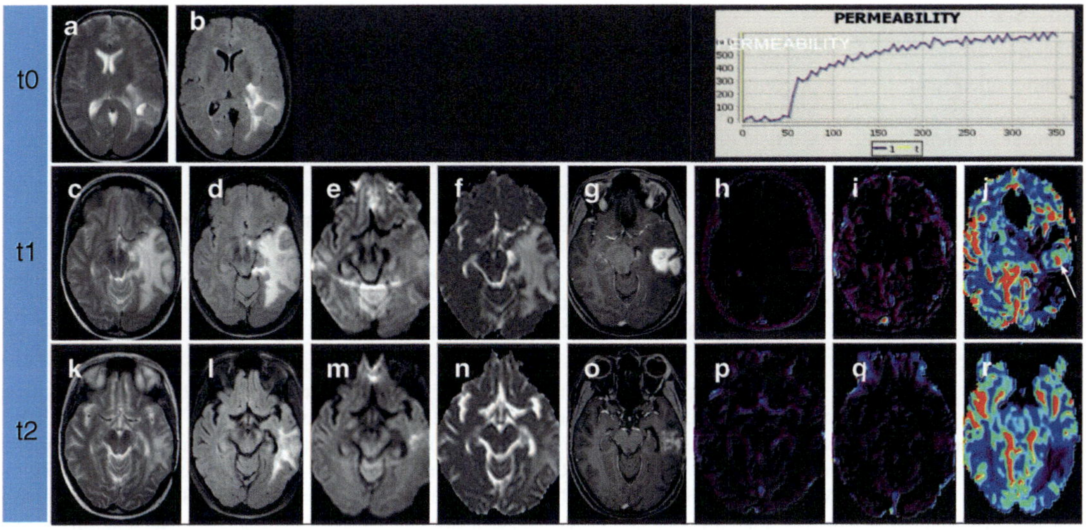

Fig. 5.4 Baseline (t0) T2-weighted (**a**), FLAIR (**b**) showing an expansive lesion in the left temporal-parietal-occipital region, resected and confirmed as cortical-subcortical high-grade glioma, treated with the Stupp protocol. Three months later (t1), a significant increase in perilesional T2 (**c**) and FLAIR (**d**) hyperintensity was observed, likely attributable to edema, extending into the thalamus, putamen, and left internal capsule. Mass effect in the deep region and on the left lateral ventricle with minimal midline shift. DWI (b1000) (**e**) and the corresponding ADC map (**f**) show no areas of diffusion restriction. Post-gadolinium T1-weighted (**g**) images demonstrate significant enhancement within the surgical cavity in the posterior left temporal region. This is accompanied by mild elevations in Vp (**h**) and Ktrans (**i**), along with a focal increase in rCBV (**j**; arrow). Additionally, a progressive increase in signal on the permeability curve is observed, raising the possibility of tumor progression versus pseudoprogression. One month later (t2), follow-up MRI shows reduced T2 (**k**) and FLAIR (**l**) hyperintensity of the anterior left temporal lesion and peritrigonal white matter. Edema is markedly reduced, with ventricular re-expansion and midline restoration. DWI (b1000) (**m**) and the corresponding ADC map (**n**) demonstrate a restoration of normal diffusion values. Post-contrast T1-weighted (**o**) images show a decrease in enhancement, with only small punctate areas persisting in the posterior region. Perfusion maps reveal a reduction in Vp (**p**), Ktrans (**q**) and rCBV (**r**) values at the site of the larger lesion, supporting a final diagnosis of pseudoprogression

Table 5.3 BM-RANO criteria for assessing brain metastases

Criteria	BM-RANO
Baseline scan	Newly diagnosed brain metastases: Pretreatment MRI is used as the baseline for assessing treatment response
Target lesions	up to 5 measurable lesions can be selected as target lesions for treatment assessment lesions should be ≥10 mm in the longest diameter to be measurable
Complete response (CR)	Disappearance of all target and nontarget lesions, no new lesions, stable or improved clinical status, and no corticosteroids.
Partial response (PR)	≥30% decrease in sum of longest diameter of target lesions compared to baseline, stable or improved nontarget lesions, no new lesions and stable or improved clinical status with corticosteroid dose that is stable or decreased.
Progressive disease (PD)	≥20% increase in sum of longest diameter of target lesions compared to nadir, progression of nontarget lesions, or appearance of new lesions
Stable disease (SD)	Neither sufficient shrinkage to qualify for PR nor sufficient increase to qualify for PD
Leptomeningeal disease	The appearance of leptomeningeal metastases is sufficient to determine PD

(continued)

Table 5.3 (continued)

Criteria	BM-RANO
Confirmation scan	A confirmation scan after ≥4 weeks is recommended to confirm CR or PR, and may also be used to confirm PD when clinically appropriate.
Clinical and steroid use	Clinical deterioration that cannot be attributed to other causes may be used to support a diagnosis of PD, especially when consistent with imaging findings. An increase in corticosteroid dose can undermine the assignment of a formal response category (e.g., PR) if radiographic improvement could reasonably be attributed to steroid effects, in which case the patient should generally be classified as SD.
Follow-up intervals	Follow-up scan after an appropriate interval (often a few months) after initial suspicious imaging may be needed to confirm true progression in equivocal cases, especially after stereotactic radiosurgery or immunotherapy.

Modified by Lin et al. [33]

This table outlines the brain metastases response assessment in neuro-oncology criteria for evaluating disease status in brain metastases. "Measurable Disease" includes metastatic lesions with specific size criteria on T1 postcontrast MRI, while "Nonmeasurable Disease" encompasses smaller or irregular lesions that do not meet these measurability thresholds. Response categories include complete response (CR), with the disappearance of all lesions; partial response (PR), with a ≥30% reduction in lesion size; stable disease (SD), without sufficient change for PR or PD; and progressive disease (PD), indicating a ≥20% increase in lesion size or new lesions. Follow-up intervals involve scanning a few months after initial suspicious findings to confirm disease progression

5.9 Imaging Features

PsP is the most common phenomenon observed in high-grade glioma patients during or shortly after the completion of concomitant CRT, as per the Stupp protocol. The imaging characteristics of PsP are as follows:

5.9.1 Conventional MRI

PsP presents as new or enlarging areas of contrast enhancement on postgadolinium T1-weighted images, typically located within the radiotherapy field. These areas often appear as ring-enhancing lesions or as nodular enhancement patterns, which are indistinguishable from progressive tumor growth. In some instances, therapy-induced enhancement patterns resembling "soap bubble" or "Swiss cheese" appearances may be observed, mimicking features of RN [34]. Surrounding the enhancing lesions, there is usually hyperintensity on T2-weighted and FLAIR images, which reflects perilesional edema and can contribute to mass effect, depending on the extent and severity of the changes. These imaging features are linked to the extravasation of contrast medium into tissues due to vascular leakage and disruption of the blood–brain barrier (BBB). Additionally, distinguishing between tumor recurrence and post-treatment radiation effects on conventional MRI is even more difficult due to the frequent histologic admixture, known as "mixed pattern", where tumor recurrence often coexists within a background of treatment-related changes [10]. This histologic heterogeneity is noted not only post-standard chemoradiation but also following immunotherapies. An interesting finding in patients treated with Regorafenib is its antiangiogenic impact, which can lead to normalized tumor vasculature and a reduction in contrast enhancement on MRI, even without an actual decrease in tumor size. In patients with glioblastoma undergoing Regorafenib treatment, MRI evaluations have revealed two distinct patterns indicative of pseudoresponse. The first (pattern A) resembles the classic progression pattern, while the second (pattern B), termed the T2-Dominant Growth Pattern, involves a marked reduction or absence of enhancing lesions on T1-weighted postcontrast images, accompanied by an increase in hyperintensity on T2/FLAIR sequences, suggesting nonenhancing tumor progression or infiltrative growth. In pattern B, DWI prominently shows hyperintensity in areas with reduced T2 signal, indicating restricted diffusion, accompanied by corresponding hypointense regions on ADC maps. SWI often reveals a thin hypointense rim surrounding the DWI hyperintense areas, likely reflecting hemosiderin deposition or microhemorrhages. PWI demonstrates reduced rCBV in these regions, indicative of decreased perfusion, and a reduction in peritumoral edema is also observed. Depending on the specific pattern, diffusion restriction may appear either more or less pronounced [35, 36]. This serves as a preliminary insight into the broader conclusion: conventional MRI, while capable of detecting changes in lesions, may not be sufficient on its own for comprehensive assessment during follow-up after brain tumor treatment. Advanced MRI techniques are increasingly necessary to provide a more complete and reliable evaluation of treatment response and tumor progression.

5.9.2 Treatment Response Assessment Maps (TRAMs)

The static permeability assessment method, known as Treatment Response Assessment Maps (TRAMs), involves subtracting 3D-T1 images obtained 5 min after contrast injection from images acquired following a delay of more than 1 h after the contrast agent administration. This technique assumes that tumor cells, which are crucial for the growth of the tumor, induce a predominantly early wash-out effect since they have a high turnover rate and are associated with increased blood vessel formation. On the other hand, the contrast medium gradually accumulates in scar tissue, indicating reduced blood vessel activity and regrowth [37]. While these maps appear to be helpful in assessing delayed treatment response in high-grade gliomas and in brain metastases after radiosurgery, as well as in monitoring GBM during immunotherapy, in the context of PsP, there are no conclusive results [38–42].

5.9.3 Advanced Imaging

In recent years, advanced imaging techniques such as Diffusion Weighted Imaging (DWI), Diffusion Tensor Imaging (DTI), Perfusion-Weighted Imaging (PWI), Magnetic Resonance Spectroscopy (MRS), and Amide Proton Transfer Chemical Exchange Saturation Transfer (APT-CEST) have shown promise in addressing this diagnostic challenge. These techniques offer enhanced capabilities to analyze tumor microenvironment characteristics, such as cellularity, vascularity, and metabolic activity, providing more accurate differentiation between PsP and TP. However, the lack of standardization in MRI scanners and settings across different institutions can lead to variability in these measurements, making it challenging to apply these methods universally in clinical practice and potentially affecting the consistency of diagnoses (Table 5.4).

5.9.3.1 Diffusion-Weighted Imaging (DWI)

Diffusion Weighted Imaging (DWI) measures the random motion of water molecules within tissues. In DWI, diffusion is quantified by applying magnetic field gradients in different directions and using different b-values, which control the strength and timing of these gradients. DWI generates images based on the degree to which water diffusion is restricted in different tissues, which can vary due to factors such as cellular density, the presence of barriers (like cell membranes), and the integrity of tissue architecture. The Apparent Diffusion Coefficient (ADC) is derived from DWI obtained by fitting the signal decay from the DWI images to a mono-exponential model and offers a quantitative measure in square millimeters per second (mm^2/s) of water diffusion in that voxel. DWI is a valuable tool in the differential diagnosis of PsP versus TP, since the latter often exhibits lower ADC values compared to PsP. In fact, true tumor growth generally has higher cellularity, restricting water movement more than the TRC seen in PsP. This evidence was confirmed in a recent meta-analysis by Yu et al., which reviewed six studies involving 214 patients and found that diffusion MRI with ADC measurements have high sensitivity (95%), specificity (83%), and an Area Under the Curve (AUC) of 0.9322, indicating excellent diagnostic accuracy. Despite this, no significant threshold effect was detected [43]. Although DWI sequences are globally ubiquitous and

Table 5.4 Overview of imaging techniques for brain tumor assessment

Imaging Technique	Pros	Cons
Structural MRI (T1, T2, FLAIR)	High-resolution anatomical images Widely available and standardized Essential for assessing tumor size, location, and enhancement patterns	Limited in distinguishing between PsP and true progression Unable to provide functional or metabolic information
Diffusion-weighted imaging (DWI)	Provides insights into cellular density Useful for identifying areas of restricted diffusion (tumor recurrence vs. necrosis) Fast acquisition and widely available	Susceptible to artifacts in areas with air-tissue interfaces or where there are artifacts from hemoglobin degradation products Less effective for tumors near the skull base
Dynamic susceptibility contrast imaging (DSC)	Measures mainly rCBV for assessing tumor vascularity Useful for distinguishing between high-grade tumors and treatment-related changes Fast and widely validated in literature	Requires gadolinium contrast Susceptibility artifacts can affect accuracy, especially in postoperative areas
Dynamic contrast-enhanced imaging (DCE)	Provides information on BBB permeability and vascular integrity Helps differentiate between true progression and PsP Complementary to DSC for a more complete assessment Less affected by susceptibility artifacts	Requires gadolinium contrast More complex postprocessing Slightly longer acquisition time compared to DSC
Arterial spin labeling (ASL)	Noncontrast perfusion technique Provides direct measurements of CBF	Lower signal-to-noise ratio than contrast-based methods Limited validation in clinical practice Sensitive to motion artifacts
Magnetic resonance spectroscopy (MRS)	Provides metabolic information, including choline and lactate levels Helps differentiate between tumor progression and necrosis Noninvasive and complementary to structural imaging	Low spatial resolution Challenging voxel placement, risking contamination from adjacent tissues
Amide proton transfer-weighted imaging is a chemical exchange saturation transfer (APT-CEST)	Detects changes in protein and peptide levels related to tumor activity Noninvasive, no need for exogenous contrast	Limited availability and requires specific sequences Still in experimental phases in many institutions
Positron emission tomography (PET) with amino acid tracers	Adds tumor metabolic assessment Overall, higher sensitivity compared to MRI (but lacks specificity) Can be combined with MRI for hybrid imaging	Expensive and involves radiation exposure Lower spatial resolution compared to MRI. Not as widely available

Each imaging modality provides unique advantages and limitations for assessing brain tumors, including differentiating between tumor progression and pseudoprogression. Structural MRI remains foundational for anatomical detail, while advanced techniques such as DSC and DCE offer insights into vascular characteristics, and DWI aids in understanding cellular density. ASL, a noncontrast method, directly measures cerebral blood flow, whereas MRS and APT-CEST offer metabolic and protein-level insights, respectively. PET with amino acid tracers complements MRI by adding metabolic information but is limited by cost and accessibility

well-standardized, ADC values can still vary significantly within a single lesion. This is partly due to the principle of standard DWI, which is based on the isotropic diffusion of water molecules, without accounting for specific diffusion directions or considering the microstructural differences within the tissue, such as those seen in TRC. In such cases, ADC measurements may reflect a mixture of necrosis, inflammation, and viable tumor cells, which can potentially lead to misinterpretation. The fifth percentile ADC values are regarded as more effective for distinguishing between TP and PsP compared to mean ADC values, as they are less influenced by the heterogeneous nature of the tumor tissue [44, 45]. Additionally, DTI measures the diffusion of water molecules in tissue in more than six directions. Key parameters derived from DTI include Fractional Anisotropy (FA) and Mean Diffusivity (MD) reflecting the directional dependence of water diffusion and the average rate of water diffusion within tissue, respectively. High FA values indicate highly organized tissue structures, while low FA values suggest disruption or loss of this organization. Areas affected by treatment may also show altered FA and MD, correlating with tumor cell density and infiltration. Lower FA values in nonenhancing peritumoral regions have been linked with eventual glioma recurrence, which can help distinguish TP from PsP [46]. Combining DTI and DSC-MRI parameters such as higher FA, low MD, and high rCBV provides a strong indication of TP compared to PsP [47]. DTI has also been applied into the evaluation of treatment effects after immunotherapy in BM. The study of Zakaria et al. found a strong correlation between high peritumoral T-cell density and low FA ($p = 0.037$). This suggests that areas with more immune cell infiltration had more disrupted white matter tracts, which could be indicative of a more active immune response [48]. Diffusion Kurtosis Imaging (DKI) provides a more detailed and accurate characterization of tissue microstructure compared to traditional diffusion techniques. Unlike conventional DWI and DTI, which assume that water diffusion in tissues follows a Gaussian distribution, DKI goes a step further by capturing the non-Gaussian properties of water diffusion. This capability allows DKI to provide additional metrics such as mean kurtosis (MK), axial kurtosis (AK), and radial kurtosis (RK), which measure the deviation of water diffusion from Gaussian behavior [49]. Several research have demonstrated the benefits of DKI. For instance, D'Amore et al. conducted a study involving 32 patients with pretreated GBM. It was found that parameters derived from diffusion MRI kurtosis maps demonstrate a high diagnostic accuracy, reaching up to 88%, in differentiating between TP and TRC [50]. DKI metrics such as relative-MK were significantly higher, and relative-MD significantly lower, in the enhancing lesions of high-grade glioma recurrence compared to PsP [51]. Nevertheless, one of the studies noticed that DKI only offered limited advantages compared to standard ADC measurements [52]. Intravoxel Incoherent Motion (IVIM) MRI separates diffusion and perfusion contributions in the signal decay of DWI. Unlike traditional diffusion MRI that assumes a single diffusion coefficient representing purely molecular diffusion, IVIM distinguishes between the microcirculatory perfusion and the diffusion of water molecules in tissues. The principle behind IVIM is that water molecules in biological tissues exhibit both true diffusion, which is the random Brownian motion of molecules, and pseudodiffusion, which is influenced by the microcirculation of blood in the capillaries [53]. By fitting the signal decay to a biexponential model, IVIM can estimate perfusion-related parameters such as the perfusion fraction (f), the pseudodiffusion coefficient (D*), and the true diffusion coefficient (D). The study conducted by Kim et al. demonstrated that the 90th percentile for (f) was significantly higher in TP compared to treatment effects, while the tenth percentile for diffusion was significantly lower in TP. The ROC curve analysis showed that the 90th percentile for (f) was a significant predictor for differentiation, with a sensitivity of 87.1% and specificity of 95.0% [54]. A comparative study of different ADC modeling approaches, including those derived from the IVIM model, effectively differentiated TP from PsP with an AUC above 0.91 [55]. Nevertheless, the usefulness of diffusion is limited in this clinical context due to the presence of magnetic susceptibility artifacts caused by hemoglobin degradation products.

5.9.3.2 Magnetic Resonance Spectroscopy (MRS)

MRS provides metabolic information about tissues, measuring the relative concentration of various metabolites in the brain tissue and offering insights into the biochemical environment of the tumor. This technique evaluates metabolites such as N-acetylaspartate (NAA), choline (Cho), creatine (Cr), lactate (Lac), and lipids. Elevated Cho, particularly when reflected in increased Cho/Cr or Cho/NAA ratios, typically indicates high cellular proliferation, suggesting TP, while stable or decreased Cho ratios may reflect treatment effects rather than new tumor growth. Additionally, the presence of lipids indicates necrosis and may suggest TRC, while increased Lac suggests hypoxia, common in both TP and TRC [56, 57]. In a systematic review and meta-analysis by Van Dijken et al., including 203 patients across 9 studies, a pooled sensitivity of 91% and specificity of 95% was reported for MRS [58]. In another meta-analysis, Zhang et al. examined 455 patients from 18 articles and found a pooled sensitivity and specificity of 83% and 83% for Cho/Cr, with an AUC of 0.9, and 88% and 86% for Cho/NAA, also with an AUC of 0.9 [59]. However, no definitive cut-off values have been established. Some studies used a Cho/NAA ratio > 1.8 as a strong indicator of TP [60–62]. In PsP, MRS may reveal a variable decrease in NAA levels relative to a baseline scan, likely due to transient neuroaxonal dysfunction, and a lack of significant elevation in Cho levels, which is more commonly seen in TP. On the other hand, some research indicates that MRS may have a limited role in differentiating between tumor recurrence and treatment effects. Increased Cho/Cr ratio combined with a normal or decreased NAA/Cr ratio may be also indicative of inflammatory lesions [63, 64]. Rock et al. reported that while MRS can differentiate pure necrosis from tumor tissue, it fails to reliably distinguish a mixture of residual or recurrent tumor from RN [65]. The relatively large voxel sizes may result in partial volume effects, potentially blending recurrent tumor tissue with changes induced by treatment [66]. One of the primary limitations of MRS is its technical complexity. The acquisition and interpretation of MRS data require specialized equipment and expertise, which are not always available in all clinical settings. The accuracy of MRS relies heavily on the quality of the spectral data, which can be affected by several factors, including patient movement, voxel selection, and the magnetic field strength of the MRI scanner. Additionally, contamination from necrotic tissue and, more critically, the presence of hemorrhage can further compromise the spectral analysis, leading to potential misinterpretations of the metabolic profile [67]. Nevertheless, the role of MRS in the routine follow-up of brain tumors under treatment is not firmly established and remains center- and protocol-dependent. [68]. For example, incorporating MRS with PWI techniques can enhance diagnostic accuracy to as high as 90% [69]. Nevertheless, the role of MRS in the follow up of brain tumors under treatment is not established.

5.9.3.3 Perfusion-Weighted Imaging (PWI)

In brain tumors, the vasculature is often characterized by increased perfusion, blood volume, and permeability compared to normal brain tissue due to angiogenesis. This altered vasculature leads to increased perfusion metrics in imaging studies. On the other hand, chemoradiation, the most common treatment approach, targets tumor growth by damaging the DNA of cancer cells and disrupting their blood supply, significantly affecting these vascular characteristics [70].

PWI is a valuable tool in the monitoring of high-grade gliomas and brain metastases. Dynamic susceptibility contrast (DSC) primarily measures the relative cerebral blood volume (rCBV), which has been validated clinically to assess tumor growth and response to treatment. It is sensitive to vascular proliferation, a hallmark of tumor recurrence. Dynamic contrast-enhanced (DCE) measures vessel permeability and perfusion, providing additional insights into the BBB's integrity. Arterial Spin Labeling (ASL) measures perfusion without the need for contrast agents, offering a direct assessment of cerebral blood flow (CBF). It is particularly useful in environments where contrast agent use is limited, and it provides absolute perfusion measurements at the tissue level, while DSC-derived rCBV can be affected by BBB leakage and susceptibility effects [53]. Kim et al. noted that the addition of

DSC (as well as DCE) to conventional imaging and DWI significantly increased the AUC on the receiver operating characteristic curve for two readers' prediction of recurrent disease [71]. One significant drawback of PWI is the variability in acquisition protocols such as the choice of sequence, field strength, temporal resolution, and postprocessing techniques used across different institutions leading to inconsistencies in the results obtained, making it difficult to compare perfusion parameters across studies and centers. As a result, it is challenging to establish universal cut-off values to differentiate between tumor recurrence and treatment effects like PsP. Consensus recommendations for a standardized brain tumor imaging protocol have been proposed to address the variability in perfusion imaging. These recommendations aim to maintain tight control and standardization of image acquisition parameters in multicenter clinical trials. Key elements include establishing a uniform dosage and injection rate for gadolinium-based contrast agents (GBCA) to ensure consistency across studies, adopting standardized imaging sequences and parameters such as slice thickness, repetition time (TR), echo time (TE), and flip angles to minimize variability in data acquisition [72]. Anzalone et al. proposed an MRI protocol to standardize image acquisition parameters and ensure consistency across different centers, thereby improving reliability and comparability in multicenter clinical trials, enhancing the quantitative assessment of brain gliomas and demonstrating the robustness of these techniques when carried out at more than one medical institution [73]. In light of these considerations, future efforts should also focus on implementing reliable quantitative measures and improving post-processing techniques. Evidence suggests that the ROI-based method of measuring perfusion parameters is subjective and insufficient for accurately capturing the full characteristics of tumors due to their significant variability and the considerable changes in vascular architecture caused by chemoradiation [74]. It may be useful to segment the enhancing lesion to refine the extraction, quantification, and analysis of features such as shape, texture, contrast, and homogeneity within and around the tumor. This involves sophisticated computational analysis techniques, such as radiomics [75]. The challenge of extracting data from images or parameter maps remains significant, and a promising approach is to evaluate lesion histograms by analyzing changes in metrics like skewness and kurtosis [76]. Lastly, multiecho perfusion sequences, like SPICE or SAGE, measure gradient echo (GRE) and/or spin echo (SE) at multiple echo times (TEs) [77]. This capability allows for the implicit correction of T1 leakage effects and enables the generation of perfusion parameter maps for both DSC-MRI and DCE-MRI. Although these technologies are still under development, they hold great promise for providing valuable information for monitoring treatment in brain tumors [78].

Dynamic Susceptibility Contrast (DSC)

DSC involves the rapid acquisition of MRI images following the injection of GBCA. The contrast agent causes a transient decrease in signal intensity on T2*-weighted images, which can be analyzed to derive quantitative perfusion metrics. The AUC of the concentration–time curve is used to calculate the rCBV, measured in mL/100 mL/min or mL/100 g/min, extensively applied as a biomarker for angiogenesis and widely used in diagnosing and monitoring brain tumors [79]. Normalization of relative cerebral blood volume (rCBV ratio) is a critical step in ensuring the reproducibility of perfusion measurements. It is done by selecting reference regions that include normal-appearing white matter which are assumed to have relatively stable perfusion characteristics. Several larger-scale investigations have also clarified how well DSC performs as a diagnostic tool in distinguishing treatment effect from recurrence with pooled sensitivity and specificity above 80% [58, 80]. In the post-treatment setting for gliomas, recurrent or residual tumors typically exhibit higher rCBV values compared to PsP or RN. Sugahara et al. observed that lesions with a rCBV ratio < 0.6 were more likely to represent TRC while lesions with a ratio > 2.6 were more likely to be PD [81]. A meta-analysis by Patel et al. highlighted the use of DSC-MRI and in a subset of 13 studies evaluating gliomas after radiation and/or chemotherapy, reporting a pooled sensitivity and specificity of 89% (95% CI, 0.83–0.94) and 80% (95% CI, 0.72–0.86) respectively for rCBV, in discriminating PsP for rCBV. However, the meta-analysis also pointed out the wide variability in the reported rCBV thresholds across different studies, which ranged from 0.9 to 2.15 for mean rCBV ratio [82]. Similar results were presented in a recent meta-analysis by Gu et al., which included 21 studies enrolling 879 patients with 888 lesions focusing on HGG. rCBV diagnostic results were reported in 20 of the analyzed studies. The pooled sensitivity, specificity, positive likelihood ratio, and negative likelihood ratio values were 86% (95% CI, 0.81–0.89), 83% (95% CI, 0.77–0.87), 4.94 (95% CI, 3.61–6.75), and 0.18 (95% CI, 0.13–0.23), respectively, for these 20 studies. The corresponding AUC value was 0.91 (95% CI, 0.88–0.93) [83].

As part of a phase II clinical trial employing TMZ, Boxerman et al. examined a subset of patients with HGG. At the first follow-up visit, they found no statistically significant difference between PsP and PD in terms of the change in absolute mean rCBV (2.35 vs. 2.17; $P = 0.67$). One notable difference between PsP and PD was the change in rCBV at the immediately following visit, which was −0.84 vs. 0.84 ($P = 0.001$) [84]. However, the concept of a user-defined ROI inside the contralateral normal appearing parenchyma is prone to notable variability in rCBV measurements [85]. Early tumor growth might be accurately predicted by calculating the percentage changes in skewness and kurtosis of rCBV histograms. Aside from that, the rCBV histogram had the best independent prediction accuracy [86]. DSC is susceptible to artifacts, particularly near air-tissue interfaces such as the sinuses and skull base, due to magnetic field inhomogeneities and vascular injury in the post-treatment setting. For instance, telangiectasias and aneurysms can increase rCBV, while radiotherapy-induced microbleeding in recurrent tumors may lead to decreased rCBV [87]. One major disadvantage of DSC is its underlying assumption that the BBB stays intact without any contrast leakage or recirculation. Contrast leakage can produce overshooting on the DSC time curve. A preload bolus approach, used either alone or in combination with post-processing leakage correction or with DCE imaging, helps to mitigate this problem. [88].

Dynamic Contrast-Enhanced (DCE)

Dynamic Contrast-Enhanced (DCE) MRI assesses tissue perfusion and vascular permeability by dynamic T1-weighted imaging after intravenous administration of a GBCA. The Tofts model is a pharmacokinetic model frequently utilized in DCE imaging to analyze contrast agent kinetics. It quantifies parameters related to tissue perfusion and permeability, such as the volume transfer constant (Ktrans), plasma volume (Vp), and the fractional volume of the extravascular-extracellular space (Ve). Compared to DSC, fewer studies have evaluated DCE imaging for glioma follow-up. The meta-analysis conducted by Patel et al. included 11 DCE studies, revealing a pooled sensitivity of 89% and a specificity of 85% [82]. Ktrans is the most commonly used parameter to measure vascular permeability. It tends to be lower in areas affected by radiation necrosis and in cases of PsP but reported thresholds vary significantly, ranging from 0.05 to 0.347 [89, 90]. The same variables that were previously highlighted in relation to DSC investigations are responsible for this variability. A single-center retrospective study investigated DCE in 37 glioblastoma patients who exhibited tumor-like contrast enhancement within and beyond the 3-month time window. The study found that PsP had lower Vp and Ktrans compared to TP. Specifically, a Vp threshold greater than 3.9 had a specificity of 92% and a sensitivity of 85% for detecting TP. Meanwhile, a Ktrans(mean) threshold greater than 3.6 had a specificity of 79% and a sensitivity of 69%. It is important to note that these findings highlight the significance of BBB damage in the differentiation between PsP and TP [91]. Qiu et al. conducted a meta-analysis that included 11 studies covering 616 patients. The results showed that the pooled sensitivity, specificity, and diagnostic odds ratio of DCE were 0.792 (95% confidence interval [CI] 0.707–0.857), 0.779 (95% CI 0.715–0.832), and 16.219 (97.5% CI 9.123–28.833), respectively [92]. They emphasized the high sensitivities (>0.6) and low false positive rates (<0.5) of DCE in distinguishing PsP from TP in most of the included studies. The evidence regarding the role of DCE in assessing PsP during immunotherapy is scarce. However, in a study involving patients with BM from melanoma undergoing immunotherapy, PsP exhibited significantly lower rVp90 on DCE compared with TP [93]. One significant advantage of DCE is its reduced artifacts compared to DSC, providing a higher SNR and better spatial resolution, especially near air-tissue interfaces like the skull base and sinuses, or in the presence of hemorrhage.

Arterial Spin Labeling (ASL)

ASL is a completely noninvasive MR imaging method based on magnetic labeling of inflowing protons, which subsequently are measured in the brain parenchyma, mainly for measurement of cerebral blood flow (CBF) by subtraction of background nonlabeled tissue. Based on the labeling method, ASL techniques are divided into continuous ASL (CASL) and pulsed ASL (PASL), which apply a long or short train of continuous RF pulse to invert the magnetization of arterial blood flowing through a labeling plane, respectively. A modified approach to CASL, known as pseudocontinuous ASL (pCASL), was developed to improve labeling efficiency. This technique uses a sequence of short RF pulses delivered in quick succession along with gradient fields, generating a stream of labeling pulses that mimic continuous labeling. This method combines the high signal-to-noise ratio of CASL with the shorter acquisition times associated with PASL, offering an optimized balance between signal quality and scanning efficiency. A crucial parameter in this technique is the postlabel delay (PLD) time, the interval between the labeling of arterial blood and the acquisition of imaging data. If the PLD is too short, the labeled blood may not reach the imaging slice, leading to underestimation of CBF, particularly in regions with longer arterial transit times. Conversely, if the PLD is too long, the signal from the labeled blood will decay due to T1 relaxation, reducing the SNR and potentially underestimating CBF in regions with shorter transit times. In clinical practice, a fixed PLD is often used for simplicity, but this compromise may not suit all patients or brain regions. The recommended PLD is 1500 milliseconds for pediatric populations and 2000 milliseconds for adult clinical populations [94, 95]. While the advised use of ASL is at a field strength of 3 T, some evidence suggests it can also be effectively conducted at 1.5 T [96]. Despite the lack of consensus regarding the optimal ASL technique for brain tumor evaluation, current recommendations suggest choosing a 3D pCASL sequence. This allows for improved evaluation, especially in areas strongly affected by susceptibility artifacts, and simpler clinical implementation [97, 98]. Meta-analyses demonstrated the utility of pCASL for preoperative glioma grading, in differentiating HGG from brain solitary metastases and primary central nervous system lymphoma [99–101]. Moreover, it is reliable in improving agreement in neuroradiologists' clinical interpretations of posttreatment HGG surveillance [102]. Manning et al. found that absolute ASL-CBF measurements were significantly higher in the PD group compared to the PsP group, with a cut-off value of 64.2 mL/100 g/min yielding a sensitivity of 1.000 and specificity of 0.880. For normalized-CBF (with normalization using a contralateral ROI), a cut-off value of 1.570 yielded a sensitivity of 0.920 and specificity of 0.857 [103]. Moreover, when comparing the CBF measurements obtained via ASL to those acquired using the DSC technique, ASL demonstrated the highest AUC and misclassified the fewest cases. To differentiate between radiation-induced brain injury and glioma recurrence, Wang et al. indicated that the optimal cut-off values for CBF and nCBF were 36.86 mL/100 g/min (74.3% sensitivity, 82.4% specificity, and 78.3% accuracy) and 1.86 (68.6% sensitivity, 91.2% specificity, and 79.7% accuracy), respectively [104]. Similar results were found by Xu et al., with optimal cut-off values for CBF and nCBF being 32.32 mL/100 g/min (88.2% sensitivity, 58% specificity, and 75.9% accuracy) and 1.11 (100% sensitivity, 75% specificity, and 89.7% accuracy), respectively [105] Although the use of a single absolute ASL-

CBF cut-off value for differentiation of TP from PsP is appealing, caution is advised because measurements are dependent on many factors including differences between scanners, ASL technique choice, and postprocessing analysis method. In fact, a recent study of Flies et al. found a poor diagnostic value of ASL in differentiating PD and TRC in irradiated HGG with radiologic progression within 6 months after radiation therapy (AUC 0.520). In radiologic progression after 6 months, the diagnostic value was better (AUC 0.587) [106]. The authors attribute the results to more inflammatory and apoptotic modifications of PsP in the initial months following RT, causing many false positives, in contrast to more uniform vascular changes of RN observed later. Overall, a meta-analysis of 20 studies with 939 patients evaluating PWI in post-treatment glioma found 79% and 78% sensitivity and specificity for ASL with an AUC of 0.88 [80]. In conclusion, ASL stands out as an interesting MRI technique due to its noncontrast nature for directly measuring CBF. ASL also avoids issues related to contrast leakage and BBB breakdown, and it provides improved lesion visualization with reduced susceptibility artifacts compared to DSC. This is particularly valuable in brain tumor treatment response assessment, where prominent susceptibility artifacts often arise from post-treatment changes, including residual blood products along the surgical cavity [107–109].

5.9.3.4 Endogenous Chemical Exchange Saturation Transfer

Chemical Exchange Saturation Transfer (CEST) is a sophisticated MRI technique that enhances image contrast based on the exchange of protons between different molecular environments, particularly between water and amide groups (APT) in proteins and peptides. The core physical principle of APT-CEST relies on the concept of selective saturation and chemical exchange. In APT-CEST, a radiofrequency (RF) pulse is applied at the specific resonance frequency of the amide protons. This RF pulse saturates the amide protons(i.e. their magnetization is selectively reduced), leading to a loss of their signal. Once these amide protons are saturated, they undergo a process called chemical exchange with the surrounding water protons. This exchange occurs because amide protons can transfer between their original molecular environment (amide groups) and the water molecules. When the saturated amide protons transfer to water, they effectively reduce the magnetization of the water protons, leading to a decrease in the overall MRI signal from water. The MRI scanner then measures the signal from water protons both with and without the saturation pulse. The difference in these signals is analyzed to create a CEST contrast image. This contrast is indicative of the relative concentration of amide protons, providing information about protein and peptide content in the tissue [110, 111]. To date the use of CEST to distinguish between TP and TRC has little data, mostly due to sample size. However, given the high reported accuracy (AUC, 0.88–0.98) in many investigations, it is possible that APT may significantly increase the diagnostic utility of MRI for this particular clinical issue [112]. In a recent study conducted by Kroh et al., MT_{const} (AUC = 0.79, $p < 0.01$) showed a stronger association with RANO response assessment and enabled differentiation of participants with PsP ($n = 8$) from those with TP (AUC = 0.79, $p = 0.02$) [113]. The preliminary results may be justified due to the observation that treatment-related alterations in tissues often lead to decreased cell density and cytoplasm disintegration. These changes result in a reduced concentration of proteins in the affected areas when compared to recurrent tumors [114]. Essed et al. conducted a systematic review and meta-analysis on the current literature, analyzing 15 studies, of which 12 were included in the meta-analysis. The study evaluates the diagnostic accuracy of APT in distinguishing TP from TRC, including PsP, in both gliomas and metastases. The results show that APT imaging performs well in gliomas, with a pooled sensitivity of 0.88 and specificity of 0.84. However, its performance was less effective in brain metastases, with a sensitivity of 0.64 and specificity of 0.56, probably due to an underrepresentation of BM in this study. Moreover, the combination of APT-CEST with PWI and/or conventional MRI techniques seems to offer superior diagnostic performance, surpassing the effectiveness of each imaging modality on its own [115].

5.10 Positron Emission Tomography

5.10.1 18F-Fluorodeoxyglucose Positron Emission Tomography

18F-fluorodeoxyglucose positron emission tomography (FDG-PET) operates on the principle of detecting metabolic activity in tissues by using a radiolabeled glucose analog. In TP, malignant cells continue to proliferate and exhibit high rates of glucose metabolism, leading to increased uptake and accumulation of FDG and indicating active tumor growth. Conversely, TRC generally has decreased glucose metabolism, resulting in lower FDG uptake [116]. Even with this apparent distinction, many lesions in practice exhibit indeterminate FDG uptake. The natural heterogeneity of the treated lesions is probably partially to blame for these inconsistent results, but more importantly the specificity of FDG-PET can be limited due to the high basal glucose uptake in normal brain tissues [117] or other alterations such as subclinical seizure activity [118]. Moreover, in PsP, there is significant inflammation and edema, leading to FDG uptake that may result in potential false positives and limit its specificity. The RANO working group confirms this, pointing out that due to enhanced FDG metabolism in inflammatory tissue, FDG has limited specificity for differentiating gliomas from other non-neoplastic diseases [119]. Overall, robust evidence for a substantial additional benefit of FDG-PET over advanced MRI techniques remains limited. According to some studies, FDG-PET does not significantly enhance diagnostic accuracy or clinical outcomes compared to advanced MRI alone, often showing lower specificity, which ranges from 40% to 94% [120, 121]. For this reason, in recent years, amino acid radiotracers are increasingly being used. They have significant advantages over FDG, including greater sensitivity, specificity, and tumor-to-background uptake ratio.

5.10.2 Amino Acid PET

Amino acid (AA) PET tracers, such as 11C-methionine (MET), 18F-fluoroethyltyrosine (FET), and 18F-fluorodopa (18F-FDOPA), exploit the elevated amino acid transport in tumor cells. Amino acid transporters, primarily the L-type amino acid transporter 1 (LAT1), take up these tracers, which are overexpressed in brain tumors. LAT1 is responsible for the transport of large neutral AAs across the cell membrane [122]. Tumor cells often have increased LAT1 expression to meet their heightened demands for AAs, which are necessary for rapid growth and proliferation. Unlike contrast-enhanced MRI, BBB rupture is not necessary for radiotracer intratumoral localization [123]. By using tracers that are substrates for LAT1, AA-PET imaging provides a more specific indication of tumor activity, reducing the likelihood of false positives associated with inflammatory or non-neoplastic processes. Active transport of AA tracers into PsP tissue should be equal to or less than that into normal brain tissue. Therefore, any increased uptake in PsP tissue likely results from passive influx and exhibits lower intensity compared to uptake in TP [124].

Evidence in the literature suggests that the most commonly used AA-PET tracers all demonstrate similar diagnostic performance to differentiate between TP and TRC [125]. MET has demonstrated excellent value in identifying PsP with diagnostic accuracy ranging from 0.89 to 0.92 [126, 127]. In a prospective study by Skvortsova involving 72 patients with treated cerebral glioma, MET-PET was used to investigate glioma progression. The analysis identified a TBRmax threshold value of greater than 1.9 for differentiating between glioma TP and PsP, achieving a sensitivity of 83.5% and a specificity of 97.0%. MET has certain limitations primarily due to the nature of its production and properties. Particularly, its short half-life of approximately 20 min, which necessitates the presence of an on-site cyclotron for production. For this reason, other radiopharmaceuticals such as FET and 18F-FDOPA have been developed. These alternatives have longer half-lives around 110 min, allowing for wider distribution and use in clinical practice. Relative simplicity, low cost of production, and absence of physiologic absorption in the striatum define the benefits of FET. Several studies have reported a TBRmax threshold range of 1.9–2.65, which detected PsP with a diagnostic accuracy of up to 99% within the RANO-defined window [128–131]. Moreover, the long half-life of FET allows for dynamic PET scans, which can provide valuable information about the kinetics of tracer uptake in tissues. TP often shows a rapid initial uptake followed by a plateau or increase, while PsP and treatment-related changes tend to have a slower, more gradual uptake. In these studies, a time to peak of 32.5 min accurately differentiates TP from PsP [132]. When combined with static parameters, diagnostic accuracy is further improved [133]. For instance, FET-PET may reveal BEV therapy failure sooner than MRI [122]. 18F-FDOPA PET is known to be more effective than MRI in detecting low-grade gliomas (LGG), providing better tumor delineation and aiding in the differentiation between LGG and HGG [134]. Although 18F-FDOPA has differential tumor absorption, its resemblance to dopamine causes preferential accumulation in the striatum, making it difficult to distinguish brain lesions in this location [135]. A systematic review of the literature conducted by Somme et al. show significant potential in detecting TP, with all PET indices being significantly higher in progressive patients than in nonprogressive ones [136]. Interestingly, semiquantitative image analysis did not enhance accuracy compared to visual 18F-FDOPA PET image analysis, with the AUC ranging from 0.77 to 0.82 versus 0.82 for visual analysis [137]. As a result, determining the threshold becomes more complex. Nonetheless, one study of Zaragory et al. identified a TBR cut-off of 1.61 as useful for differentiation [138].

Overall, PET imaging, especially with amino acid radiotracers, has shown good diagnostic value in distinguishing TRC from TP, complementing MRI in glioma management, although results on performance are controversial or unknown in the setting of PsP [139]. Additionally, the recent joint recommendations by the European Association of Nuclear Medicine (EANM) and the European Association of Neuro-Oncology (EANO), along with the guidelines from the RANO working group, have proposed PET imaging as a criterion for managing glioma, complementing MRI [140].

Despite the potential advantages of AA PET, few studies have thoroughly examined its diagnostic utility in the context of BM. By consolidating findings from various research, Schlurmann et al. conducted a meta-analysis including 12 studies with a total of 547 lesions in 397 patients. The pooled sensitivity and specificity are 82% and 84%, respectively, suggesting a high diagnostic accuracy for AA PET also in this context. However, the Authors note that the sensitivity is slightly lower compared to gliomas. This variation is attributed to differences in AA transporter expression and the potential impact of systemic therapies on tracer uptake. Similarly to gliomas, AA PET's specificity for BM is not perfect. Reactive astrocytosis brought on by radiation treatment or immunotherapy can cause tracer absorption higher than found in normal brain tissue, sometimes producing false-positive results [141, 142].

5.11 Conclusion

Distinguishing PsP from TP is critical in neuro-oncology, as misdiagnosis can lead to unnecessary treatment changes, delayed interventions, and compromised patient outcomes. MRI imaging techniques such as DWI and PWI are not merely supplementary—they are indispensable for accurate tumor evaluation. Contrast-free techniques like ASL and postcontrast methods such as DSC and DCE imaging improve diagnostic accuracy. Moreover, if available, amino acid PET further enhance diagnostic capabilities, offering a comprehensive assessment of tumor activity. As a consequence, advanced imaging is no longer optional. Nevertheless, conventional imaging should not be underestimated, as it represents a cornerstone of clinical practice and has the advantage of being widely available across healthcare facilities. It provides essential information on the lesion's morphology and changes.

The latest RANO criteria offer a robust framework for combining imaging with clinical insights, providing consistent, reliable evaluations of treatment response.

References

1. Abbasi AW, Westerlaan HE, Holtman GA, Aden KM, van Laar PJ, van der Hoorn A. Incidence of tumour progression and Pseudoprogression in high-Grade gliomas: a systematic review and meta-analysis. Clin Neuroradiol. 2018;28(3):401–11. https://doi.org/10.1007/s00062-017-0584-x.
2. Ludmir EB, et al. Increased risk of pseudoprogression among pediatric low-grade glioma patients treated with proton versus photon radiotherapy. Neuro-Oncology. 2019;21(5):686–95. https://doi.org/10.1093/neuonc/noz042.
3. Romano A, et al. Radiosurgery for brain metastases: challenges in imaging interpretation after treatment. Cancers (Basel). 2023;15(20):5092. https://doi.org/10.3390/cancers15205092.
4. Skeie BS, et al. A simple score to estimate the likelihood of pseudoprogression vs. recurrence following stereotactic radiosurgery for brain metastases: the Bergen criteria. Neurooncol Adv. 2020;2(1). https://doi.org/10.1093/noajnl/vdaa026.
5. Dworkin M, et al. Increase of pseudoprogression and other treatment related effects in low-grade glioma patients treated with proton radiation and temozolomide. J Neuro-Oncol. 2019;142(1):69–77. https://doi.org/10.1007/s11060-018-03063-1.
6. Brandsma D, Stalpers L, Taal W, Sminia P, van den Bent MJ. Clinical features, mechanisms, and management of pseudoprogression in malignant gliomas. Lancet Oncol. 2008;9(5):453–61. https://doi.org/10.1016/S1470-2045(08)70125-6.
7. Chambrelant I, Eber J, Antoni D, Burckel H, Noël G, Auvergne R. Proton therapy and gliomas: a systematic review. Radiation. 2021;1(3):218–33. https://doi.org/10.3390/radiation1030019.
8. Hegi ME, et al. *MGMT* gene silencing and benefit from Temozolomide in glioblastoma. N Engl J Med. 2005;352(10):997–1003. https://doi.org/10.1056/NEJMoa043331.
9. Li Y, et al. Advanced imaging techniques for differentiating Pseudoprogression and tumor recurrence after immunotherapy for glioblastoma. Front Immunol. 2021;12. https://doi.org/10.3389/fimmu.2021.790674.
10. Thust SC, van den Bent MJ, Smits M. Pseudoprogression of brain tumors. J Magn Reson Imaging. 2018;48(3):571–89. https://doi.org/10.1002/jmri.26171.
11. Blakstad H, et al. Incidence and outcome of pseudoprogression after radiation therapy in glioblastoma patients: a cohort study. Neurooncol Pract. 2024;11(1):36–45. https://doi.org/10.1093/nop/npad063.
12. Castellano A, Anzalone N. Radiation and chemotherapy induced injury. In: Clinical neuroradiology. Cham: Springer; 2019. p. 1–29. https://doi.org/10.1007/978-3-319-61423-6_68-1.
13. Bernhardt D, et al. DEGRO practical guideline for central nervous system radiation necrosis part 2: treatment. Strahlenther Onkol. 2022;198(11):971–80. https://doi.org/10.1007/s00066-022-01973-8.
14. Liao G, Khan M, Zhao Z, Arooj S, Yan M, Li X. Bevacizumab treatment of radiation-induced brain necrosis: a systematic review. Front Oncol. 2021;11. https://doi.org/10.3389/fonc.2021.593449.
15. Cruz N, et al. Highlighted advances in therapies for difficult-to-treat brain tumours such as glioblastoma. Pharmaceutics. 2023;15(3):928. https://doi.org/10.3390/pharmaceutics15030928.
16. Caccese M, et al. REGOMA-OSS: a large, Italian, multicenter, prospective, observational study evaluating the efficacy and safety of regorafenib in patients with recurrent glioblastoma. ESMO Open. 2024;9(4):102943. https://doi.org/10.1016/j.esmoop.2024.102943.
17. Lombardi G, et al. Regorafenib compared with lomustine in patients with relapsed glioblastoma (REGOMA): a multicentre, open-label, randomised, controlled, phase 2 trial. Lancet Oncol. 2019;20(1):110–9. https://doi.org/10.1016/S1470-2045(18)30675-2.
18. Wu W, et al. Glioblastoma multiforme (GBM): an overview of current therapies and mechanisms of resistance. Pharmacol Res. 2021;171:105780. https://doi.org/10.1016/j.phrs.2021.105780.
19. Ahluwalia M, et al. Laser ablation after stereotactic radiosurgery: a multicenter prospective study in patients with metastatic brain tumors and radiation necrosis. J Neurosurg. 2019;130(3):804–11. https://doi.org/10.3171/2017.11.JNS171273.
20. Sankey EW, et al. Time to steroid independence after laser interstitial thermal therapy vs medical management for treatment of biopsy-proven radiation necrosis secondary to stereotactic radiosurgery for brain metastasis. Neurosurgery. 2022;90(6):684–90. https://doi.org/10.1227/neu.0000000000001922.
21. Woodworth G, McGirt MJ, Samdani A, Garonzik I, Olivi A, Weingart JD. Accuracy of frameless and frame-based image-guided stereotactic brain biopsy in the diagnosis of glioma: comparison of biopsy and open resection specimen. Neurol Res. 2005;27(4):358–62. https://doi.org/10.1179/016164105X40057.
22. Otsuji R, et al. Liquid biopsy for glioma using cell-free DNA in cerebrospinal fluid. Cancers (Basel). 2024;16(5):1009. https://doi.org/10.3390/cancers16051009.
23. Wadden J, Ravi K, John V, Babila CM, Koschmann C. Cell-free tumor DNA (cf-tDNA) liquid biopsy: current methods and use in brain tumor

immunotherapy. Front Immunol. 2022;13. https://doi.org/10.3389/fimmu.2022.882452.
24. Bagley SJ, et al. Clinical utility of plasma cell-free DNA in adult patients with newly diagnosed glioblastoma: a pilot prospective study. Clin Cancer Res. 2020;26(2):397–407. https://doi.org/10.1158/1078-0432.CCR-19-2533.
25. Raza IJ, Tingate CA, Gkolia P, Romero L, Tee JW, Hunn MK. Blood biomarkers of glioma in response assessment including Pseudoprogression and other treatment effects: a systematic review. Front Oncol. 2020;10. https://doi.org/10.3389/fonc.2020.01191.
26. Macdonald DR, Cascino TL, Schold SC, Cairncross JG. Response criteria for phase II studies of supratentorial malignant glioma. J Clin Oncol. 1990;8(7):1277–80. https://doi.org/10.1200/JCO.1990.8.7.1277.
27. Wen PY, et al. Updated response assessment criteria for high-Grade gliomas: response assessment in neuro-oncology working group. J Clin Oncol. 2010;28(11):1963–72. https://doi.org/10.1200/JCO.2009.26.3541.
28. Ellingson BM, et al. A Neuroradiologist's guide to operationalizing the response assessment in neuro-oncology (RANO) criteria version 2.0 for gliomas in adults. Am J Neuroradiol. 2024. https://doi.org/10.1007/s13311-016-0507-6.
29. Ellingson BM, et al. A Neuroradiologist's guide to operationalizing the response assessment in neuro-oncology (RANO) criteria version 2.0 for gliomas in adults. Am J Neuroradiol. 2024; https://doi.org/10.3174/ajnr.A8396.
30. Louis DN, Perry A, Wesseling P, et al. The 2021 WHO Classification of Tumors of the Central Nervous System: a summary. Neuro Oncol. 2021;23(8):1231–51. https://doi.org/10.1093/neuonc/noab106.
31. Wen PY, et al. RANO 2.0: update to the response assessment in neuro-oncology criteria for high- and low-grade gliomas in adults. J Clin Oncol. 2023;41(33):5187–99. https://doi.org/10.1200/JCO.23.01059.
32. Okada H, et al. Immunotherapy response assessment in neuro-oncology: a report of the RANO working group. Lancet Oncol. 2015;16(15):e534–42. https://doi.org/10.1016/S1470-2045(15)00088-1.
33. Lin NU, et al. Response assessment criteria for brain metastases: proposal from the RANO group. Lancet Oncol. 2015;16(6):e270–8. https://doi.org/10.1016/S1470-2045(15)70057-4.
34. Katsura M, Sato J, Akahane M, Furuta T, Mori H, Abe O. Recognizing radiation-induced changes in the central nervous system: where to look and what to look for. Radio Graphics. 2021;41(1):224–48. https://doi.org/10.1148/rg.2021200064.
35. Gaudino S, et al. Regorafenib in glioblastoma recurrence: how to Deal with MR imaging treatments changes. Front Radiol. 2022;1. https://doi.org/10.3389/fradi.2021.790456.
36. Mansour M, Vitale V, Lombardi G, Riva G, Pancheri F, Zanusso M. Modification of MRI pattern of high-grade glioma pseudoprogression in regorafenib therapy. J Med Imaging Radiat Oncol. 2022;66(3):414–8. https://doi.org/10.1111/1754-9485.13267.
37. Zach L, et al. Delayed contrast extravasation MRI: a new paradigm in neuro-oncology. Neuro-Oncology. 2015;17(3):457–65. https://doi.org/10.1093/neuonc/nou230.
38. Cuccarini V, et al. Response assessment of GBM during immunotherapy by delayed contrast treatment response assessment maps. Front Neurol. 2024;15. https://doi.org/10.3389/fneur.2024.1374737.
39. Peker S, et al. The use of treatment response assessment maps in discriminating between radiation effect and persistent Tumoral lesion in metastatic brain tumors treated with gamma knife radiosurgery. World Neurosurg. 2021;146:e1134–46. https://doi.org/10.1016/j.wneu.2020.11.114.
40. Zach L, et al. Delayed contrast extravasation MRI for depicting tumor and non-Tumoral tissues in primary and metastatic brain tumors. PLoS One. 2012;7(12):e52008. https://doi.org/10.1371/journal.pone.0052008.
41. Müller SJ, Khadhraoui E, Ganslandt O, Henkes H, Gihr GA. MRI treatment response assessment maps (TRAMs) for differentiating recurrent glioblastoma from radiation necrosis. J Neuro-Oncol. 2024;166(3):513–21. https://doi.org/10.1007/s11060-024-04573-x.
42. Tsang K, Pang C, Butler S. Static permeability assessment method to distinguish brain tumour recurrence from pseudoprogression. Neuro-Oncology. 2021;23(Supplement 4):iv25. https://doi.org/10.1093/neuonc/noab195.064.
43. Yu Y, Ma Y, Sun M, Jiang W, Yuan T, Tong D. Meta-analysis of the diagnostic performance of diffusion magnetic resonance imaging with apparent diffusion coefficient measurements for differentiating glioma recurrence from pseudoprogression. Medicine. 2020;99(23):e20270. https://doi.org/10.1097/MD.0000000000020270.
44. Song YS, et al. True progression versus Pseudoprogression in the treatment of glioblastomas: a comparison study of normalized cerebral blood volume and apparent diffusion coefficient by histogram analysis. Korean J Radiol. 2013;14(4):662. https://doi.org/10.3348/kjr.2013.14.4.662.
45. Chu HH, et al. Differentiation of true progression from Pseudoprogression in glioblastoma treated with radiation therapy and concomitant Temozolomide: comparison study of standard and high- *b* -value diffusion-weighted imaging. Radiology. 2013;269(3):831–40. https://doi.org/10.1148/radiol.13122024.
46. Bette S, et al. Local fractional anisotropy is reduced in areas with tumor recurrence in glioblastoma. Radiology. 2017;283(2):499–507. https://doi.org/10.1148/radiol.2016152832.

47. Wang S, et al. Differentiating tumor progression from Pseudoprogression in patients with glioblastomas using diffusion tensor imaging and dynamic susceptibility contrast MRI. Am J Neuroradiol. 2016;37(1):28–36. https://doi.org/10.3174/ajnr.A4474.
48. Zakaria R, et al. T-cell densities in brain metastases are associated with patient survival times and diffusion tensor MRI changes. Cancer Res. 2018;78(3):610–6. https://doi.org/10.1158/0008-5472.CAN-17-1720.
49. Jensen JH, Helpern JA, Ramani A, Lu H, Kaczynski K. Diffusional kurtosis imaging: the quantification of non-gaussian water diffusion by means of magnetic resonance imaging. Magn Reson Med. 2005;53(6):1432–40. https://doi.org/10.1002/mrm.20508.
50. D'Amore F, et al. Combined 18F-FET PET and diffusion kurtosis MRI in posttreatment glioblastoma: differentiation of true progression from treatment-related changes. Neurooncol Adv. 2021;3(1). https://doi.org/10.1093/noajnl/vdab044.
51. Wu X, et al. Differentiating high-grade glioma recurrence from pseudoprogression: comparing diffusion kurtosis imaging and diffusion tensor imaging. Eur J Radiol. 2021;135:109445. https://doi.org/10.1016/j.ejrad.2020.109445.
52. Chakhoyan A, et al. Mono-exponential, diffusion kurtosis and stretched exponential diffusion MR imaging response to chemoradiation in newly diagnosed glioblastoma. J Neuro-Oncol. 2018;139(3):651–9. https://doi.org/10.1007/s11060-018-2910-9.
53. Henriksen OM, et al. High-grade glioma treatment response monitoring biomarkers: a position statement on the evidence supporting the use of advanced MRI techniques in the clinic, and the latest bench-to-bedside developments. Part 1: perfusion and diffusion techniques. Front Oncologia. 2022;12. https://doi.org/10.3389/fonc.2022.810263.
54. Kim HS, Suh CH, Kim N, Choi C-G, Kim SJ. Histogram analysis of Intravoxel incoherent motion for differentiating recurrent tumor from treatment effect in patients with glioblastoma: initial clinical experience. Am J Neuroradiol. 2014;35(3):490–7. https://doi.org/10.3174/ajnr.A3719.
55. Liao D, Liu Y-C, Liu J-Y, Wang D, Liu X-F. Differentiating tumour progression from pseudoprogression in glioblastoma patients: a monoexponential, biexponential, and stretched-exponential model-based DWI study. BMC Med Imaging. 2023;23(1):119. https://doi.org/10.1186/s12880-023-01082-7.
56. Horská A, Barker PB. Imaging of brain tumors: MR spectroscopy and metabolic imaging. Neuroimaging Clin N Am. 2010;20(3):293–310. https://doi.org/10.1016/j.nic.2010.04.003.
57. Brandão LA, Castillo M. Adult brain tumors. Magn Reson Imaging Clin N Am. 2016;24(4):781–809. https://doi.org/10.1016/j.mric.2016.07.005.
58. van Dijken BRJ, van Laar PJ, Holtman GA, van der Hoorn A. Diagnostic accuracy of magnetic resonance imaging techniques for treatment response evaluation in patients with high-grade glioma, a systematic review and meta-analysis. Eur Radiol. 2017;27(10):4129–44. https://doi.org/10.1007/s00330-017-4789-9.
59. Zhang H, Ma L, Wang Q, Zheng X, Wu C, Xu B. Role of magnetic resonance spectroscopy for the differentiation of recurrent glioma from radiation necrosis: a systematic review and meta-analysis. Eur J Radiol. 2014;83(12):2181–9. https://doi.org/10.1016/j.ejrad.2014.09.018.
60. Weybright P, et al. Differentiation between brain tumor recurrence and radiation injury using MR spectroscopy. Am J Roentgenol. 2005;185(6):1471–6. https://doi.org/10.2214/AJR.04.0933.
61. Nakajima T, et al. Differential diagnosis between radiation necrosis and glioma progression using sequential proton magnetic resonance spectroscopy and methionine positron emission tomography. Neurol Med Chir (Tokyo). 2009;49(9):394–401. https://doi.org/10.2176/nmc.49.394.
62. Anbarloui MR, et al. Accuracy of magnetic resonance spectroscopy in distinction between radiation necrosis and recurrence of brain tumors. Iran J Neurol. 2015;14(1):29–34.
63. Zeng Q-S, Li C-F, Zhang K, Liu H, Kang X-S, Zhen J-H. Multivoxel 3D proton MR spectroscopy in the distinction of recurrent glioma from radiation injury. J Neuro-Oncol. 2007;84(1):63–9. https://doi.org/10.1007/s11060-007-9341-3.
64. Rabinov JD, et al. In vivo 3-T MR spectroscopy in the distinction of recurrent glioma versus radiation effects: initial experience. Radiology. 2002;225(3):871–9. https://doi.org/10.1148/radiol.2253010997.
65. Rock JP, et al. Associations among magnetic resonance spectroscopy, apparent diffusion coefficients, and image-guided histopathology with special attention to radiation necrosis. Neurosurgery. 2004;54(5):1111–9. https://doi.org/10.1227/01.NEU.0000119328.56431.A7.
66. Dhermain FG, Hau P, Lanfermann H, Jacobs AH, van den Bent MJ. Advanced MRI and PET imaging for assessment of treatment response in patients with gliomas. Lancet Neurol. 2010;9(9):906–20. https://doi.org/10.1016/S1474-4422(10)70181-2.
67. Maudsley AA, et al. Advanced magnetic resonance spectroscopic neuroimaging: experts' consensus recommendations. NMR Biomed. 2021;34(5). https://doi.org/10.1002/nbm.4309.
68. Artzi M, et al. Differentiation between vasogenic-edema versus tumor-infiltrative area in patients with glioblastoma during bevacizumab therapy: a longitudinal MRI study. Eur J Radiol. 2014;83(7):1250–6. https://doi.org/10.1016/j.ejrad.2014.03.026.
69. Seeger A, et al. Comparison of three different MR perfusion techniques and MR spectroscopy for multiparametric assessment in distinguishing recurrent high-Grade gliomas from stable disease.

Acad Radiol. 2013;20(12):1557–65. https://doi.org/10.1016/j.acra.2013.09.003.
70. Ahir BK, Engelhard HH, Lakka SS. Tumor development and angiogenesis in adult brain tumor: glioblastoma. Mol Neurobiol. 2020;57(5):2461–78. https://doi.org/10.1007/s12035-020-01892-8.
71. Kim HS, Goh MJ, Kim N, Choi CG, Kim SJ, Kim JH. Which combination of MR imaging modalities is best for predicting recurrent glioblastoma? Study of diagnostic accuracy and reproducibility. Radiology. 2014;273(3):831–43. https://doi.org/10.1148/radiol.14132868.
72. Ellingson BM, Smits M. The path forward: the standardized brain tumor imaging protocol (BTIP) for multicenter trials. In: Glioma imaging. Cham: Springer; 2020. p. 267–82. https://doi.org/10.1007/978-3-030-27359-0_17.
73. Anzalone N, et al. Brain gliomas: multicenter standardized assessment of dynamic contrast-enhanced and dynamic susceptibility contrast MR images. Radiology. 2018;287(3):933–43. https://doi.org/10.1148/radiol.2017170362.
74. Zhang J, et al. Clinical applications of contrast-enhanced perfusion MRI techniques in gliomas: recent advances and current challenges. Contrast Media Mol Imaging. 2017;2017:1–27. https://doi.org/10.1155/2017/7064120.
75. Tiwari P, et al. Computer-extracted texture features to distinguish cerebral Radionecrosis from recurrent brain tumors on multiparametric MRI: a feasibility study. AJNR Am J Neuroradiol. 2016;37(12):2231–6. https://doi.org/10.3174/ajnr.A4931.
76. Baek HJ, Kim HS, Kim N, Choi YJ, Kim YJ. Percent change of perfusion skewness and kurtosis: a potential imaging biomarker for early treatment response in patients with newly diagnosed glioblastomas. Radiology. 2012;264(3):834–43. https://doi.org/10.1148/radiol.12112120.
77. Paulson ES, Prah DE, Schmainda KM. Spiral perfusion imaging with consecutive echoes (SPICE™) for the simultaneous mapping of DSC- and DCE-MRI parameters in brain tumor patients: theory and initial feasibility. Tomography. 2016;2(4):295–307. https://doi.org/10.18383/j.tom.2016.00217.
78. Sanvito F, et al. Simultaneous quantification of perfusion, permeability, and leakage effects in brain gliomas using dynamic spin-and-gradient-echo echoplanar imaging MRI. Eur Radiol. 2023;34(5):3087–101. https://doi.org/10.1007/s00330-023-10215-z.
79. Kessler AT, Bhatt AA. Brain tumour post-treatment imaging and treatment-related complications. Insights Imaging. 2018;9(6):1057–75. https://doi.org/10.1007/s13244-018-0661-y.
80. Wang L, et al. Evaluation of perfusion MRI value for tumor progression assessment after glioma radiotherapy. Medicine. 2020;99(52):e23766. https://doi.org/10.1097/MD.0000000000023766.
81. Sugahara T, et al. Posttherapeutic intraaxial brain tumor: the value of perfusion-sensitive contrast-enhanced MR imaging for differentiating tumor recurrence from nonneoplastic contrast-enhancing tissue. AJNR Am J Neuroradiol. 2000;21(5):901–9.
82. Patel P, et al. MR perfusion-weighted imaging in the evaluation of high-grade gliomas after treatment: a systematic review and meta-analysis. Neuro-Oncology. 2017;19(1):118–27. https://doi.org/10.1093/neuonc/now148.
83. Gu X, He X, Wang H, Li J, Chen R, Liu H. Dynamic susceptibility contrast-enhanced perfusion-weighted imaging in differentiation between recurrence and Pseudoprogression in high-Grade glioma: a meta-analysis. J Comput Assist Tomogr. 2024;48(2):303–10. https://doi.org/10.1097/RCT.0000000000001543.
84. Boxerman JL, et al. Longitudinal DSC-MRI for distinguishing tumor recurrence from Pseudoprogression in patients with a high-grade glioma. Am J Clin Oncol. 2017;40(3):228–34. https://doi.org/10.1097/COC.0000000000000156.
85. Hoxworth JM, et al. Performance of standardized relative CBV for quantifying regional histologic tumor burden in recurrent high-Grade glioma: comparison against normalized relative CBV using image-localized stereotactic biopsies. Am J Neuroradiol. 2020;41(3):408–15. https://doi.org/10.3174/ajnr.A6486.
86. Śledzińska-Bebyn P, Furtak J, Bebyn M, Serafin Z. Beyond conventional imaging: advancements in MRI for glioma malignancy prediction and molecular profiling. Magn Reson Imaging. 2024;112:63–81. https://doi.org/10.1016/j.mri.2024.06.004.
87. Santarosa C, et al. Dynamic contrast-enhanced and dynamic susceptibility contrast perfusion MR imaging for glioma grading: preliminary comparison of vessel compartment and permeability parameters using hotspot and histogram analysis. Eur J Radiol. 2016;85(6):1147–56. https://doi.org/10.1016/j.ejrad.2016.03.020.
88. Leu K, et al. Bidirectional contrast agent leakage correction of dynamic susceptibility contrast (DSC)-MRI improves cerebral blood volume estimation and survival prediction in recurrent glioblastoma treated with bevacizumab. J Magn Reson Imaging. 2016;44(5):1229–37. https://doi.org/10.1002/jmri.25227.
89. Hamilton JD, et al. Dynamic contrast-enhanced perfusion processing for Neuroradiologists: model-dependent analysis may not be necessary for determining recurrent high-Grade glioma versus treatment effect. Am J Neuroradiol. 2015;36(4):686–93. https://doi.org/10.3174/ajnr.A4190.
90. Morabito R, et al. DCE and DSC perfusion MRI diagnostic accuracy in the follow-up of primary and metastatic intra-axial brain tumors treated by radiosurgery with cyberknife. Radiat Oncol. 2019;14(1):65. https://doi.org/10.1186/s13014-019-1271-7.

91. Thomas AA, et al. Dynamic contrast enhanced T1 MRI perfusion differentiates pseudoprogression from recurrent glioblastoma. J Neuro-Oncol. 2015;125(1):183–90. https://doi.org/10.1007/s11060-015-1893-z.
92. Qiu J, et al. Diagnostic accuracy of dynamic contrast-enhanced magnetic resonance imaging for distinguishing pseudoprogression from glioma recurrence: a meta-analysis. Chin Med J. 2021;134(21):2535–43. https://doi.org/10.1097/CM9.0000000000001445.
93. Umemura Y, et al. DCE-MRI perfusion predicts pseudoprogression in metastatic melanoma treated with immunotherapy. J Neuro-Oncol. 2020;146(2):339–46. https://doi.org/10.1007/s11060-019-03379-6.
94. Haller S, Zaharchuk G, Thomas DL, Lovblad K-O, Barkhof F, Golay X. Arterial spin labeling perfusion of the brain: emerging clinical applications. Radiology. 2016;281(2):337–56. https://doi.org/10.1148/radiol.2016150789.
95. Iutaka T, et al. Arterial spin labeling: techniques, clinical applications, and interpretation. Radiographics. 2023;43(1). https://doi.org/10.1148/rg.220088.
96. Baas KPA, Petr J, Kuijer JPA, Nederveen AJ, Mutsaerts HJMM, van de Ven KCC. Effects of acquisition parameter modifications and field strength on the reproducibility of brain perfusion measurements using arterial spin-labeling. Am J Neuroradiol. 2021;42(1):109–15. https://doi.org/10.3174/ajnr.A6856.
97. Alsop DC, et al. Recommended implementation of arterial spin-labeled perfusion MRI for clinical applications: a consensus of the ISMRM perfusion study group and the European consortium for ASL in dementia. Magn Reson Med. 2015;73(1):102–16. https://doi.org/10.1002/mrm.25197.
98. Grade M, Hernandez Tamames JA, Pizzini FB, Achten E, Golay X, Smits M. A neuroradiologist's guide to arterial spin labeling MRI in clinical practice. Neuroradiology. 2015;57(12):1181–202. https://doi.org/10.1007/s00234-015-1571-z.
99. Xu W, Wang Q, Shao A, Xu B, Zhang J. The performance of MR perfusion-weighted imaging for the differentiation of high-grade glioma from primary central nervous system lymphoma: a systematic review and meta-analysis. PLoS One. 2017;12(3):e0173430. https://doi.org/10.1371/journal.pone.0173430.
100. Fu M, Han F, Feng C, Chen T, Feng X. Based on arterial spin labeling helps to differentiate high-grade gliomas from brain solitary metastasis. Medicine. 2019;98(19):e15580. https://doi.org/10.1097/MD.0000000000015580.
101. Fu J, Li L, Wang X, Zhang M, Zhang Y, Li Z. Clinical utility of arterial spin labeling for preoperative grading of glioma. Biosci Rep. 2018;38(4). https://doi.org/10.1042/BSR20180507.
102. Yamin G, et al. Arterial spin-labeling and DSC perfusion metrics improve agreement in neuroradiologists' clinical interpretations of posttreatment high-Grade glioma surveillance MR imaging—an institutional experience. Am J Neuroradiol. 2024;45(4):453–60. https://doi.org/10.3174/ajnr.A8190.
103. Manning P, et al. Differentiation of progressive disease from pseudoprogression using 3D PCASL and DSC perfusion MRI in patients with glioblastoma. J Neuro-Oncol. 2020;147(3):681–90. https://doi.org/10.1007/s11060-020-03475-y.
104. Wang Y-L, et al. Differentiation between radiation-induced brain injury and glioma recurrence using 3D pCASL and dynamic susceptibility contrast-enhanced perfusion-weighted imaging. Radiother Oncol. 2018;129(1):68–74. https://doi.org/10.1016/j.radonc.2018.01.009.
105. Xu Q, et al. Tumor recurrence versus treatment effects in glioma. Medicine. 2017;96(50):e9332. https://doi.org/10.1097/MD.0000000000009332.
106. Flies CM, et al. The differentiation between progressive disease and treatment-induced effects with perfusion-weighted arterial spin-labeling in high-grade gliomas. Am J Neuroradiol. 2024;45(7):920–6. https://doi.org/10.3174/ajnr.A8336.
107. Paulson ES, Schmainda KM. Comparison of dynamic susceptibility-weighted contrast-enhanced MR methods: recommendations for measuring relative cerebral blood volume in brain tumors. Radiology. 2008;249(2):601–13. https://doi.org/10.1148/radiol.2492071659.
108. Boxerman JL, Schmainda KM, Weisskoff RM. Relative cerebral blood volume maps corrected for contrast agent extravasation significantly correlate with glioma tumor grade, whereas uncorrected maps do not. AJNR Am J Neuroradiol. 2006;27(4):859–67.
109. Järnum H, et al. Perfusion MRI of brain tumours: a comparative study of pseudo-continuous arterial spin labelling and dynamic susceptibility contrast imaging. Neuroradiology. 2010;52(4):307–17. https://doi.org/10.1007/s00234-009-0616-6.
110. Zhou J, Heo H, Knutsson L, van Zijl PCM, Jiang S. APT-weighted MRI: techniques, current neuro applications, and challenging issues. J Magn Reson Imaging. 2019;50(2):347–64. https://doi.org/10.1002/jmri.26645.
111. Wu B, et al. An overview of CEST MRI for non-MR physicists. EJNMMI Phys. 2016;3(1):19. https://doi.org/10.1186/s40658-016-0155-2.
112. Okuchi S, Hammam A, Golay X, Kim M, Thust S. Endogenous chemical exchange saturation transfer MRI for the diagnosis and therapy response assessment of brain tumors: a systematic review. Radiol Imaging Cancer. 2020;2(1):e190036. https://doi.org/10.1148/rycan.2020190036.
113. Kroh F, et al. Semi-solid MT> and APTw CEST-MRI predict clinical outcome of patients with glioma early after radiotherapy. Magn Reson Med. 2023;90(4):1569–81. https://doi.org/10.1002/mrm.29746.
114. Zhang P, et al. A preliminary quantitative proteomic analysis of glioblastoma pseudoprogres-

sion. Proteome Sci. 2015;13(1):12. https://doi.org/10.1186/s12953-015-0066-5.
115. Essed RA, Prysiazhniuk Y, Wamelink IJ, Azizova A, Keil VC. Performance of amide proton transfer imaging to differentiate true progression from therapy-related changes in gliomas and metastases. Eur Radiol. 2024. https://doi.org/10.1007/s00330-024-11004-y.
116. Mabray MC, Barajas RF, Cha S. Modern brain tumor imaging. Brain Tumor Res Treat. 2015;3(1):8. https://doi.org/10.14791/btrt.2015.3.1.8.
117. Guedj E, et al. Correction to: EANM procedure guidelines for brain PET imaging using [18F] FDG, version 3. Eur J Nucl Med Mol Imaging. 2022;49(6):2100–1. https://doi.org/10.1007/s00259-022-05755-3.
118. Karunanithi S, et al. 18F-FDOPA PET/CT for detection of recurrence in patients with glioma: prospective comparison with 18F-FDG PET/CT. Eur J Nucl Med Mol Imaging. 2013;40(7):1025–35. https://doi.org/10.1007/s00259-013-2384-0.
119. Albert NL, et al. Response assessment in Neuro-Oncology Working Group and European Association for Neuro-Oncology recommendations for the clinical use of PET imaging in gliomas. Neuro-Oncology. 2016;18(9):1199–208. https://doi.org/10.1093/neuonc/now058.
120. Youland RS, et al. Prospective trial evaluating the sensitivity and specificity of 3,4-dihydroxy-6-[18F]-fluoro-l-phenylalanine (18F-DOPA) PET and MRI in patients with recurrent gliomas. J Neuro-Oncol. 2018;137(3):583–91. https://doi.org/10.1007/s11060-018-2750-7.
121. Langleben DD, Segall GM. PET in differentiation of recurrent brain tumor from radiation injury. J Nucl Med. 2000;41(11):1861–7.
122. Hughes KL, O'Neal CM, Andrews BJ, Westrup AM, Battiste JD, Glenn CA. A systematic review of the utility of amino acid PET in assessing treatment response to bevacizumab in recurrent high-grade glioma. Neurooncol Adv. 2021;3(1). https://doi.org/10.1093/noajnl/vdab003.
123. Puranik AD, et al. Brain FET PET tumor-to-white mater ratio to differentiate recurrence from post-treatment changes in high-grade gliomas. J Neuroimaging. 2021;31(6):1211–8. https://doi.org/10.1111/jon.12914.
124. Pöpperl G, Götz C, Rachinger W, Gildehaus F-J, Tonn J-C, Tatsch K. Value of O-(2-[18F]fluoroethyl)- L-tyrosine PET for the diagnosis of recurrent glioma. Eur J Nucl Med Mol Imaging. 2004;31(11):1464–70. https://doi.org/10.1007/s00259-004-1590-1.
125. Lapa C, et al. Comparison of the amino acid tracers ^{18} F-FET and ^{18} F-DOPA in high-Grade glioma patients. J Nucl Med. 2014;55(10):1611–6. https://doi.org/10.2967/jnumed.114.140608.
126. Bag AK, et al. 11C-methionine PET for identification of pediatric high-Grade glioma recurrence. J Nucl Med. 2022;63(5):664–71. https://doi.org/10.2967/jnumed.120.261891.
127. Ouyang Z-Q, et al. Diagnostic accuracy of glioma pseudoprogression identification with positron emission tomography imaging: a systematic review and meta-analysis. Quant Imaging Med Surg. 2023;13(8):4943–59. https://doi.org/10.21037/qims-22-1340.
128. Werner J-M, et al. Diagnosis of pseudoprogression following lomustine–temozolomide chemoradiation in newly diagnosed glioblastoma patients using FET-PET. Clin Cancer Res. 2021;27(13):3704–13. https://doi.org/10.1158/1078-0432.CCR-21-0471.
129. Kebir S, et al. Late pseudoprogression in glioblastoma: diagnostic value of dynamic O-(2-[18F] fluoroethyl)-L-tyrosine PET. Clin Cancer Res. 2016;22(9):2190–6. https://doi.org/10.1158/1078-0432.CCR-15-1334.
130. Galldiks N, Langen K-J, Pope WB. From the clinician's point of view – what is the status quo of positron emission tomography in patients with brain tumors? Neuro-Oncology. 2015;17(11):1434–44. https://doi.org/10.1093/neuonc/nov118.
131. Bashir A, et al. Recurrent glioblastoma versus late posttreatment changes: diagnostic accuracy of O-(2-[18F]fluoroethyl)-L-tyrosine positron emission tomography (18F-FET PET). Neuro-Oncology. 2019;21(12):1595–606. https://doi.org/10.1093/neuonc/noz166.
132. Prather KY, et al. A systematic review of amino acid PET in assessing treatment response to temozolomide in glioma. Neurooncol Adv. 2022;4(1):vdac008. https://doi.org/10.1093/noajnl/vdac008.
133. Werner J-M, et al. Differentiation of treatment-related changes from tumour progression: a direct comparison between dynamic FET PET and ADC values obtained from DWI MRI. Eur J Nucl Med Mol Imaging. 2019;46(9):1889–901. https://doi.org/10.1007/s00259-019-04384-7.

134. Smith JS, et al. Serial diffusion-weighted magnetic resonance imaging in cases of glioma: distinguishing tumor recurrence from postresection injury. J Neurosurg. 2005;103(3):428–38. https://doi.org/10.3171/jns.2005.103.3.0428.
135. Cicone F, et al. Volumetric assessment of recurrent or progressive gliomas: comparison between F-DOPA PET and perfusion-weighted MRI. Eur J Nucl Med Mol Imaging. 2015;42(6):905–15. https://doi.org/10.1007/s00259-015-3018-5.
136. Somme F, Bender L, Namer IJ, Noël G, Bund C. Usefulness of 18F-FDOPA PET for the management of primary brain tumors: a systematic review of the literature. Cancer Imaging. 2020;20(1):70. https://doi.org/10.1186/s40644-020-00348-5.
137. Herrmann K, et al. Comparison of visual and semiquantitative analysis of 18F-FDOPA-PET/CT for recurrence detection in glioblastoma patients. Neuro-Oncology. 2014;16(4):603–9. https://doi.org/10.1093/neuonc/not166.
138. Zaragori T, et al. Use of static and dynamic [18F]-F-DOPA PET parameters for detecting patients with glioma recurrence or progression. EJNMMI Res. 2020;10(1):56. https://doi.org/10.1186/s13550-020-00645-x.
139. Brandes AA, et al. Disease progression or pseudoprogression after concomitant radiochemotherapy treatment: pitfalls in neurooncology. Neuro-Oncology. 2008;10(3):361–7. https://doi.org/10.1215/15228517-2008-008.
140. Law I, et al. Joint EANM/EANO/RANO practice guidelines/SNMMI procedure standards for imaging of gliomas using PET with radiolabelled amino acids and [18F]FDG: version 1.0. Eur J Nucl Med Mol Imaging. 2019;46(3):540–57. https://doi.org/10.1007/s00259-018-4207-9.
141. Piroth MD, et al. Uptake of O-(2-[18F] fluoroethyl)-L-tyrosine in reactive astrocytosis in the vicinity of cerebral gliomas. Nucl Med Biol. 2013;40(6):795–800. https://doi.org/10.1016/j.nucmedbio.2013.05.001.
142. Schlürmann T, et al. Utility of amino acid PET in the differential diagnosis of recurrent brain metastases and treatment-related changes: a meta-analysis. J Nucl Med. 2023;64(5):816–21. https://doi.org/10.2967/jnumed.122.264803.

6 Iatrogenic Progressive Multifocal Leukoencephalopathy

Marialuisa Zedde, Simonetta Gerevini, and Rosario Pascarella

6.1 Introduction

Progressive multifocal leukoencephalopathy (PML) is a rare and potentially fatal disease induced by the JC virus (JCV), which primarily affects the central nervous system (CNS). While the virus typically remains asymptomatic in healthy individuals, it can become active when the immune system is weakened [1, 2]. PML gained widespread attention in the 1980s as a severe complication of AIDS, marked by rapid progression and a poor prognosis. Magnetic Resonance Imaging (MRI) often shows multiple areas of demyelination, and the presence of the JCV in cerebrospinal fluid (CSF) can be detected through polymerase chain reaction (PCR), offering a definitive diagnosis. Historically, autopsies were necessary to confirm the pathology.

M. Zedde (✉)
Neurology Unit, Stroke Unit, Azienda Unità Sanitaria Locale-IRCCS di Reggio Emilia, Reggio Emilia, Italy
e-mail: zedde.marialuisa@ausl.re.it

S. Gerevini
UOC Neuroradiologia, ASST Papa Giovanni XXIII, Bergamo, Italy

R. Pascarella
Neuroradiology Unit, Ospedale Santa Maria della Misericordia, AULSS 5 Polesana, Rovigo, Italy
e-mail: rosario.pascarella@aulss5.veneto.it

In 2005, cases of PML were reported in patients with multiple sclerosis (MS) undergoing treatment with disease-modifying therapies (DMTs) [3–5]. Since then, PML has been identified as a significant adverse effect of certain immunosuppressive and immunomodulatory medications that was already know for some rheumatologic diseases for instance [6–9]. However, unlike PML associated with AIDS, drug-induced PML can often be managed more effectively, and this is more specific for Natalizumab induced PML. This form of the disease tends to have a slower progression and is frequently associated with lower JC viral loads, with some immune function still present in the host i.e. benign persistent infection in the urinary tract. These characteristics are commonly seen in age-related immune suppression and in PML cases with an unknown cause of profound immunosuppression.

Early detection of PML is vital, though MRI may not always provide clear results, especially in the early stages where pathological changes are less evident. Additionally, the JC viral genome may be absent in CSF due to low viral replication, meaning a negative PCR, by in situ technique, result does not exclude PML [10]. In these instances, a brain biopsy may be required, but the tissue sample can be small and may fail to show the hallmark JC virus-infected cells with enlarged nuclei. Furthermore, inflammatory responses are often present, and other condi-

M. Zedde, R. Pascarella (eds.), Neuroimaging of Treatment-Related Conditions in the Brain,
https://doi.org/10.1007/978-3-032-23618-0_6

tions such as malignant lymphoma, vasculitis, and other demyelinating diseases must be considered in the differential diagnosis.

Prior to the AIDS epidemic, PML was an uncommon complication, primarily observed in individuals with immunosuppression due to lymphoproliferative disorders. The onset of the AIDS epidemic marked a dramatic rise in PML cases. However, the widespread implementation of highly effective antiretroviral therapies (ART) significantly reduced the incidence of PML in individuals with HIV, though HIV infection remains the leading contributor to global PML cases. In recent years, a smaller but notable increase in PML incidence has been linked to advancements in therapies for cancer, organ transplantation, and chronic inflammatory diseases. This trend is particularly evident with the use of Natalizumab in MS treatment. Collectively, HIV, lymphoproliferative disorders, and DMTs for MS are responsible for the majority of PML cases worldwide [11].

Currently, there are no antiviral treatments available for JCV infection or PML. Management of the disease heavily relies on reversing the underlying immunosuppression. Emerging research suggests that novel immunotherapeutic strategies aimed at enhancing antiviral immune responses could provide new avenues for treatment, particularly in cases where immunosuppression cannot be easily reversed.

6.2 The Role of Polyomaviruses

Human polyomavirus 2 (HPyV-2), previously known as JC Polyomavirus (JCPyV or JCV), is a member of the Polyomaviridae family, genus Polyomavirus. It was first isolated in 1971 from a patient with Hodgkin's lymphoma who succumbed to PML [1, 12]. The virus's genome consists of a 5.13 kb supercoiled circular double-stranded DNA, which includes three primary regions: the early coding region, the late coding region, and the noncoding control region (NCCR). The early region encodes two alternatively spliced transforming proteins, the large tumor antigen (T-Ag) and small tumor antigen (t-Ag), both essential for viral replication. The late region encodes the capsid proteins VP1, VP2, and VP3, and a regulatory protein called agnoprotein, which appears to aid in trafficking capsid proteins to the nucleus [13, 14]. The NCCR, a critical sequence for viral replication, separates the early and late coding regions. This sequence exists in two forms: the nonrearranged, nonpathogenic archetype form, typically found in the urine of healthy individuals, and the rearranged, more virulent prototype form, which is often detected in CSF, brain tissue, and blood of PML patients. The neurotropic pathogenic form features duplications of promoter/enhancer elements and deletions of suppressor elements, rearrangements that contribute to the development of PML.

HPyV-2 is a human-specific virus with a preference for infecting glial cells, kidney epithelial cells, and B lymphocytes. Primary infection mechanisms remain unclear, but between 50% and 90% of the adult population (depending on age and geographical region) have antibodies against JCPyV, suggesting that the virus commonly causes asymptomatic infections in childhood [15]. The virus enters target cells via the serotoninergic 5HT-2a receptor and an N-linked glycoprotein with α(2, 6)-linked sialic acid, which is present on various human cell types. Once inside the cells, JCPyV establishes a latent infection in the kidneys and lymphoid system. In cases of immunosuppression, the virus reactivates, replicating in the bloodstream and crossing the blood–brain barrier [16]. Neurotropic variants of JCPyV specifically target oligodendrocytes, where viral replication leads to the accumulation of viral particles, nuclear enlargement, neuronal apoptosis, and multifocal demyelination [15].

6.3 Pathogenesis

PML is an exceptionally rare occurrence in immunocompetent individuals, underscoring the critical role of prolonged cellular immune impairment in enabling JCV reactivation. CD8+ T cells are central to both preventing and resolving PML, with their activity closely linked to disease outcomes. Deficiencies in CD4+ T cells, such as those observed in HIV infection, are strongly associated with PML, with CD4+ T cell counts serving as a key prognostic indicator [2, 17–19]. Even in the absence of clinical PML, patients receiving immunosuppressive therapies may exhibit JCV reactivation and viraemia, reflecting an impaired cellular immune response to the virus [20, 21].

This reactivation often corresponds to increased variability in noncoding control region (NCCR) rearrangements, which accumulate through replication-driven mutations [22–24]. However, the uneven distribution of PML among immunocompromised patients suggests additional factors influence susceptibility. Mutations in viral proteins, such as VP1, have been implicated in heightened neurovirulence and aggressive disease progression [25–28]. Similarly, host genetic factors play a role: the HLA-DRB1*0401 allele, which impairs robust antiviral responses [29], and p53 polymorphisms that alter viral gene expression [30], are notable examples. Whole-exome sequencing has also identified rare germline variants in 17 immune-related genes that contribute to PML risk [31].

Underlying diseases and specific immunosuppressive drugs remain the most significant risk factors for PML [32–37]. For instance, during the AIDS epidemic, PML developed in up to 5% of HIV-infected individuals, potentially driven by synergistic interactions between HIV and JCV. Experimental studies have shown that the HIV transactivator protein Tat enhances JCV transcription and replication, contributing to viral latency escape [38, 39].

The cytokine environment shaped by underlying diseases also influences JCV reactivation. Several transcription factors involved in JCV replication, including NF-κB, NFAT4, and C/EBP-β, are activated by proinflammatory cytokines such as tumor necrosis factor (TNF) [40]. Features of B cells, particularly in B cell lymphoproliferative disorders, further facilitate JCV replication. For example, Spi-B, a transcription factor critical for B cell maturation, regulates JCV gene expression and promotes NCCR rearrangements via recombinase enzymes RAG1 and RAG2 [41, 42]. Treatments like natalizumab, which mobilize CD34+ hematopoietic precursors and CD19+ B cell precursors, may also contribute to JCV reactivation and dissemination [43].

Table 6.1 Stages of PML pathogenesis

Stage	Features
1	Persistent infection with nonpathogenic JCV archetypes occurs in the kidneys and potentially other secondary sites
2	Prolonged cellular immune impairment allows viral reactivation, leading to NCCR rearrangements and the emergence of neuropathogenic JCV variants. The virus may access the brain during this stage or earlier
3	Clinical PML develops, characterized by typical MRI findings and JCV DNA detection in cerebrospinal fluid (CSF) or brain tissue

Once JCV replication is unchecked by T cells, neurotropic quasispecies may emerge, independent of disease-specific cofactors [15]. This understanding supports a three-stage model of PML pathogenesis [44] (Table 6.1).

With the advent of immune reconstitution therapies, a potential fourth stage can be proposed, where equilibrium between host immunity and the virus is re-established. Some survivors exhibit persistent low-level viral detection in the CSF, raising concerns about PML recurrence [45–47]. This stage underscores the need for continued vigilance and long-term monitoring of PML survivors.

The virus could gain access to the brain during stage 1 or stage 2. Stage 3 is the clinical manifestation of PML [48].

6.4 Diagnosis

The diagnostic approach for PML has evolved considerably since its initial description in 1958 [49]. Initially, diagnosis relied primarily on brain histopathology, as there were no clinical, laboratory, or radiographic markers to confirm the condition. The hallmark histopathology of PML was characterized by a triad of demyelination, bizarre astrocytes, and oligodendroglial nuclear inclusions. The uniqueness of these findings drew attention to the disorder's distinct nature [49]. Following the discovery of JC virus, the causative polyomavirus, in 1971 [50], diagnostic advances included the use of electron microscopy and immunohistochemistry to detect the virus in tissue samples [51]. Further progress came with the establishment of PCR techniques to amplify JC virus DNA from brain tissue and CSF [52].

The etiology of PML is linked to JCV, a ubiquitous polyomavirus that infects more than 50% of the adult population worldwide. However, PML remains an extraordinarily rare complication in otherwise healthy individuals and almost always occurs in the context of immunosuppressive conditions. Recent studies have highlighted that JC virus can cause other neurological disorders, including granule cell neuronopathy in the cerebellum [53] and a fulminant encephalopathy involving cortical pyramidal neurons [54]. In some cases, the pathological findings in PML overlap with those seen in these other disorders, suggesting the potential for viral mutations or variations [55, 56].

Although the virus can be detected in the brains of otherwise healthy individuals, its mere presence, whether in tissue or CSF, is not sufficient for diagnosing PML. Thus, a multifactorial diagnostic approach, integrating clinical, imaging, and virologic evidence, is essential.

No single criterion can definitively diagnose PML. A comprehensive diagnostic framework incorporates multiple factors:

- Histopathologic Evidence: The presence of the classic triad of demyelination, bizarre astrocytes, and enlarged oligodendroglial nuclei, along with the detection of JC virus by in situ technique, is considered diagnostic.
- Clinical and Imaging Findings: Clinical symptoms and imaging manifestations consistent with PML, coupled with exclusion of other diagnoses, help strengthen the case for PML.
- Virological Evidence: PCR detection of JC virus in CSF further supports the diagnosis. it is diagnostic in the presence of consistent clinical radiological picture.

A German multidisciplinary working group proposed a case definition specifically for PML in the context of monoclonal antibody treatments [57]. However, this definition has some shortcomings, such as:

- Its focus solely on monoclonal antibody treatments, excluding broader risk factors.
- Heavy reliance on PCR for detecting JC virus in CSF without fully addressing the test's sensitivity and specificity.
- Underappreciation of cranial MRI abnormalities that may precede clinical symptoms.

The criteria for excluding PML in cases with concurrent neurological diseases are too lenient.

In 2013, a consensus statement for PML diagnostic criteria was published by members of the Neuroinfectious Disease Section of the American Academy of Neurology (AAN). Diagnostic classification distinguishes between definite, probable, and possible PML. The current diagnostic criteria for definite PML are stringently based on the demonstration of JCV in brain tissue or, in the context of a typical MRI and clinical presentation, the demonstration of JCV DNA in the CSF [44]. A summary of the diagnostic criteria is provided in Table 6.2.

Table 6.2 Diagnostic criteria of PML [44]

Pathology available	Diagnostic features	Definite PML	Probable PML	Possible PML	Not PML
Yes	Histopathological triad (demyelination, bizarre astrocytes, and enlarged oligodendroglial nuclei) JCV protein detected in focal brain lesions by immunohistochemistry or electron microscopy JCV DNA detected in focal brain lesions by in situ hybridization or PCR	Histopathological triad with detection of JCV protein and/or JCV DNA	Histopathological triad only	Detection of JCV protein only	No histopathological evidence of JCV infection
No	Clinical: progressive neurological symptoms Imaging: MRI features Laboratory: JCV DNA detected in the CSF by PCR	JCV DNA detected in the CSF, and both imaging features and clinical features present	JCV DNA detected in the CSF and either imaging or clinical features present	Imaging and clinical features only, or only detection of JCV DNA in the CSF	Isolated clinical or imaging features

The evolving understanding of PML and its diagnostic criteria highlights the need for a more nuanced and comprehensive approach to diagnosis, incorporating clinical, radiological, pathological, and virological data.

6.5 Clinical Manifestations

Over time, PML has evolved alongside the emergence of new at-risk populations, leading to variations in its clinical presentation. These presentations exist on a spectrum shaped predominantly by the patient's immune response. On one end is "classic PML," characterized by a lack of significant antiviral immune activity, as seen in its earliest documented cases. Moving along the spectrum, intermediate cases show varying degrees of immune preservation or reconstitution, described here as "inflammatory PML." At the extreme end lies "PML immune reconstitution inflammatory syndrome" (PML IRIS), marked by intense inflammation that can result in immune-mediated tissue damage. Notably, PML IRIS is most often associated with clinical deterioration linked to inflammation, although a universal definition for this condition across patient populations is yet to be established.

Then, though there is no unified classification system for the clinical subtypes of PML, Cortese et al. [1] identified several distinct phenotypes: "classical PML," "inflammatory PML," and "PML IRIS." The one described as classical form is related to the first description of PML in immunodeficient setting, so it is a specific setting, and it is frequently seen once the lesion is grown and developed affecting both supratentorial and infratentorial regions, with neurological symptoms depending on the areas involved. Common symptoms include cognitive and behavioral changes, sensory and motor deficits, seizures, ataxia, and aphasia, while inflammation-related symptoms is generally absent since the established failure of immune system of the host. In contrast, inflammatory PML, that can evolve or be present as IRIS, it is characterized by the possibility of an immune reaction, therefore inflammation in some cases can be severe, uncontrolled inflammation, which may be fatal in the acute phase. Additional pathological manifestations of JCPyV infection include granule cell neuronopathy, fulminant encephalopathy, and JCPyV meningitis [1]. Today, classic PML remains the most severe and prevalent form of the disease, that can develop only in specific immune depressed setting.

PML can have a variable clinical presentation being related to the site of the developing lesion: subacute cognitive and neuropsychiatric alterations (36–54%), visual disturbances (19–41%), motor (33–45%), or sensory (7–19%) dysfunctions, coordination, and gait difficulties (13–35%), to epileptic seizures (5–14%) [44] have been described. Specific ataxic symptoms in case of early infection of granule cells of the cerebellum [58], can be present.

PML typically does not involve the optic nerve. Visual deficits in PML patients are usually a result of damage to the optic radiations, rather than the optic nerve itself. While spinal cord involvement by PML has been reported in pathological specimens, it is extremely rare, and myelopathic (spinal cord-related) clinical features have not been commonly observed. The lack of recognition of myelopathic signs and symptoms may be due to the more prominent brain involvement in these atypical cases. Importantly, PML does not affect the peripheral nervous system [59].

6.6 Laboratory Data

The vast majority of HIV-infected patients with PML have CD4 lymphocyte counts below 200 cells/mm^3. In separate series of AIDS-related PML, the mean CD4 count ranged from 84 to 104 cells/mm^3 [60, 61]. However, in the largest series of HIV-associated PML [60], more than 10% of patients had CD4 lymphocyte counts exceeding 200 cells/mm^3. In the era of highly active antiretroviral therapy (HAART), the percentage of HIV-associated PML with CD4 counts exceeding 200 cells/mm^3 may be higher.

CSF examination is very helpful in excluding other diagnoses. Cell counts are usually less than 20 cells/mm^3, the median cell count being 2 cells/mm^3 and the mean one 7.7 cells/mm^3 [60], with 55% of patients having an abnormally elevated CSF protein (mean value 66.5 mg/dL). Hypoglycorrhachia was observed in less than 15%.

The greatest value of the CSF examination is demonstrating the presence of JCV PCR. Several studies have shown a high sensitivity and specificity of CSF PCR for JC virus in PML [61–64]. Prior to the development of ultrasensitive PCR techniques for JCV, the sensitivity of this test was around 75% [61]. However, with newer ultrasensitive techniques, sensitivity has increased to over 95%.

Although the amplification of the virus from the CSF in the absence of PML is very unlikely, a low copy number of JC virus was reported in 2 of 515 CSF samples from patients without PML using ultrasensitive techniques [65]. Since JCV viremia can occur in healthy individuals, any contamination of the CSF with blood could potentially lead to a false-positive result. Despite the high sensitivity of the PCR assay, a negative PCR does not rule out PML, and in some cases, biopsy of the brain with PCR amplification from brain tissue has been used to establish the diagnosis [66]. In patients with MS and other autoimmune diseases, the viral loads are often lower, and the sensitivity of the assay becomes critical for establishing the diagnosis.

6.7 Risk Factors for PML

The incidence of PML increased initially in patients with hematological or solid tumors, followed by a significant rise during the AIDS epidemic of the 1980s, when individuals with HIV accounted for 50–80% of PML cases. However, following the widespread introduction of highly active antiretroviral therapy (HAART), the number of PML cases in this population declined, and cases in individuals with autoimmune diseases or those receiving immunosuppressive or targeted therapies became more prominent [12, 16].

Among drug-induced cases of PML, Natalizumab, a monoclonal antibody targeting α-4 integrin, is most commonly associated with the disease. However, an increasing body of evidence now implicates other immunosuppressants and biologic drugs. MS patients receiving immunosuppressive treatments currently represent a significant proportion of drug-induced PML cases. Other drugs have been explored for their potential role in PML development or have included PML as a potential risk in their prescribing information. These include Alemtuzumab, Brentuximab Vedotin, Dimethyl fumarate, Efalizumab, Fingolimod, Ibrutinib, Obinutuzumab, Ocrelizumab, Ofatumumab, Glatiramer acetate, Dalfampridine, and Rituximab [6, 67].

The distribution of PML cases varies across different patient populations. PML is not a reportable disease, which complicates efforts to determine precise incidence rates within these groups. Over the last 40 years, HIV infection has been the dominant cause of PML, accounting for approximately 80% of cases [1]. However, recent data indicate a declining proportion of PML cases linked to HIV, suggesting a shifting trend [1].

Patients with hematological malignancies, particularly non-Hodgkin lymphoma and chronic lymphocytic leukemia (CLL), comprise the second-largest group, responsible for roughly 10% of PML cases. Another significant risk group includes individuals treated with Natalizumab, primarily for MS, which accounts for less than 5% of all PML cases.

The remaining ~10% of cases are distributed among individuals with other identifiable immunosuppressive conditions, such as organ transplant recipients and patients with chronic inflammatory or rheumatological diseases. Rarely, PML arises in individuals without an apparent predisposing condition. This phenomenon is more frequently observed in elderly patients, hinting at potential age-related immune vulnerabilities.

There is an expanding list of drugs associated with PML risk, many of which carry specific label warnings [1]. These medications contribute to PML risk in vulnerable populations. Examples include immunosuppressive treatments for conditions like chronic graft-versus-host disease (cGVHD), rheumatoid arthritis (RA), systemic lupus erythematosus (SLE), ulcerative colitis (UC), and Wegener granulomatosis (WG), among others. Notably, drugs such as Natalizumab, used for relapsing-remitting MS (RRMS) and primary progressive MS (PPMS), underscore the interplay between therapeutic advances and increased PML risk.

This evolving landscape of risk factors emphasizes the importance of ongoing vigilance in managing immunosuppressive therapies and monitoring susceptible populations.

6.8 Drug-Induced PML

The FDA Adverse Event Reporting System (FAERS) has reported 7220 cases of PML [68].

A recent systematic review and metanalysis addressed the issue of drug-induced PML [69], aiming to answer the following question: "what is the incidence of drug-induced PML in patients under the age of 80 years, affected by pathologies requiring immunosuppressant treatment, but not affected by HIV, primary immunodeficiencies or malignancies?". Only observational studies and randomized controlled trials (RCTs) were considered eligible. Then, isolated case reports or case series were not considered. Overall, there were 1017 PML events, reported in 42.71% of the included studies (n = 44). Among these, 70.45% included natalizumab in their treatment regimen (n = 31). The incidence of PML cases among patients diagnosed with MS who were undergoing Natalizumab treatment was 0.4 cases/100 persons (95% CI 0.36–0.44, I2 = 94%; $p < 0.001$), for a median observation period of 36 months (IQR 24–60 months) (mean 45.7, SD 28). The incidence of PML under fingolimod treatment was 0.01 cases/100 persons (95% CI 0.00–0.01, I2 = 91.9%; $p < 0.001$), for a median observation period of 47.6 months (IQR 31.62–53.85 months) (mean 44.5, SD 17.6). The incidence of PML under rituximab treatment was 0.01 cases/100 persons (95% CI −0.08 to 0.09, I2 = 20.4%; $p = 0.255$), for a median observation period of 23.5 months (IQR 22.1–42.1 months) (mean 28.1, SD 12.9). The incidence of PML under dimethyl fumarate treatment was 0.17 cases/100 persons (95% CI 0.12–0.22, I2 = 64.4%; $p = 0.06$), for a median observation period of 36.1 months (IQR 24–77.8 months) (mean 45.9, SD 28.2).

No study included in this review reported cases of PML during follow-up or treatment with ocrelizumab, vedolizumab, abrilumab, ontamalimab, teriflunomide, daclizumab, inebilizumab, basiliximab, tacrolimus, belimumab, infliximab, firategrast, disulone, azathioprine, or danazole. However, there are reports in the literature of PML occurring during treatment with some of these drugs. For example, cases of PML have been documented in patients treated with ocrelizumab, tacrolimus, and Inebilizumab [70, 71]. Notably, Inebilizumab was listed as the possible cause of PML in a deceased patient during a clinical trial [72].

For dimethyl fumarate, it is important to note that the reported findings may be influenced by the results of single studies. Although this drug appears relatively safe in terms of PML risk, the necessary data on specific known risk factors, such as absolute lymphocyte count, were not reported for all reported cases of PML [73].

In addition, nine cases of PML were reported after treatment with mycophenolate mofetil and four cases after treatment with belatacept.

Using Natalizumab, despite limited data, it appears that there may be a difference in PML risk based on the infusion protocol used, as shown by our meta-analysis comparing standard interval dosing with extended interval dosing. When considering only patients treated with extended or standard interval dosing, the risk of PML is lower in those receiving extended interval dosing: 0.07 cases/100 persons (95% CI 0.0–0.15%) for a mean observation period of 48.2 months (SD 19.6) and a mean of 35.1 doses (SD 14.5), compared to 0.3 cases/100 persons (95% CI 0.25–0.34%) for a mean observation period of 33.7 months (SD 11.1) and a mean of 32.0 doses (SD 9.1) [69].

In a recently published cohort [74], the features of PML associated with sphingosine-1-phosphate receptor modulators (S1P-RM; fingolimod, siponimod, ozanimod) were described. S1P-RM patients were more prone to show symptoms at diagnosis (100 vs 80.6%, $p = 0.035$), had more disseminated lesions (80% vs 34.9%, $p = 0.002$), and had higher gadolinium enhancement (65% vs 39.1%, $p = 0.042$) than natalizumab-related PML with a similar prognosis.

6.9 Pathology

In 2013, the American Academy of Neurology (AAN) established a consensus set of diagnostic criteria for PML [44]. According to these guidelines, a definitive diagnosis can be made if a pathological examination reveals a histopathological triad: demyelination, the presence of bizarre astrocytes, and oligodendrocytes with enlarged nuclei [11]. However, unlike autopsies, which allow for an extensive analysis of the entire brain, biopsy samples are generally small and may not capture the full triad. As a result, there is no universally accepted diagnostic standard for brain biopsy cases due to the limited number of pathological findings available. Selecting the correct biopsy location and being familiar with the early pathological features of PML are essential for an accurate diagnosis [75].

The mechanism of viral replication within the affected brain was explored by comparing longitudinal MRI with postmortem brain tissue from an autopsy case [76]. It is hypothesized that PML lesions develop in three stages: initiation, extension/expansion, and fusion. The first stage, initiation, involves the formation of small viral proliferation foci, typically located at the corticomedullary junction within the frontotemporal lobe. The JC virus reaches the brain via the bloodstream, initiating these foci. In the second stage, extension, these small foci spread along nerve fibers in a discontinuous manner, eventually converging deep within the white matter, where nerve fibers intersect. The final stage, fusion, occurs when these proliferating viral foci meet, causing extensive tissue damage. Thus, the

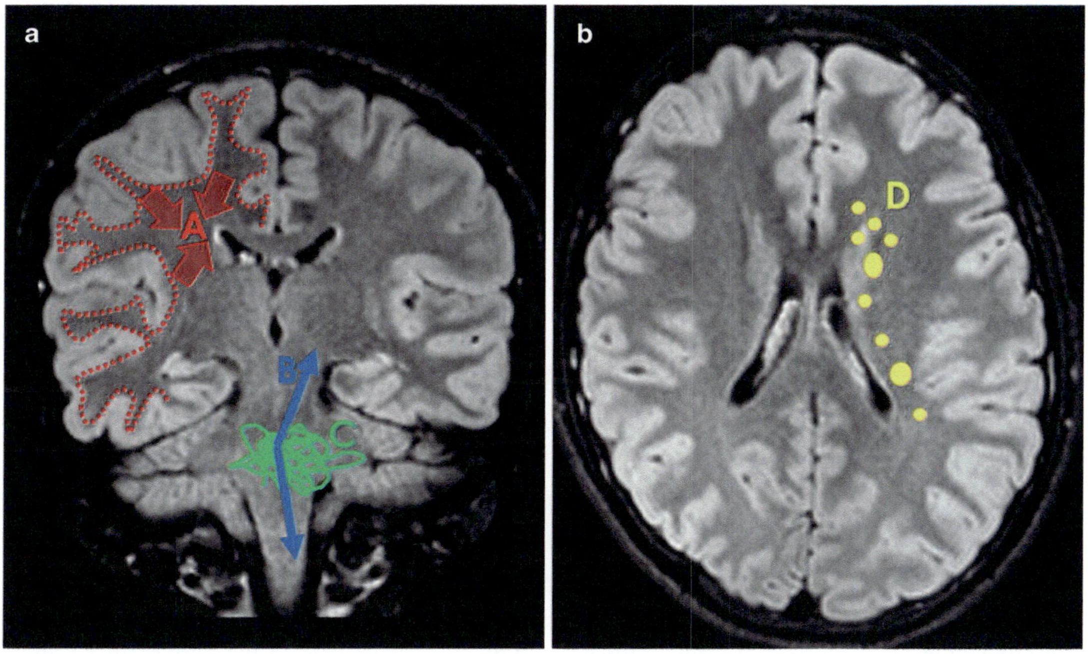

Fig. 6.1 Some examples of patterns and progression pathways of PML lesions along axons, represented on coronal and axial FLAIR slices of a normal brain MRI. All these patterns may occur simultaneously and/or in combination and the progression might follow vertical tract of fibers in both directions (coronal plana in panel (**a**) and axial plane in panel (**b**). (*A*) Supratentorial cortical lesions; (*B*) vertical extension into deep gray matter and the brainstem; (*C*) infratentorial lesions affecting the cerebellum and brainstem; (*D*) deep white matter lesions with punctate MRI patterns

progression of PML lesions is closely linked to neural tracts.

A pathological attempt [77] to transfer the pathways of virus spreading into MRI patterns does not allow a convincing explanation of the whole MRI spectrum of PML (Fig. 6.1). PML has frequently being described once "grown up," therefore as established lesion involving the deep white matter, with multiple foci, extending through corpus callosum, involving supra end infratentorial regions. These MRI patterns are commonly observed across various forms of immunosuppression and throughout the clinical progression of the disease. The patterns might occur in combination [78].

At the onset of the lesion, the newborn PML, clearly seen in patient with MS during DMT, can appear as punctate lesion (milky way appearance) both on T2/FLAIR and as enhancing dot spots on T1 postcontrast images [79, 80]. Furthermore, JCV-infected glial cells are frequently located at the gray matter–white matter junction or within the gray matter, causing demyelinating lesions within cortical areas [81].

While FLAIR images can be highly sensitive in detecting gliosis and histiocytic infiltration, they may not always indicate an active PML lesion.

Biopsy should focus on active sites where JCV proliferation is occurring. Potential biopsy targets include the leading edge of expanding lesions, that can be evident as hyperintense rim seen on diffusion-weighted imaging (DWI) compared with T2/FLAIR hyperintensities. In case of an immune competent patient, therefore able to react with and inflammatory setting, the interface between T1 hypointense areas, and peripheric regions can exhibit contrast enhancement on MRI that may also serve as a viable biopsy target. MRI plays a crucial role in identifying the location and progression of expanding PML lesions [82–84], but careful and expert analysis is essential for accurate interpretation.

The identification of JCV-infected oligodendrocytes is essential for an accurate pathological diagnosis. Infected cells typically display enlarged, spherical nuclei filled with amphophilic viral inclusions when stained with hematoxylin and eosin (HE). The JC viral antigen can be detected throughout the entire nucleus, forming a full inclusion pattern in immunohistochemical staining. However, during the early stages of infection, JCV-infected cells may be absent or hard to identify due to low viral copy numbers, resulting in relatively small nuclei in the infected cells. JCV replicates within a distinct intranuclear region, known as promyelocytic leukemia bodies (PML-NBs). As a result, JCV progeny accumulate in PML-NBs in the initial stages, forming dot-like inclusions. Upon JCV infection, the cell cycle is activated, leading to the enlargement of PML-NBs. Within these expanding PML-NBs, the virus replicates and forms dot-shaped inclusions in medium-to-large-sized nuclei. In immunohistochemistry, these cells are typically positive for Ki-67/MIB-1.

A systematic review of 47 studies covering 52 cases of natalizumab-associated PML from 2005 to 2016 revealed that approximately 80% of cases exhibited contrast enhancement on MRI [77]. This finding reflects the presence of antiviral host inflammatory responses, typically involving T cells, B cells, plasma cells, and macrophages infiltrating the brain tissue. A host inflammatory response is often associated with a better prognosis due to suppression of viral replication. However, the degree of inflammation varies widely between cases. In most instances, inflammatory responses are mild, with a low viral copy number [85–87]. In some cases, severe inflammation has been observed, showing pathological features that resemble malignant lymphoma, which could lead to misdiagnosis [87]. Fortunately, high-dose methotrexate (MTX) therapy has been shown to effectively reduce inflammation [87]. Therefore, when conducting a biopsy, it is crucial to evaluate both the qualitative and quantitative aspects of the host inflammatory response to accurately assess the patient's condition.

In cases of PML with moderate inflammatory reactions, diagnosing the condition can be challenging due to the absence of characteristic JCV -infected cells. However, the prognosis tends to be more favorable given the low viral load. For instance, a case was reported in which pathological examination initially revealed perivascular and parenchymal lymphocyte infiltration, reactive gliosis, and numerous foamy macrophages. The proportion of CD4+ cells was 70.4%, and CD8+ cells made up 24.1%, leading to an initial diagnosis of inflammatory demyelinating disease. However, JC virus infection was later confirmed through in situ hybridization (ISH), resulting in a diagnosis of CD4 + -dominant PML-IRIS [89].

In PML cases with inflammatory reactions, plasma cell infiltration is commonly observed around JC virus-infected cells. CD20+ B cells typically accumulate in the perivascular region, often forming a cuff-like structure. In contrast, CD79+ B cells and CD138+ plasma cells tend to accumulate in the outer regions of these cuffs or infiltrate the parenchyma diffusely. Interestingly, these perivascular cuffs may resemble lymphoid follicles, suggesting a role in B cell maturation. In cases of severe inflammation, plasma cell activation is evident, with binucleated plasma cells being present [88]. These findings support the role of B-cell and plasma cell-mediated immunity in the host's defense against JCV.

IRIS is clinically characterized as a "paradoxical deterioration" of the condition following immune reconstitution. In the context of PML, IRIS occurs when the restored immune system begins to recognize JC virus antigens, leading to exacerbated inflammation. Initially identified in AIDS patients undergoing antiretroviral therapy (ART), PML-IRIS involves a robust immune response triggered by the recovery of CD4+ cells, often resulting in death. Similar immune responses have been observed in other clinical settings, such as after bone marrow transplantation or cessation of immunosuppressive treatments.

The prognosis for PML-IRIS in AIDS patients during the 1990s was poor, but more recent reports, particularly in drug-associated PML cases after 2005, indicate better outcomes. As a result, there is ongoing debate about whether inflammatory reactions in PML signal a favorable prognosis or a poor one [90]. Diagnostic criteria for PML-IRIS remain undetermined, though it is typically diagnosed through the observation of rapidly enlarging lesions with contrast enhancement on MRI but associated with an abrupt clinical deterioration: it is a clinic radiological definition, therefore MRI imaging should be acquired in conjunction with clinical worsening. However, chronic, low-grade inflammation may persist even after the resolution of acute PML-IRIS, suggesting that the host's immune response can vary over time. The correlation between pathological findings and PML-IRIS remains under investigation.

When a brain biopsy is performed on contrast-enhanced lesions seen on MRI, pathological analysis typically reveals a polymorphic antiviral host inflammatory response, which includes CD4+ and CD8+ T cells, B cells, and plasma cells [91].

Progressive multifocal leukoencephalopathy in HIV-1 infection. In these cases, the prognosis is usually favorable. In contrast, autopsy studies of fatal PML-IRIS cases often report a predominance of CD8+ T cells in the immune response [92, 93]. A fatal case of PML-IRIS in an MS patient treated with natalizumab exhibited a monomorphic immune response dominated by CD8+ T lymphocytes, with minimal or absent CD4+ T cells, B cells, and plasma cells. Monoclonal T cell expansion was also detected in the bone marrow and spleen. These findings suggest that the fatality of PML-IRIS may be linked to a monomorphic CD8+ T cell response in the absence of CD4+ T cells.

6.10 Neuroimaging Findings

In the appropriate clinical setting, brain imaging can provide strong evidence supporting the diagnosis of PML. CT scans of the brain typically reveal hypodense lesions in the affected white matter. If in the more frequent immune depressed setting, these lesions do not cause mass effect and rarely show contrast enhancement. When the subcortical arcuate fibers are involved, a "scalloped" appearance beneath the cortex may be observed [94] (old radiological sing). However, brain MRI is significantly more sensitive than CT in detecting PML-related white matter lesions [94]. MRI typically shows hyperintense lesions on T2-weighted and fluid-attenuated inversion recovery (FLAIR) images in the affected areas. On T1-weighted images, these lesions appear hypointense. With CT scans, faint contrast enhancement, often at the periphery, may be seen in 5–10% of cases [94]. Gadolinium enhancement is found in approximately 15% of patients with HIV-associated PML [60] and 40% of those with natalizumab-associated PML at the time of diagnosis [95–98].

PML lesions can appear anywhere in the brain and are typically multifocal, in case of established disease. Since they are early detected, in cases of natalizumab-associated PML, the lesions are often monofocal, with a tendency for the frontal lobe to be predominantly affected [98]. In radiographic studies of PML, the frontal lobes and parieto-occipital regions are most commonly affected, likely due to their larger volume. However, involvement of the basal ganglia, external capsule, and posterior fossa structures (including the cerebellum and brainstem) can also be observed [94]. Some examples are illustrated in Figs. 6.2, 6.3, 6.4, 6.5, and 6.6.

Diffusion-weighted imaging (DWI) may be useful in differential diagnosis, since at the onset PML lesion can be mistaken with acute cerebrovascular insult. On T2W imaging, the affected tissue of PML has a "ground glass" appearance. Approximately 50% of PML cases associated with natalizumab, where inflammation is common, exhibit gadolinium enhancement, which may present as a faint rim or speckled interior enhancement.

The role of other neuroimaging techniques, such as magnetization transfer MRI, magnetic resonance spectroscopy, SPECT, and PET, is limited. Magnetization transfer MRI studies have been suggested for monitoring the degree of demyelination in PML [99]. Magnetic resonance spectroscopy reveals a decrease in

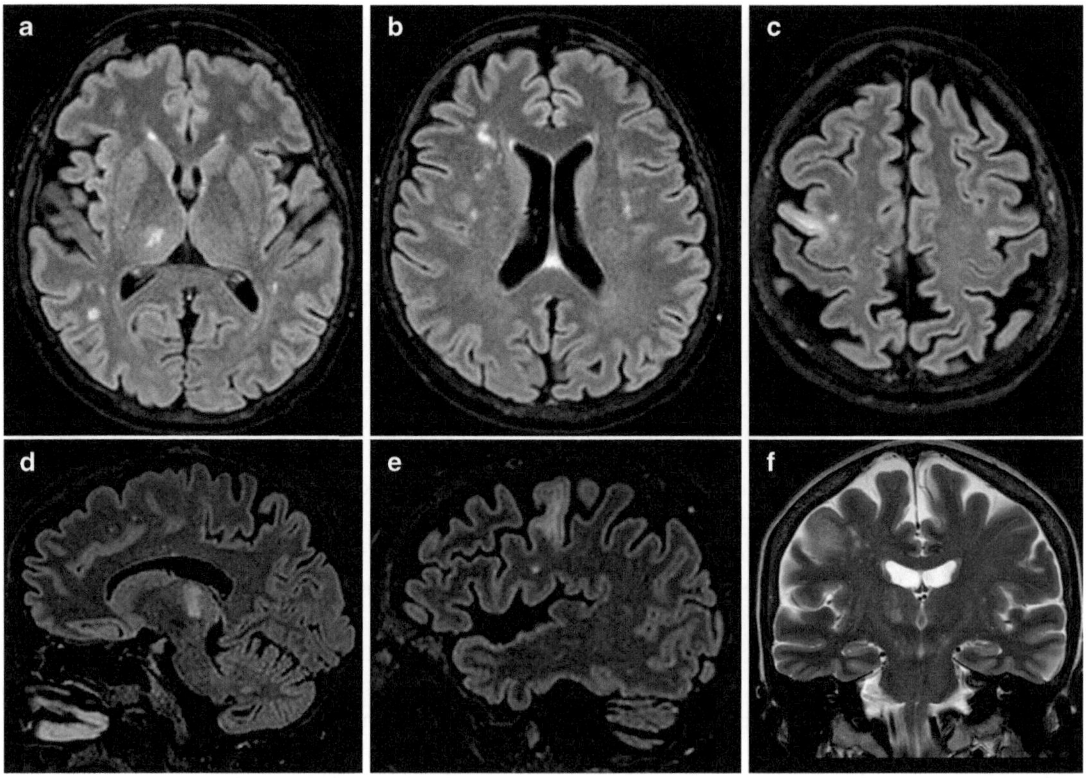

Fig. 6.2 T2-FLAIR MRI of a patient with PML. Panels (**a**–**c**) show axial FLAIR with involvement (hyperintense lesions) of right thalamus and bilateral cortico-subcortical region of the precentral gyrus affecting the U-fibers. Isolated scattered white matter hyperintensities in the right centrum semiovale are also represented. Panels (**d**, **e**) show sagittal FLAIR centered on the right thalamus and on the right precentral gyrus lesions. Panel (**f**) shows coronal T2W MRI

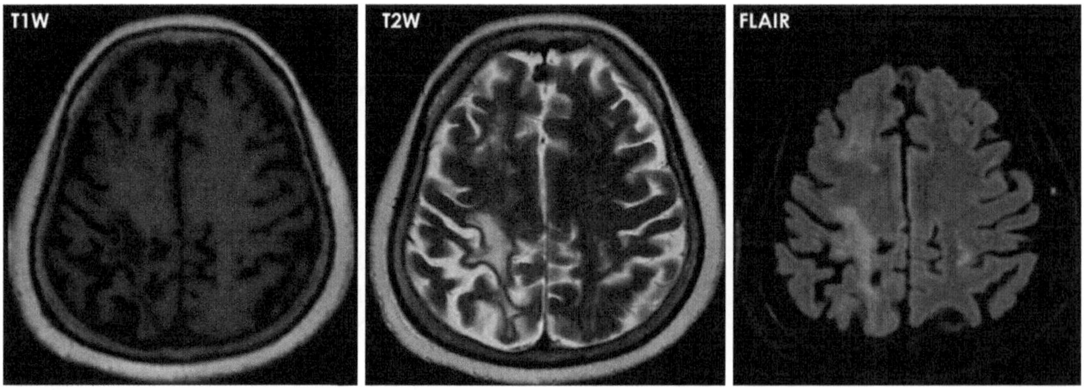

Fig. 6.3 Different signal features in white mater of a patient with PML on MRI. The involved white matter appears hypointense on T1W sequence and hyperintense on T2W and T2-FLAIR sequences

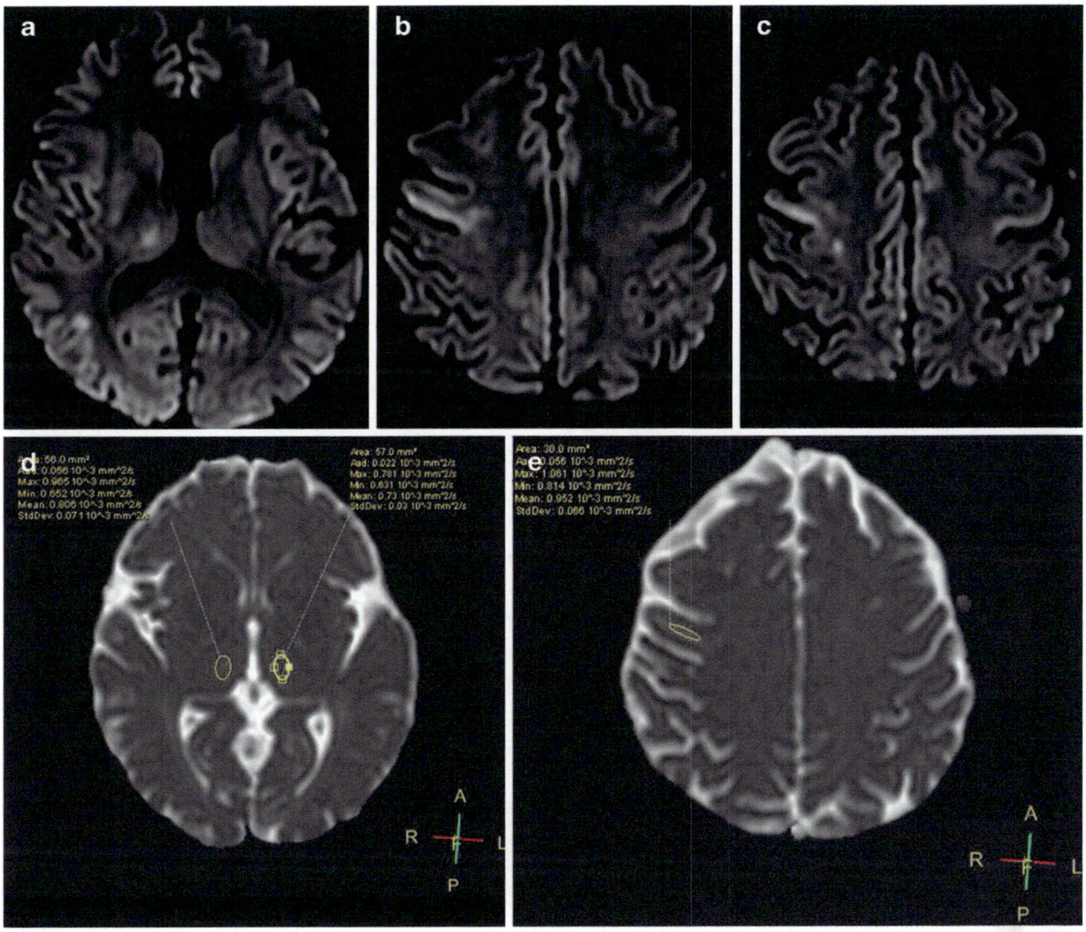

Fig. 6.4 DWI/ADC in the same patient as in Fig. 6.2. The lesions hyperintense in FLAIR are also hyperintense on DWI (thalamus and both precentral gyri) (panels **a**–**c**). ADC values are reported in panels **d** and **e**

N-acetylaspartate and creatine, along with increased choline products, myo-inositol, and lactate in the lesions of PML [100]. These changes likely reflect neuronal loss and cell membrane and myelin breakdown. Cerebral angiography is not routinely performed, but it exhibited arteriovenous shunting and a parenchymal blush in the absence of contrast enhancement on MRI in 4 out of 6 patients in one study [101]. Pathologic studies suggested that small-vessel proliferation and perivascular inflammation explained these unexpected angiographic features.

Summarizing, MRI findings highly suggestive of PML typically present as T2 hyperintense lesions located within the juxtacortical and deep white matter, often crossing the boundary between white matter and adjacent cortical gray matter (leukocortical lesions) (Fig. 6.2). The appearance of these lesions evolves with disease progression, presenting as T1 isointense lesions in early stages or as hypointense lesions in advanced stages due to irreversible demyelination, in comparison to unaffected white matter (Fig. 6.3). In lesions with active viral replication, DWI may reveal areas of hyperintense signal intensity, particularly at the lesion borders, reflecting oligodendrocyte swelling from lytic infection, with varying ADC values, including low, normal, or high measurements (Fig. 6.4) [98, 99]. Additionally, multiple small T2 hyperintense lesions, with or without contrast enhancement,

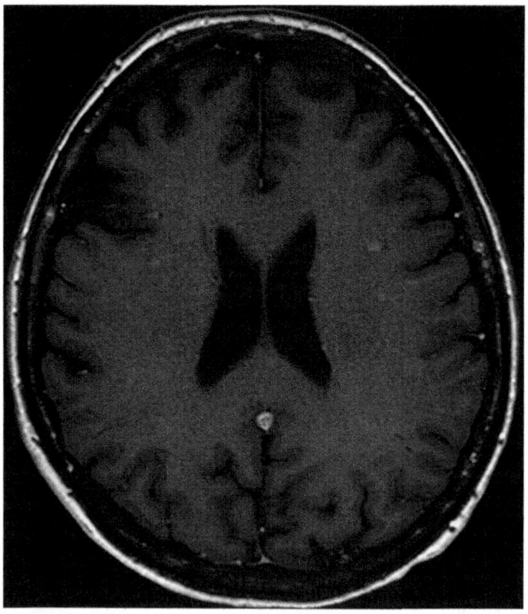

Fig. 6.5 Postcontrast T1W in axial plane in the same patient as in Figs. 6.2 and 6.3, showing punctate contrast enhancement (Milky Way) in the white matter and isolated linear enhancement in the iuxtacortical white matter

are often observed near primary PML lesions, forming an imaging pattern described as a "punctuate pattern" or "milky way appearance" (MWA) [79, 102]. This punctate pattern of T2 lesions can be observed in the presymptomatic stage of PML before the emergence of larger PML lesions [93, 103] (Fig. 6.5) since they are considered to be the newborn PML lesion.

Initial imaging findings in PML can vary based on the degree of inflammatory or antiviral immune activity. In HIV-associated PML among cART-naive individuals or in cases linked to hematologic malignancies with limited JCV-specific immune response, contrast enhancement is typically absent at presentation, referred to as classical PML, as unable to have an immune reaction and therefore signs of inflammation at MRI. Conversely, in HIV-associated PML treated with cART or in DMT-related PML, such as Natalizumab-associated PML in MS patients, the immune system often retains

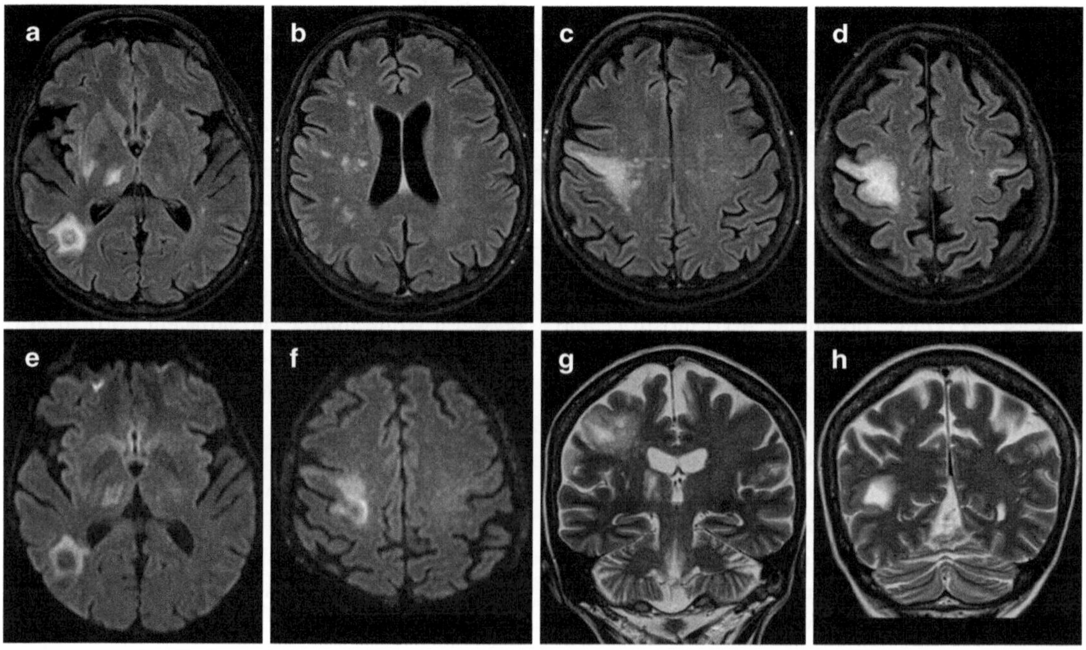

Fig. 6.6 Follow-up MRI in the same patient described in Figs. 6.2, 6.3, and 6.4. (**a–d**) Show axial FLAIT with enlarges and extended hyperintense lesions in the right precentral gyrus, actually affecting the white matter up to the centrum semiovale and a cavitated lesion in the right occipito-temporal transition. (**e**, **f**) Show the corresponding DWI hyperintense signal (with the hypointense signal of the cavitation). (**g**, **h**) Show ground glass appearance of lesions on T2W imaging

partial functionality. In these cases, even early MRI findings may display active inflammation, including gadolinium enhancement and perilesional edema [82, 104].

PML can also affect infratentorial structures [80, 105]. A recent study focusing on patients with Natalizumab-associated PML reported an initial infratentorial presentation in 33% of cases, with a third of these patients exhibiting exclusive infratentorial involvement. The most common symptoms in these patients included ataxia, dysmetria, dysarthria, cerebellar deficits, and paresis, primarily due to the involvement of the cerebellum and pons [106, 107].

In addition, in CNS JCV infection at least five radiological entities have been described [108]: classic PML (or anergic), inflammatory PML, JCV granule cell neuronopathy, meningeal, and encephalopathic JC variants. More recently, deep gray matter (DGM) and pyramidal tract involvement have also been described as other possible locations of disease [109]. The MRI findings of PML should be interpreted depending on the supposed spreading pathways of JCV and on the stage of the disease, particularly in drug-related PML (Fig. 6.7). In fact, how lesions evolve and why certain anatomical locations are more frequently affected remains unknown [109] (Figs. 6.8 and 6.9).

Early and correct identification of PML remains a challenge [110], in particular in presymptomatic stage, where almost all the evidence is related to NTZ-PML [80, 84, 110–112] and agrees that linear hyperintensity (T2-FLAIR-DWI) of subcortical U-fibers and punctate T2 hyperintense lesions ("punctate pattern" or milky way pattern) are highly predictive features. Hematogenous spread to the CNS appears to be of great importance in the pathophysiology of the disease and this would explain, at least partially, the special tropism of JCV for highly vascularized areas such as the subcortical white matter, as supported by a recent demonstration of cortical lesions and immediate subcortical involvement in a patient assessed on high-field MRI (7 Tesla) after several negative scans in 3 Tesla [112]. A similar finding (linear hyperintensity on FLAIR sequence along the corticomedullary junction) was supported by a neuropathological study documenting small demyelinating lesions at the cortical gray matter and juxtacortical white matter in a 52-year-old man who died 170 days after PML diagnosis [76] and pathologic changes in the cerebral cortex were specifically described at autopsy brain tissue of 13 patients (83).

Furthermore, the gray matter may be the initial site of JCV injury barely visible with conventional sequences until advanced stages.

Although the "punctate pattern" has been described in NTZ-PML, it was as well reported in PML related to other etiologies [113]. Moreover, if the punctate lesions are more than 20 and they are close to a larger PML lesion, it is designated as "MWA." Hodel et al. [105] observed the MWA in 11 of 20 patients during symptomatic PML, but only occasionally in presymptomatic stage. The histopathological correlation of MWA was provided by Ono et al. [76] as presence of early and small demyelinating perivascular lesions with edema in corticomedullary border all over the brain without a central vein.

There is a direct correlation between the size and spread of PML lesions at the symptomatic stage of the disease, which could support the extension features of PML [114]. Although we do not know how the virus spreads within the CNS, some evidence supports the migration of JCV through association or projections fibers [115, 116]. Only few pathological studies focus on the dynamic nature of PML. An "extension" stage was described in which demyelinating lesions spread to another anatomical site in a tract-dependent manner (involvement of the corpus callosum in relation to deep white matter lesions, and pontine tegmentum damage extending to the thalamus through the midbrain, including reticular formation and involvement of the trigemino-thalamic tract) [76]. In the series of Ruiz Romagnoli et al. [117], lesions in commissural and projection fibers were found with a relatively high frequency (corpus callosum 38.4% and internal capsule 46%, respectively), in association with involvement of the pyramidal tract, including crossed lesions.

The tendency to affect the pons, middle cerebellar peduncle, and cerebellar hemisphere,

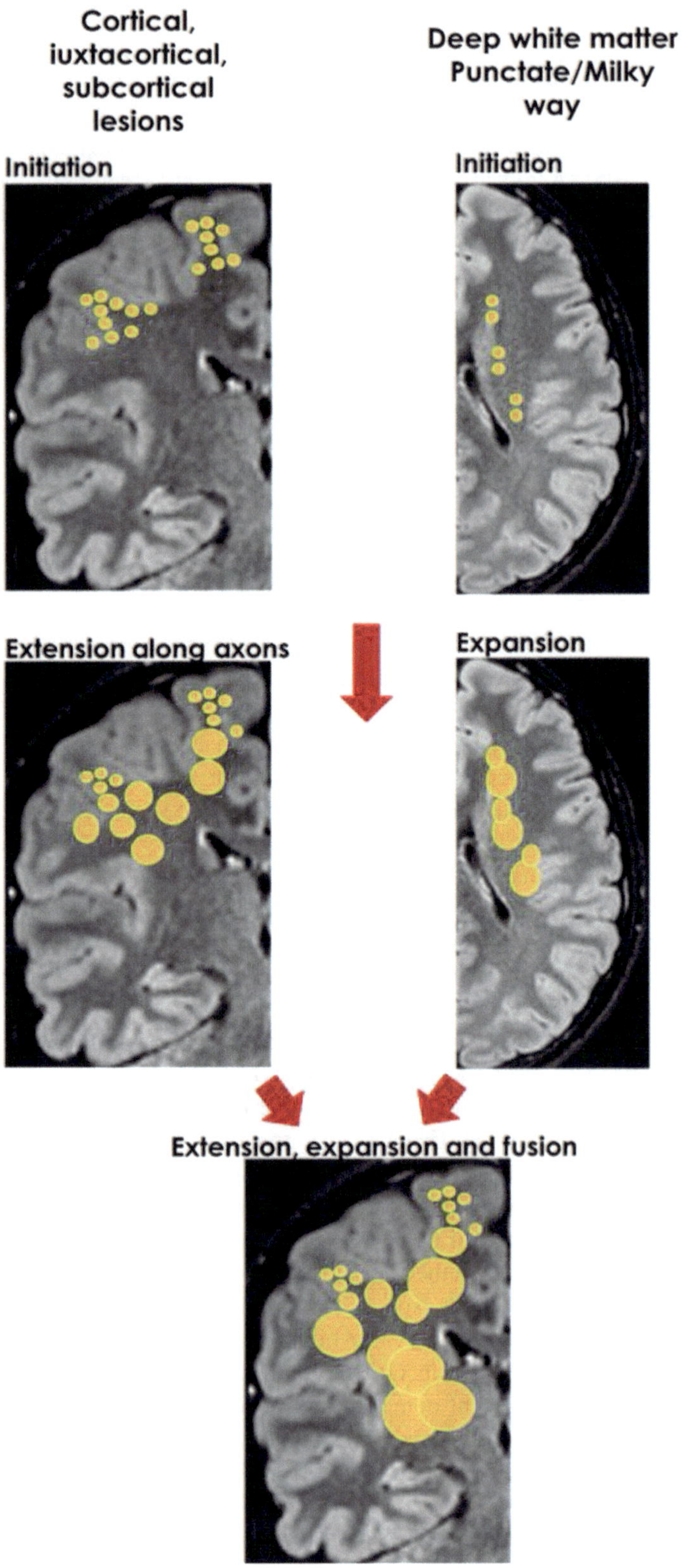

Fig. 6.7 Pathways of evolution of lesions in PML though the gray and white matter in classic PML. PML lesions evolve through distinct patterns, often described as "initiation," "extension," and "fusion." Early, small demyelinating lesions typically emerge in vascular-rich regions, such as the cortical gray matter, juxtacortical and subcortical white matter, and basal ganglia. These areas serve as primary sites for the onset of demyelination. Over time, lesions spread discontinuously along nerve fibers or expand locally. Eventually, smaller lesions merge (a process termed "fusion") to form larger, more extensive demyelinating regions

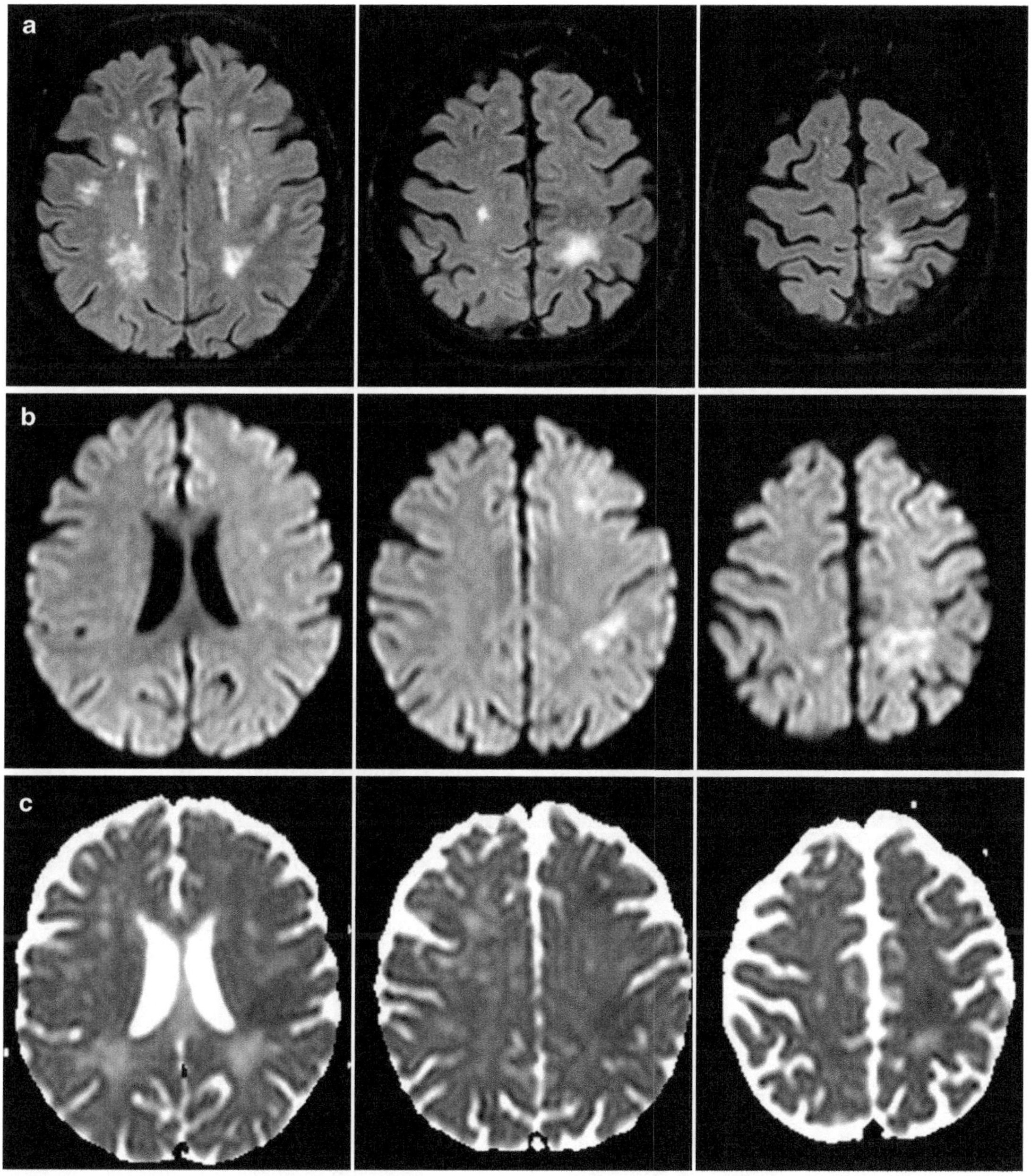

Fig. 6.8 Baseline MRI on FLAIR (panel **a**), DWI (panel **b**) and ADC (panel **c**) in the same patient described in Figs. 6.2, 6.3, and 6.4. The white matter subcortical confluent lesions in the left frontal posterior lobe have a faint DWI hyperintense signal and an ADC hypointensity

described as typical sites of affect, suggest that these anatomical locations deserve special attention in the semiographic evaluation of MRI. Moreover, there are some patients with the DGM pattern (the only gray matter structure affected was the thalamus) [117] and the associated infratentorial anatomical structures involved appear to be other than those described as typical (dentate nuclei, red nuclei). In infratentorial involvement, there are few studies of the

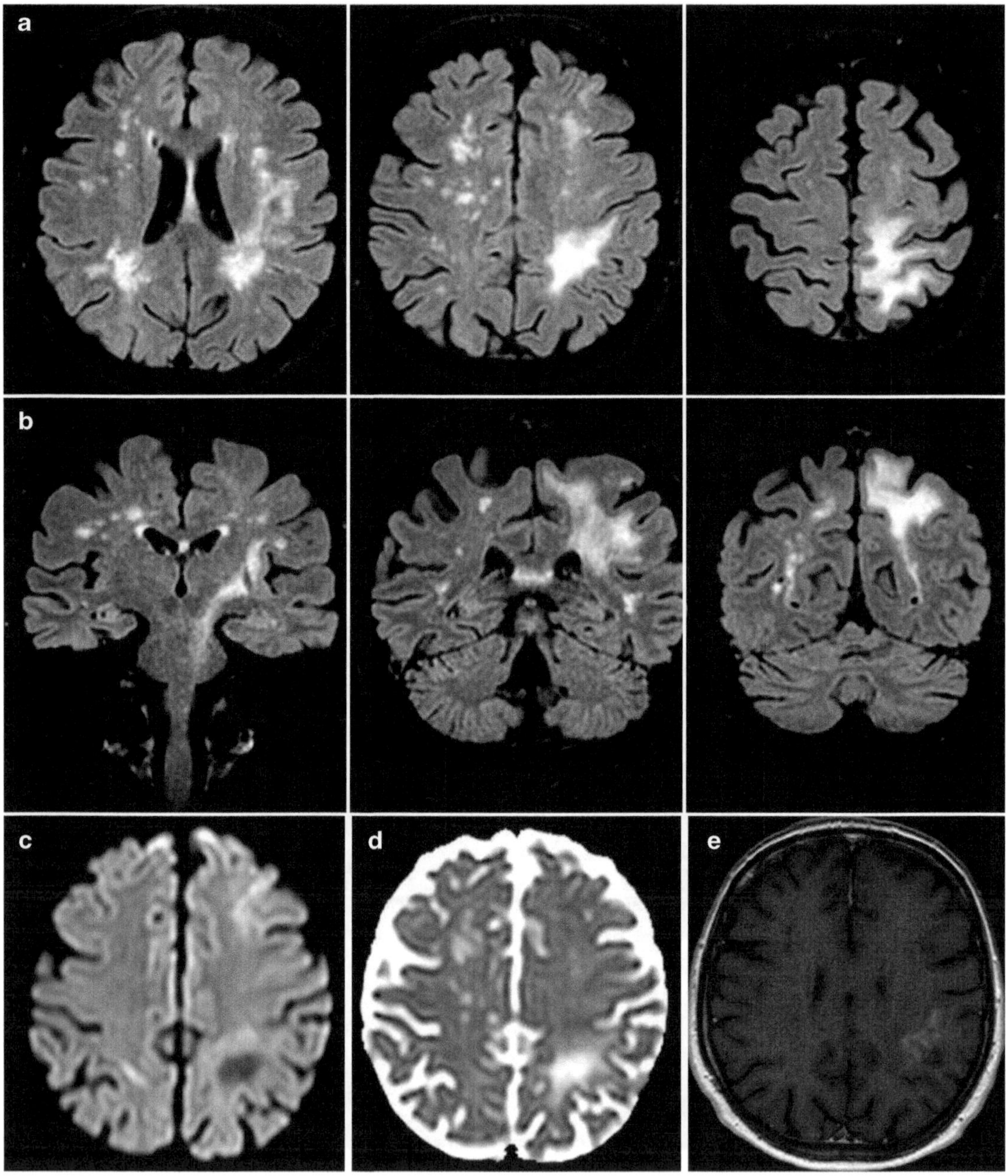

Fig. 6.9 Follow-up MRI in the same patient as in Fig. 6.7. (**a**) Shows sequential axial FLAIR slices, with a significant extension of the previously highlighted left-sided white matter lesion. (**b**) Shows coronal FLAIR, where the involvement of the left pyramidal tract is evident and the comparison of a iuxtacortical white matter lesion in the right parietal lobe is highlighted. (**c, d**) Shows a change in DWI/ADC signal in comparison with the baseline MRI, with DWI hypointensity and ADC hyperintensity. In the same panels, the new right white matter lesion has a hyperintense signal o DWI. (**e**) Shows postcontrast axial T1 with punctate contrast enhancement ate the borders of the left white matter lesion

diagnostic specificity of pontocerebellar findings on MRI in PML [118–121]. The hot cross bun sign, a cruciform T2 hyperintense signal in the midpons, has been noted late in the course of PML, affecting posterior fossa structures, when both the brainstem and the cerebellum have lost considerable volume (olivopontocerebellar atrophy). The hot cross bun sign was described initially in the cerebellar subtype of multiple system atrophy [121] and is also seen in spinocerebellar ataxia, particularly spinocerebellar ataxia 1 and 2, and in variant Creutzfeldt-Jakob disease and cerebral vasculitis [122–125]. The shrimp sign was first proposed as a marker of cerebellar PML as a well-defined T2- or FLAIR-hyperintense and T1-hypointense lesion in the cerebellar white matter that abuts-but-spares the dentate nucleus and has the shape of a shrimp. It may also involve the hilum of the dentate nucleus. On axial MRI, the well-defined white matter lesion outlines the serrated, curvilinear-shaped dentate nucleus. The MRI shrimp sign was proposed as having a sensitivity 0.85, specificity 1, positive predictive value 1, and negative predictive value 0.93 [126].

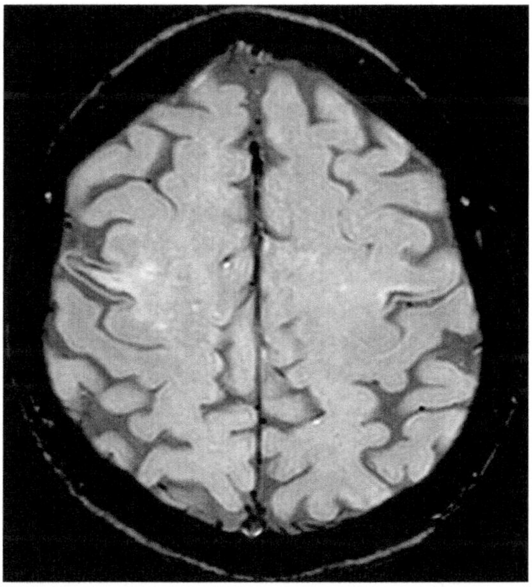

Fig. 6.10 SWI (same patient of the Figs. 6.2, 6.3, 6.4, and 6.5) showing a linear bandlike hypointense rim on both precentral gyri

Another MRI marker of evoluted stages of PML is the thin, uniformly linear, gyriform SWI-hypointense rim in the paralesional U-fibers (Fig. 6.10). It might represent an end-point stage of the neuroinflammatory process in long-term survivors [127]. The data based on quantitative susceptibility mapping of the lesions suggested a paramagnetic (blood product or nonheme iron deposits) effect [128]. However, the mechanism that led to the susceptibility change remains unclear, because no histologic correlation was performed. In general, contrast enhancement was not observed in the region of SWI-hypointense rim [128]. In one patient, there is a pathological support of a lower number of PML-infected cells than in the patient without an SWI rim, much more prominent astrogliosis and microglial activation in the deep cortical layers and at the cortical-subcortical junction, including the U-fibers and also in areas without focal lesions, but with diffuse white matter pallor and moderate gliosis. Iron deposits were detected within actively demyelinating lesions and in the pericapillary cells. The detection of the linear hypointense rim in the region of the U-fibers on SWI sequences is not specific of PML, being found also in chronic cerebral infarction and after encephalitis [129]. Several morphologic phenomena occur at the edges of a PML lesion and beneath juxtacortical areas, mainly primary oligodendroglial dysfunction by JCV infection and consequent myelin degeneration, microglial activation, astroglial proliferation, and axonal impairment. Axonal damage can produce retrograde neuronal degeneration and lead to progressive cortical atrophy. It is known that PML also involves the U-fibers. Chronically activated glial cells and microglia/macrophages may contain high levels of iron and pigment within their cytoplasm. In addition, blood-brain barrier disruption caused by PML may lead to leakage of heme products into the perivascular space.

A similar but less prominent SWI-hypointense rim was observed in the deep cortical layers of the precentral gyrus in patients with amyotrophic lateral sclerosis. On histopathologic studies, intracellular deposits of iron (in the form of ferritin) were confirmed in reactive microglial cells, located in the middle and deep layers of the motor cortex, in areas that were affected by neuronal loss and axonal degeneration [130]. In recently published studies [131, 132], a bandlike T2*-hypointense cortical rim was observed on 7 T in a subset of patients with Alzheimer disease, which was believed to be derived from increased myelin-associated, nonheme iron in the middle layers of the cortex and Baillarger lines and was also found in disintegrated axons and microglial cells.

One possible explanation for the specific location of iron deposition is the fact that subcortical U-fibers have a greater iron content than both cerebral gray and white matter, due to the high density of iron-rich oligodendrocytes, and are considered slow metabolic fibers with a slow myelin turnover. In addition, the region of U-fibers has long medullary arterioles and venules in a gyriform distribution [133]. Ferritin accumulation could be a nonspecific, acute-phase reactant in response to inflammation. It seems that accumulating iron in proliferated microglial cells is not a specific finding in any of the above-mentioned neurodegenerative diseases, but rather a pattern in progressive and long-standing neuroinflammation [134].

In addition, in a recently published study, a T1WI-hyperintense cortical signal on MRI has been reported in 61.2% of patients with PML [59]. A hyperintense cortical signal was detected adjacent to subcortical PML lesions on precontrast T1-weighted MR images and resembled the SWI-hypointense rim seen in our patients. In addition, atrophy of the cortical area affected was reported in 96.7% of cases with hyperintense cortical signal. SWI was available in 15 of 49 patients in that particular study, and none of them had any SWI abnormality. On histology, hyperintense cortical signal areas were associated with striking JCV-associated demyelination of the cortical and subcortical U-fibers, heavy macrophage infiltration, and a pronounced reactive gliosis in the deep cortical layers [59].

6.11 Phenotypes of PML

The description of several phenotypes of PML comes from a growing literature about the different manifestations of a rare disease. Currently, the better knowledge of the disease makes the differentiation of phenotypes less useful because the main features are overlapping. As a matter of fact, it is a continuum from no inflammation to high inflammation due to clinical contest and/or immunosuppressive status.

6.11.1 Classic (Immunocompromised Patient) PML

Classic PML typically affects the brain's supratentorial or infratentorial regions, manifesting as progressive neurological decline. The spinal cord and optic nerves are generally spared. Symptoms vary depending on lesion locations but commonly include cognitive and behavioral changes, motor and sensory deficits, ataxia, aphasia, and cortical visual impairments. Seizures occur in 20–44% of cases during the disease course [135–137].

Pathologically, PML is characterized by multifocal demyelination, oligodendrocytes with enlarged hyperchromatic nuclei, and bizarre astrocytes with irregular, lobulated nuclei [44]. The JCV primarily infects oligodendrocytes, with viral genome levels in the brain 100–1000 times higher than in the kidney [138]. Although rare, astrocytes and neurons can also harbor viral particles. Lesions in classic PML exhibit a zonal structure. At the periphery, swollen oligodendrocytes containing viral particles show partial loss of myelin-associated proteins, with axons preserved. The lesion core, in contrast, reveals extensive loss of myelin and axons, accompanied by phagocytic activity clearing debris. Lymphocytes and plasma cells are scarce in this region, which also shows gliotic changes and disrupted parenchymal architecture. PML lesions extend beyond subcortical white matter into cortical and deep gray matter, accounting for the disease's mixed cortical and subcortical symptomatology [60, 76, 139–144].

MRI, particularly T2WI and T2-FLAIR sequences, is invaluable in identifying PML lesions. At presentation, multifocal lesions are common, and follow-up imaging often reveals asynchronous enlargement, coalescence, or the emergence of new lesions. Classic PML lesions typically appear hyperintense on T2-weighted FLAIR sequences and involve subcortical and juxtacortical white matter. Their borders are sharply defined at the cortical margin. On T1W imaging, lesions vary in intensity depending on the degree of tissue necrosis, with advanced destruction resulting in marked hypointensity. Survivors often develop neurodegenerative changes, including focal atrophy and CSF space dilation. Inflammation-associated imaging features, such as mass effect, are rare but faint peripheral contrast enhancement has been observed in 9% of HIV-related PML cases from the pre-cART era, even without histological evidence of inflammation [99].

Restricted diffusion at active lesion margins, attributed to swelling of dying oligodendrocytes and astrocytes, is frequently observed. Additionally, paramagnetic shifts and T2* signal changes at the gray-white matter junction, potentially linked to iron deposition, have been reported, though their clinical significance remains unclear [129, 145]. Cortical and deep gray matter lesions, however, are challenging to visualize using standard MRI protocols.

6.11.2 Inflammatory PML

The advent of cART in the mid-1990s marked a transformative shift in the clinical management of HIV-related PML. Not only did cART reduce the overall incidence of PML in individuals with HIV, but it also altered the spectrum of clinical manifestations. As immune function was restored, new pathological and radiological features emerged, particularly those linked to inflammation. This change in disease presentation coincided with a significant increase in survival rates, with approximately 60% of patients surviving for at least 1 year [146].

Successful immune reconstitution allows for the detection of JCV-specific CD8+ and CD4+ T cells in the peripheral blood of survivors. Detailed epitope mapping has shown that the capsid protein VP1 of the JC virus elicits the strongest immune response. The presence of these cellular antiviral responses correlates with viral clearance and is a stronger prognostic marker for survival than CD4+ T cell counts alone [147]. The role of humoral immune responses in PML remains less clear, although a rising antibody level to JCV has become a reliable biomarker for viral reactivation in natalizumab-treated patients with MS, helping to identify those at the greatest risk for developing PML [148].

The partial or full immune reconstitution driven by cART can also unmask previously hidden opportunistic infections, triggering an inflammatory response to these asymptomatic infections. Initially described as "immune reconstitution syndrome," this phenomenon was later renamed IRIS [149, 150]. When it occurs in the context of PML related to HIV, IRIS is defined by the restoration of immune function—evidenced by an increase in CD4+ T cell count or a decrease in plasma HIV RNA levels—coupled with a sudden worsening of neurological symptoms. Two forms of IRIS are recognized: paradoxical IRIS, where symptoms of a known infection worsen, and unmasked IRIS, where subclinical infections become clinically apparent due to the inflammatory response. IRIS occurs in 4–42% of patients with HIV-related PML [151–154]. Although clinical manifestations are typically mild, severe inflammatory responses—often seen in patients with the greatest increase in CD4+ T cell counts—can be life-threatening, with mortality rates ranging from 5% to 28% [155–157]. Generally, the presence of inflammatory features in PML is associated with better survival outcomes [157, 158], although some studies suggest this is not always the case.

Immune reconstitution in PML patients is frequently associated with distinct MRI features that indicate inflammation, including contrast enhancement within PML lesions

(56–87%), edema (30%), and mass effect (24%) [99, 159]. These features are rarely seen in classic PML, where contrast enhancement occurs in fewer than 3% of cases [156]. However, the sensitivity of these MRI features in detecting inflammation may be limited, and contrast enhancement may not always be visible on MRI, even in cases of pathologically confirmed inflammatory PML [146, 160]. More sensitive imaging techniques, such as magnetic resonance spectroscopy [161], arterial spin labeling [162], and 18F-fluorodeoxyglucose PET [163], have been proposed to better visualize active inflammation in PML.

The pathological hallmark of PML IRIS is an intense perivascular lymphocytic infiltration, predominantly composed of CD8+ T cells [156]. CD20+ B cells and CD138+ plasma cells are also present in large numbers, whereas macrophage and microglial populations remain similar to those seen in classic PML [164]. Interestingly, PML IRIS tends to exhibit fewer JCV-infected cells compared to classic PML, suggesting a successful reduction of viral load [164, 165].

6.11.3 Iatrogenic PML

It should be clear that these are not a single phenotype of PML, since they include both non inflammatory and inflammatory PML form and we have to keep in mind that Natalizumab PML is different from RTX PML form. This as a statement and iatrogenic PML can present in either its classic or inflammatory form, depending on the severity of pharmacological immunosuppression and the potential for immune recovery. The association of rituximab, a CD20 monoclonal antibody approved by the FDA in 1997 [166], with PML was first documented in 2002, with cases reported in patients with non-Hodgkin lymphoma. At that time, it was difficult to isolate the impact of rituximab alone due to confounding factors such as prior treatments and co-morbidities that independently elevate the risk of PML. However, in 2005, alarming cases of PML in otherwise immunocompetent patients began to emerge, marking a new chapter in iatrogenic PML. This year saw the first reports of PML in patients treated with Natalizumab, an α4 integrin monoclonal antibody that had been approved the previous year for MS treatment and Crohn's disease. This was followed by cases of PML in patients with systemic lupus erythematosus treated with rituximab, and in 2008, PML was reported in patients with rheumatoid arthritis [167].

At least 18 FDA-approved medications carry warnings about the risk of PML [48]. While the overall risk of PML with these drugs is generally low, there are notable exceptions such as natalizumab, with an overall risk of approximately 1 in 1000, and the CD11a monoclonal antibody efalizumab, which had an estimated risk of 1 in 400 before it was withdrawn from the market in 2009 following four reported cases of PML [168]. Both of these drugs affect lymphocyte trafficking but do not directly suppress the immune system, making them distinct from traditional immunosuppressive agents. The risk of PML with these drugs is particularly associated with prolonged exposure, typically more than 2 years.

Natalizumab was briefly withdrawn in 2005 after the first cases of PML were reported, but it was reintroduced in 2006 for the treatment of MS under a strict pharmacovigilance program. Despite this, the number of natalizumab-associated PML cases continued to rise. In the post-cART era, and among patients with autoimmune diseases, the levels of JCV in CSF are often below detection limits. Therefore, many cases that don't meet current diagnostic criteria may go unreported, suggesting that the true number of PML cases is likely higher.

Early imaging studies of natalizumab-associated PML revealed that around 40% of patients had contrast-enhancing lesions at diagnosis [98, 99]. This frequency was notably higher compared to other forms of PML, and the enhancement patterns observed—linear, punctate, or rim-like—are thought to reflect the unique immune dysregulation induced by natalizumab. Additionally, a new MRI feature, referred to as the MWA, has been described in 72% of patients with natalizumab-associated PML. This feature consists of small perilesional T2 hyperintensities, often enhanced by contrast material, which may indicate an early immune response in perivascular spaces, possibly linked to active JCV replication [83, 84]. Similar findings have been observed in other PML cases involving immune dysregulation, including HIV-related PML [156, 157].

In almost all cases of natalizumab-associated PML, PML IRIS occurs after discontinuation of natalizumab therapy. This typically happens within days to a few weeks after plasma exchange or immunoabsorption treatments are used to accelerate the clearance of the drug. Similar to PML IRIS in HIV, this syndrome is marked by contrast enhancement, edema, and mass effect [98]. The survival rate for patients with natalizumab-associated PML is approximately 77%, which is higher than in other PML patient populations. This is likely due to the restoration of antiviral immunity following the discontinuation of the medication [95].

The overall estimated risk of developing PML in patients treated with natalizumab is 1 in 1000. However, several factors, when combined, can significantly increase the risk. These include the presence of JCV antibodies, treatment duration beyond 2 years, and prior use of immunosuppressive agents. For patients in the highest-risk group, based on these factors, the estimated incidence of PML increases to 11.1 cases per 1000 per year, while patients who are antibody-negative face a much lower risk (0.09 cases per 1000 per year) [169]. Evidence supporting the utility of JCV antibody testing as a screening tool comes from the observation that the incidence of PML among natalizumab-treated patients decreased by approximately 50% within 18 months after the introduction of the JCV antibody assay [170]. The JCV antibody index is now routinely used to further stratify risk among patients treated with natalizumab who have not previously received immunosuppressive therapy [171]. Emerging evidence also suggests that extending the dosing interval of natalizumab (more than 4 weeks) may reduce the risk of PML in patients who are positive for JCV antibodies or who have a history of immunosuppressive treatment [172].

For all PML patients, the success of immune reconstitution as a treatment for PML is often limited by the fact that the disease is usually diagnosed only after neurological symptoms appear, by which time an effective antiviral immune response may be too late to improve the outcome. However, pharmacovigilance programs associated with natalizumab use, which include monitoring JCV antibody levels and conducting frequent MRIs, have led to earlier identification of PML, even in its preclinical, asymptomatic stages [173]. This early detection contributes to the relatively better prognosis seen in natalizumab-associated PML compared to other forms of the disease.

6.11.4 Subclinical PML

In HIV infection, the duration of subclinical PML before it is unmasked by antiretroviral therapy is not well understood. In patients treated with natalizumab, asymptomatic PML lesions have been identified retrospectively as long as 9 months before the clinical diagnosis [173–176]. In rare instances, PML has been discovered at autopsy in individuals with no prior neurological symptoms [177]. This evidence supports the notion that PML may initially develop more slowly than its rapid, end-stage clinical course suggests, potentially providing an opportunity for early diagnosis and intervention.

MRI findings of subclinical PML tend to be more localized, with 68% of affected individuals presenting with lesions in a single lobe, most commonly in the frontal lobe (78%). Inflammation is observed in 40% of people with subclinical PML, either as contrast-enhanced lesions or as the punctate perilesional MWA. Up to 40% of asymptomatic patients may not exhibit diffusion restriction at the lesion edges, possibly indicating limited tissue damage [178].

Survival rates after discontinuation of natalizumab treatment are significantly higher in asymptomatic patients (96%) compared to symptomatic patients (75%) [179]. In cases of asymptomatic PML, JCV is often undetectable in CSF, which is consistent with the observation that smaller lesion volumes may correlate with low levels of JCV DNA [180]. The inability to detect JCV in the initial CSF examination can delay a definitive diagnosis and appropriate management, creating a diagnostic challenge given the current criteria that require virus detection [11, 181]. Notably, up to 20% of patients monitored in pharmacovigilance programs who developed confirmed PML had undetected JCV in the CSF during their first diagnostic evaluation. This highlights the importance of assay sensitivity for improving early diagnosis [44].

6.12 Management

The development of antiviral strategies for JCV has been hindered by the lack of an animal model for PML and challenges in propagating the virus in culture. Furthermore, the rarity and severity and also heterogeneity of presentation: different underlying disease, degree of virus replication, host response, time of diagnosis, possibility of reversing immunosuppression, etc. of the disease have presented methodological, ethical and market-related obstacles to clinical investigations. Also the. Severity: often also fast progression that may prevent enrolment in clinical trials/experimental treatments, despite initially planned. As a result, research into treatments for PML has been limited to small case series. Broadly, two therapeutic approaches have been investigated: direct antiviral therapies and indirect strategies aimed at restoring antiviral immune responses.

However, none of these strategies have convincingly prolonged survival or reduced neurological disability in clinical trials. In fact, most studies were terminated early due to lack of benefit or excessive toxicity [182–186]. Consequently, immune reconstitution remains the most effective treatment strategy for PML. The success of this approach depends on early diagnosis, limited disease progression, and rapid and effective immune restoration. In its simplest form, immune reconstitution can be achieved through the initiation of cART in HIV-related PML or discontinuation of immunosuppressive therapy in non-HIV-related PML. In natalizumab-associated PML, plasma exchange or immunoadsorption is commonly used to accelerate drug clearance, although some evidence suggests these treatments may not improve outcomes and could be associated with more severe IRIS [187, 188].

Some immune reconstitution strategies have been tested in larger patient cohorts and show promise. One such strategy is the use of checkpoint inhibitors. Persistent viral infections are often associated with immune exhaustion, which involves the progressive loss of lymphocyte effector functions. This mechanism limits immune-mediated injury in chronic inflammation but can impair viral clearance. Checkpoint inhibitors target pathways involved in immune exhaustion and can rejuvenate antiviral immunity. Evidence from 18 patients with refractory immunosuppression suggests that targeting programmed cell death protein 1 (PD1) can restore the anti-JCV activity of CD4+ and CD8+ T cells, yielding clinical and radiological benefits in some patients [189]. This approach appears most promising for individuals with detectable anti-JCV cellular immune responses before treatment, as antiviral responses are reinvigorated after one or two monthly drug administrations. However, advanced PML and profound immune compromise are typically associated with poor responses to this therapy [190]. In a recently described retrospective cohort, aiming to assess the real-world effectiveness of immune checkpoint inhibitors for treatment of PML (19% with IRIS), the development of contrast enhancement on follow-up MRI at least once during follow-up was associated with 1-year survival (OR = 3.16, 95% confidence interval = 1.20–8.72, p = 0.02), but the mortality remains high [191].

Another promising therapeutic strategy for PML is adoptive immunotherapy using virus-specific T cells generated from related or unrelated donors [192, 193]. This is much more promising, but very difficult and time-requiring to organize [194, 195]. This approach can be useful in early and well defined patients (disposable high compatibility of the donor and of the cells that should be used). Some results have been suggested with the use of Interleukin-7 (IL 7) [195].

All immune reconstitution strategies carry the risk of triggering IRIS. Managing IRIS presents a dilemma, as it requires balancing the need to suppress inflammatory responses while also preventing PML progression if inflammation is overly suppressed, even if it is actually well known that if IRIS is present is a good prognostic sign.

6.13 Conclusion

PML is a rare and life-threatening CNS infection caused by reactivation of JCV. PML occurs when JCV reactivates in people with weakened immune systems. No antiviral treatments exist, making the reversal of immunosuppression essential for survival. Advances in immunotherapy, including checkpoint inhibitors and T cell transfer (that seems to be more promising than checkpoint inhibitors), show potential in treating PML but require caution to avoid IRIS, that, on the other hand, should not be consider a limit of this approach. Modern immunosuppressive therapies, such as natalizumab for MS, have increased PML cases by fostering conditions for JCV reactivation. PML remains a serious threat due to the expanding use of immunosuppressive therapies and unresolved questions about its pathobiology. Developing more effective strategies to boost antiviral immune responses is critical.

Acknowledgments The authors acknowledge Prof. Paola Cinque for her relevant work on PML pathophysiology and treatment.

References

1. Cortese I, Reich DS, Nath A. Progressive multifocal leukoencephalopathy and the spectrum of JC virus-related disease. Nat Rev Neurol. 2021;17:37–51.
2. Ferenczy MW, Marshall LJ, Nelson CDS, Atwood WJ, Nath A, Khalili K, et al. Molecular biology, epidemiology, and pathogenesis of progressive multifocal leukoencephalopathy, the JC virus-induced demyelinating disease of the human brain. Clin Microbiol Rev. 2012;25:471–506.
3. Langer-Gould A, Atlas SW, Green AJ, Bollen AW, Pelletier D. Progressive multifocal leukoencephalopathy in a patient treated with natalizumab. N Engl J Med. 2005;353:375–81.
4. Kleinschmidt-DeMasters BK, Tyler KL. Progressive multifocal leukoencephalopathy complicating treatment with natalizumab and interferon beta-1a for multiple sclerosis. N Engl J Med. 2005;353:369–74.
5. Berger JR, Koralnik IJ. Progressive multifocal leukoencephalopathy and natalizumab–unforeseen consequences. N Engl J Med. 2005;353:414–6.
6. Oshima Y, Tanimoto T, Yuji K, Tojo A. Drug-associated progressive multifocal leukoencephalopathy in multiple sclerosis patients. Mult Scler J. 2019;25:1141–9.
7. Maas RPPWM, Muller-Hansma AHG, Esselink RAJ, Murk JL, Warnke C, Killestein J, et al. Drug-associated progressive multifocal leukoencephalopathy: a clinical, radiological, and cerebrospinal fluid analysis of 326 cases. J Neurol. 2016;263:2004–21.
8. Rindi LV, Zaçe D, Braccialarghe N, Massa B, Barchi V, Iannazzo R, et al. Drug-induced progressive multifocal leukoencephalopathy (PML): a systematic review and meta-analysis. Drug Saf. 2024;47:333–54.
9. Sriwastava S, Kataria S, Srivastava S, Kazemlou S, Gao S, Wen S, et al. Disease-modifying therapies and progressive multifocal leukoencephalopathy in multiple sclerosis: a systematic review and meta-analysis. J Neuroimmunol. 2021;360:577721.
10. Chiu CY, Amenta E, Chavez V, Fukuta Y, Hasbun R. Undetectable JC virus CSF PCR in patients with JC virus-induced progressive multifocal leukoencephalopathy. J Neurovirol. 2023;29:94–9.
11. Schweitzer F, Laurent S, Cortese I, Fink GR, Silling S, Skripuletz T, Metz I, Wattjes MP, Warnke C. Progressive multifocal leukoencephalopathy: pathogenesis, diagnostic tools, and potential biomarkers of response to therapy. Neurology. 2023;101(16):700–13. https://doi.org/10.1212/WNL.0000000000207622.
12. Maginnis MS, Atwood WJ. JC virus: an oncogenic virus in animals and humans? Semin Cancer Biol. 2009;19:261–9.
13. Khalili A, Craigie M, Donadoni M, Sariyer IK. Host-immune interactions in JC virus reactivation and development of progressive multifocal leukoencephalopathy (PML). J Neuroimmune Pharmacol. 2019;14:649–60.
14. Miyamura T, Jikuya H, Soeda E, Yoshiike K. Genomic structure of human polyoma virus JC: nucleotide sequence of the region containing replication origin and small-T-antigen gene. J Virol. 1983;45:73.
15. Gosert R, Kardas P, Major EO, Hirsch HH. Rearranged JC virus noncoding control regions found in progressive multifocal leukoencephalopathy patient samples increase virus early gene expression and replication rate. J Virol. 2010;84:10448–56.

16. Tan CS, Koralnik IJ. Progressive multifocal leukoencephalopathy and other disorders caused by JC virus: clinical features and pathogenesis. Lancet Neurol. 2010;9:425–37.
17. Pasquier DRA, et al. A prospective study demonstrates an association between JC virus-specific cytotoxic T lymphocytes and the early control of progressive multifocal leukoencephalopathy. Brain. 2004;127:1970–8.
18. Gheuens S, et al. Role of CD4+ and CD8+ T-cell responses against JC virus in the outcome of patients with progressive multifocal leukoencephalopathy (PML) and PML with immune reconstitution inflammatory syndrome. J Virol. 2011;85:7256–63.
19. Khanna N, Wolbers M, Mueller NJ, Garzoni C, Pasquier DRA, Fux CA, et al. JC virus-specific immune responses in human immunodeficiency virus type 1 patients with progressive multifocal leukoencephalopathy. J Virol. 2009;83:4404–11.
20. Tan CS, et al. Immune reconstitution after allogeneic hematopoietic stem cell transplantation is associated with selective control of JC virus reactivation. Biol Blood Marrow Transplant. 2014;20:992–9.
21. Wittmann T, et al. JC polyomavirus reactivation is common following allogeneic stem cell transplantation and its preemptive detection may prevent lethal complications. Bone Marrow Transpl. 2015;50:984–91.
22. Chen Y, et al. Asymptomatic reactivation of JC virus in patients treated with natalizumab. N Engl J Med. 2009;361:1067–74.
23. Pietropaolo V, et al. Human polyomavirus JC replication and non-coding control region analysis in multiple sclerosis patients under natalizumab treatment. J Neurovirol. 2015;21:653–65.
24. Bellizzi A, et al. Polyomavirus JC reactivation and noncoding control region sequence analysis in pediatric Crohn's disease patients treated with infliximab. J Neurovirol. 2011;17:303–13.
25. Zheng H-Y, et al. New sequence polymorphisms in the outer loops of the JC polyomavirus major capsid protein (VP1) possibly associated with progressive multifocal leukoencephalopathy. J Gen Virol. 2005;86:2035–45.
26. Delbue S, et al. JC virus VP1 loop-specific polymorphisms are associated with favorable prognosis for progressive multifocal leukoencephalopathy. J Neurovirol. 2009;15:51–6.
27. Sunyaev SR, Lugovskoy A, Simon K, Gorelik L. Adaptive mutations in the JC virus protein capsid are associated with progressive multifocal leukoencephalopathy (PML). PLoS Genet. 2009;5:e1000368.
28. Gorelik L, et al. Progressive multifocal leukoencephalopathy (PML) development is associated with mutations in JC virus capsid protein VP1 that change its receptor specificity. J Infect Dis. 2011;204:103–14.
29. Jelcic I, et al. T cell epitope mapping of JC polyoma virus-encoded proteome reveals reduced T cell responses in HLA-DRB1*04:01+ donors. J Virol. 2013;87:3393–408.
30. Power C, et al. AIDS- and non-AIDS-related PML association with distinct p53 polymorphism. Neurology. 2000;54:743–6.
31. Eis PS, et al. Germline genetic risk variants for progressive multifocal leukoencephalopathy. Front Neurol. 2020;11:186.
32. Shishido-Hara Y. Progressive multifocal leukoencephalopathy and promyelocytic leukemia nuclear bodies: a review of clinical, neuropathological, and virological aspects of JC virus-induced demyelinating disease. Acta Neuropathol. 2010;120:403–17.
33. Shishido-Hara Y. Progressive multifocal leukoencephalopathy: dot-shaped inclusions and virus-host interactions. Neuropathology. 2015;35:487–96.
34. Shishido-Hara Y, Ichinose S, Uchihara T. JC virus Intranuclear inclusions associated with PML-NBs. Am J Pathol. 2012;180:1095–106.
35. Shishido-Hara Y, Yazawa T, Nagane M, Higuchi K, Abe-Suzuki S, Kurata M, et al. JC virus inclusions in progressive multifocal leukoencephalopathy: scaffolding promyelocytic leukemia nuclear bodies grow with cell cycle transition through an S-to-G2-like state in enlarging oligodendrocyte nuclei. J Neuropathol Exp Neurol. 2014;73:442–53.
36. Shishido-Hara Y, Higuchi K, Ohara S, Duyckaerts C, Hauw JJ, Uchihara T. Promyelocytic leukemia nuclear bodies provide a scaffold for human polyomavirus JC replication and are disrupted after development of viral inclusions in progressive multifocal leukoencephalopathy. J Neuropathol Exp Neurol. 2008;67:299–308.
37. Shishido-Hara Y, Ichinose S, Higuchi K, Hara Y, Yasui K. Major and minor capsid proteins of human polyomavirus JC cooperatively accumulate to nuclear domain 10 for assembly into virions. J Virol. 2004;78:9890–903.
38. Tada H, et al. Trans-activation of the JC virus late promoter by the tat protein of type 1 human immunodeficiency virus in glial cells. Proc Natl Acad Sci USA. 1990;87:3479–83.
39. Daniel DC, et al. Internalization of exogenous human immunodeficiency virus-1 protein, tat, by KG-1 oligodendroglioma cells followed by stimulation of DNA replication initiated at the JC virus origin. DNA Cell Biol. 2004;23:858–67.
40. White MK, Gordon J, Khalili K. The rapidly expanding family of human polyomaviruses: recent developments in understanding their life cycle and role in human pathology. PLoS Pathog. 2013;9:e1003206.
41. Marshall LJ, Dunham L, Major EO. Transcription factor Spi-B binds unique sequences present in the tandem repeat promoter/enhancer of JC virus and supports viral activity. J Gen Virol. 2010;91:3042–52.
42. Marshall LJ, et al. Lymphocyte gene expression and JC virus noncoding control region sequences are linked with the risk of progressive multifocal leukoencephalopathy. J Virol. 2014;88:5177–83.

43. Frohman EM, et al. JC virus in CD34+ and CD19+ cells in patients with multiple sclerosis treated with natalizumab. JAMA Neurol. 2014;71:596–602.
44. Berger JR, et al. PML diagnostic criteria: consensus statement from the AAN Neuroinfectious disease section. Neurology. 2013;80:1430–8.
45. Ryschkewitsch CF, Jensen PN, Monaco MC, Major EO. JC virus persistence following progressive multifocal leukoencephalopathy in multiple sclerosis patients treated with natalizumab. Ann Neurol. 2010;68:384–91.
46. Himedan M, et al. Pathologic findings of chronic PML-IRIS in a patient with prolonged PML survival following natalizumab treatment. J Investig Med High Impact Case Rep. 2017;5:2324709617734248.
47. Crossley KM, et al. Recurrence of progressive multifocal leukoencephalopathy despite immune recovery in two HIV seropositive individuals. J Neurovirol. 2016;22:541–5.
48. Pavlovic D, Patel MA, Patera AC, Peterson I, Progressive Multifocal Leukoencephalopathy Consortium. T cell deficiencies as a common risk factor for drug associated progressive multifocal leukoencephalopathy. Immunobiology. 2018;223:508–17.
49. Astrom KE, Mancall EL, Richardson EP Jr. Progressive multifocal leuko-encephalopathy; a hitherto unrecognized complication of chronic lymphatic leukaemia and Hodgkin's disease. Brain. 1958;81:93–111.
50. Padgett BL, Walker DL, ZuRhein GM, Eckroade RJ, Dessel BH. Cultivation of papova-like virus from human brain with progressive multifocal leucoencephalopathy. Lancet. 1971;1:1257–60.
51. Aksamit AJ, Sever JL, Major EO. Progressive multifocal leukoencephalopathy: JC virus detection by in situ hybridization compared with immunohistochemistry. Neurology. 1986;36:499–504.
52. Arthur RR, Dagostin S, Shah KV. Detection of BK virus and JC virus in urine and brain tissue by the polymerase chain reaction. J Clin Microbiol. 1989;27:1174–9.
53. Koralnik IJ, Wuthrich C, Dang X, et al. JC virus granule cell neuronopathy: a novel clinical syndrome distinct from progressive multifocal leukoencephalopathy. Ann Neurol. 2005;57:576–80.
54. Wuthrich C, Dang X, Westmoreland S, et al. Fulminant JC virus encephalopathy with productive infection of cortical pyramidal neurons. Ann Neurol. 2009;65:742–8.
55. Richardson E Jr. Progressive multifocal leukoencephalopathy. N Engl J Med. 1961;265:815–23.
56. Dang X, Koralnik IJ. A granule cell neuron-associated JC virus variant has a unique deletion in the VP1 gene. J Gen Virol. 2006;87:2533–7.
57. Mentzer D, Prestel J, Adams O, et al. Case definition for progressive multifocal leukoencephalopathy following treatment with monoclonal antibodies. J Neurol Neurosurg Psychiatry. 2012;83:927–33.
58. Miskin DP, Koralnik IJ. Novel syndromes associated with JC virus infection of neurons and meningeal cells: no longer a gray area. Curr Opin Neurol. 2015;28(3):288–94. https://doi.org/10.1097/wco.0000000000000201.
59. Bernal-Cano F, Joseph JT, Koralnik IJ. Spinal cord lesions of progressive multifocal leukoencephalopathy in an acquired immunodeficiency syndrome patient. J Neurovirol. 2007;13:474–6.
60. Berger JR, Pall L, Lanska D, Whiteman M. Progressive multifocal leukoencephalopathy in patients with HIV infection. J Neurovirol. 1998;4:59–68.
61. Fong IW, Britton CB, Luinstra KE, Toma E, Mahony JB. Diagnostic value of detecting JC virus DNA in cerebrospinal fluid of patients with progressive multifocal leukoencephalopathy. J Clin Microbiol. 1995;33:484–6.
62. Marshall DW, Brey RL, Cahill WT, Houk RW, Zajac RA, Boswell RN. Spectrum of cerebrospinal fluid findings in various stages of human immunodeficiency virus infection. Arch Neurol. 1988;45:954–8.
63. McGuire D, Barhite S, Hollander H, Miles M. JC virus DNA in cerebrospinal fluid of human immunodeficiency virus-infected patients: predictive value for progressive multifocal leukoencephalopathy. Ann Neurol. 1995;37:395–9.
64. Weber T, Turner RW, Frye S, et al. Progressive multifocal leukoencephalopathy diagnosed by amplification of JC virus-specific DNA from cerebrospinal fluid. AIDS. 1994;8:49–57.
65. Iacobaeus E, Ryschkewitsch C, Gravell M, et al. Analysis of cerebrospinal fluid and cerebrospinal fluid cells from patients with multiple sclerosis for detection of JC virus DNA. Mult Scler. 2009;15:28–35.
66. Kuhle J, Gosert R, Buhler R, et al. Management and outcome of CSF-JC virus PCR-negative PML in a natalizumab-treated MS patient. Neurology. 2011;77:2010–6.
67. Hatchwell E, Smith EB, Jalilzadeh S, Bruno CD, Taoufik Y, Hendel-Chavez H, et al. Progressive multifocal leukoencephalopathy genetic risk variants for pharmacovigilance of immunosuppressant therapies. Front Neurol. 2022;13:1016377.
68. Rindi LV, Zaçe D, Braccialarghe N, Massa B, Barchi V, Iannazzo R, Fato I, De Maria F, Kontogiannis D, Malagnino V, Sarmati L, Iannetta M. Drug-induced progressive multifocal leukoencephalopathy (PML): a systematic review and meta-analysis. Drug Saf. 2024;47(4):333–54. https://doi.org/10.1007/s40264-023-01383-4.
69. Bianchi A, Ragonese P, Banco MA, Realmuto S, Vazzoler G, Portera E, et al. Four cases of progressive multifocal leukoencephalopathy in iatrogenic immunocompromised patients. eNeurologicalSci. 2020;19:100243.
70. Patel A, Sul J, Gordon ML, Steinklein J, Sanguinetti S, Pramanik B, et al. Progressive multifocal leukoencephalopathy in a patient with progressive multiple sclerosis treated with ocrelizumab monotherapy. JAMA Neurol. 2021;78:736–40.

71. FDA. Food and Drug Administration, US UPLIZNA product information. [Internet]. 2023. https://www.accessdata.fda.gov/drugsatfda_docs/label/2020/761142s000lbl.pdf
72. Jordan ALM, Yang J, Fisher CJ, Racke MK, Mao-Draayer Y. Progressive multifocal leukoencephalopathy in dimethyl fumarate-treated multiple sclerosis patients. Mult Scler J. 2022;28:7–15.
73. Blant JC, De Rossi NN, Gold R, Maurousset A, Kraemer M, Romero-Pinel L, Misu T, Ouallet JC, Pallix Guyot M, Gerevini S, Bakirtzis C, Piñar Morales R, Vlad B, Karypidis P, Moisset X, Derfuss TJ, Jelcic I, Martin-Blondel G, Ayzenberg I, McGraw C, Laplaud DA, Du Pasquier RA, Bernard-Valnet R, for CORPUS and Italian Study Groups. Presentation and outcome in S1P-RM and natalizumab-associated progressive multifocal leukoencephalopathy: a multicenter cohort study. Neurol Neuroimmunol Neuroinflamm. 2024;11(5):e200281. https://doi.org/10.1212/NXI.0000000000200281.
74. Shishido-Hara Y. Brain biopsy and pathological diagnosis for drug-associated progressive multifocal leukoencephalopathy (PML) with inflammatory reactions. Pathol Int. 2024;74(12):673–81. https://doi.org/10.1111/pin.13492.
75. Ono D, Shishido-Hara Y, Mizutani S, Mori Y, Ichinose K, Watanabe M, et al. Development of demyelinating lesions in progressive multifocal leukoencephalopathy (PML): comparison of magnetic resonance images and neuropathology of postmortem brain. Neuropathology. 2019;39:294–306.
76. Shishido-Hara Y, Kanoto M. Neuroradiological diagnosis of progressive multifocal leukoencephalopathy (PML): pathology of extending/expanding demyelinating lesions detected by MRI. Brain Nerve. 2020;72:973–86.
77. Abramson RC, Morawetz RB, Schlitt M. Multiple complications from an intracranial epidermoid cyst: case report and literature review. Neurosurgery. 1989;24:574–8.
78. Simonetta Gerevini, Ruggero Capra, Mirco Cosottini. Monitoring long-term treatment with natalizumab: clinical and neuroradiological findings from the Italian PML database. J Neurol Neurosurg Psychiatry. 2019;90(3):261–7. https://doi.org/10.1136/jnnp-2018-319208. ISBN 978 88 6756 223 7.
79. Scarpazza C, Signori A, Prosperini L, Sormani MP, Cosottini M, Capra R, Gerevini S, Italian PML Group. Early diagnosis of progressive multifocal leucoencephalopathy: longitudinal lesion evolution. J Neurol Neurosurg Psychiatry. 2019;90(3):261–7. https://doi.org/10.1136/jnnp-2018-319208.
80. Moll NM, Rietsch AM, Ransohoff AJ, Cossoy MB, Huang D, Eichler FS, Trapp BD, Ransohoff RM. Cortical demyelination in PML and MS: similarities and differences. Neurology. 2008;70(5):336–43. https://doi.org/10.1212/01.WNL.0000284601.54436.e4.
81. Baldassari LE, Wattjes MP, Cortese ICM, Gass A, Metz I, Yousry T, et al. The neuroradiology of progressive multifocal leukoencephalopathy: a clinical trial perspective. Brain. 2022;145:426–40.
82. Wattjes MP, Wijburg MT, van Eijk J, Frequin S, Uitdehaag BMJ, Barkhof F, et al. Inflammatory natalizumab-associated PML: baseline characteristics, lesion evolution and relation with PML-IRIS. J Neurol Neurosurg Psychiatry. 2018;89:535–41.
83. Wattjes MP, Wijburg MT, Vennegoor A, Witte BI, de Vos M, Richert ND, et al. MRI characteristics of early PML-IRIS after natalizumab treatment in patients with MS. J Neurol Neurosurg Psychiatry. 2016;87:879–84.
84. Nishigori R, Warabi Y, Shishido-Hara Y, Nakamichi K, Nakata Y, Komori T, et al. Inflammatory cerebellar PML with a CD4/CD8 ratio of 2.9 showed a favorable prognosis in a patient with rheumatoid arthritis. Intern Med. 2019;58:3323–9.
85. Nishiyama S, Misu T, Shishido-Hara Y, Nakamichi K, Saijo M, Takai Y, et al. Fingolimod-associated PML with mild IRIS in MS: a clinicopathologic study. Neurol Neuroimmunol Neuroinflamm. 2018;5:e415.
86. Hamaguchi M, Suzuki K, Fujita H, Uzuka T, Matsuda H, Shishido-Hara Y, et al. Successful treatment of non-HIV progressive multifocal leukoencephalopathy: case report and literature review. J Neurol. 2020;267:731–8.
87. Shishido-Hara Y, Akimoto J, Fukami S, Kohno M, Matsubayashi J, Nagao T. Pathology for severe inflammatory PML with PD1/PD-L1 expression of favorable prognosis: what's a prognostic factor for PML-IRIS? Neuropathology. 2024;44:47–58.
88. Aly L, Yousef S, Schippling S, Jelcic I, Breiden P, Matschke J, et al. Central role of JC virus-specific CD4+ lymphocytes in progressive multi-focal leucoencephalopathy-immune reconstitution inflammatory syndrome. Brain. 2011;134:2687–702.
89. Pasquier RAD, Koralnik IJ. Inflammatory reaction in progressive multifocal leukoencephalopathy: harmful or beneficial? J Neurovirol. 2003;9:25–31.
90. Cinque P, Koralnik IJ, Gerevini S, Miro JM, Price RW. Progressive multifocal leukoencephalopathy in HIV-1 infection. Lancet Infect Dis. 2009;9(10):625–36. https://doi.org/10.1016/S1473-3099(09)70226-9.
91. Martin-Blondel G, Bauer J, Cuvinciuc V, Uro-Coste E, Debard A, Massip P, et al. In situ evidence of JC virus control by CD8+ T cells in PML-IRIS during HIV infection. Neurology. 2013;81:964–70.
92. Kleinschmidt-DeMasters BK, Miravalle A, Schowinsky J, Corboy J, Vollmer T. Update on PML and PML-IRIS occurring in multiple sclerosis patients treated with natalizumab. J Neuropathol Exp Neurol. 2012;71:604–17.
93. Whiteman ML, Post MJ, Berger JR, Tate LG, Bell MD, Limonte LP. Progressive multifocal leukoencephalopathy in 47 HIV-seropositive patients: neu-

roimaging with clinical and pathologic correlation. Radiology. 1993;187:233–40.
94. Clifford DB, De Luca A, Simpson DM, Arendt G, Giovannoni G, Nath A. Natalizumab-associated progressive multifocal leukoencephalopathy in patients with multiple sclerosis: lessons from 28 cases. Lancet Neurol. 2010;9:438–46.
95. Tan IL, McArthur JC, Clifford DB, Major EO, Nath A. Immune reconstitution inflammatory syndrome in natalizumab-associated PML. Neurology. 2011;77:1061–7.
96. Yousry TA, Pelletier D, Cadavid D, et al. Magnetic resonance imaging pattern in natalizumab-associated progressive multifocal leukoencephalopathy. Ann Neurol. 2012;72:779–87.
97. Harrison DM, Newsome SD, Skolasky RL, McArthur JC, Nath A. Immune reconstitution is not a prognostic factor in progressive multifocal leukoencephalopathy. J Neuroimmunol. 2011;238:81–6.
98. Brochet B, Dousset V. Pathological correlates of magnetization transfer imaging abnormalities in animal models and humans with multiple sclerosis. Neurology. 1999;53:S12–7.
99. Chang L, Ernst T, Tornatore C, et al. Metabolite abnormalities in progressive multifocal leukoencephalopathy by proton magnetic resonance spectroscopy. Neurology. 1997;48:836–45.
100. Nelson PK, Masters LT, Zagzag D, Kelly PJ. Angiographic abnormalities in progressive multifocal leukoencephalopathy: an explanation based on neuropathologic findings. AJNR Am J Neuroradiol. 1999;20:487–94.
101. Bergui M, Bradac GB, Oguz KK, et al. Progressive multifocal leukoencephalopathy: diffusion-weighted imaging and pathological correlations. Neuroradiology. 2004;46(1):22–5. https://doi.org/10.1007/s00234-003-1115-9.
102. Wattjes MP, Barkhof F. Diagnosis of natalizumab-associated progressive multifocal leukoencephalopathy using MRI. Curr Opin Neurol. 2014;27(3):260–70. https://doi.org/10.1097/WCO.0000000000000099.
103. Wijburg MT, Witte BI, Vennegoor A, et al. MRI criteria differentiating asymptomatic PML from new MS lesions during natalizumab pharmacovigilance. J Neurol Neurosurg Psychiatry. 2016;87(10):1138–45. https://doi.org/10.1136/jnnp-2016-313772.
104. Hodel J, Darchis C, Outteryck O, et al. Punctate pattern: a promising imaging marker for the diagnosis of natalizumab-associated PML. Neurology. 2016;86:1516–23.
105. Maas RP, Muller-Hansma AH, Esselink RA, et al. Drug-associated progressive multifocal leukoencephalopathy: a clinical, radiological, and cerebrospinal fluid analysis of 326 cases. J Neurol. 2016;263:2004–21.
106. Hoepner R, Ahlbrecht J, Faissner S, et al. Clinical and paraclinical findings in natalizumab-associated infratentorial progressive multifocal leukoencephalopathy patients. J Neurol Neurosurg Psychiatry. 2014;85:1177–8.
107. Bag AK, Cure JK, Chapman PR, et al. JC virus infection of the brain. AJNR Am J Neuroradiol. 2010;31:1564–76.
108. Bartsch T, Rempe T, Leypoldt F, et al. The spectrum of progressive multifocal leukoencephalopathy: a practical approach. Eur J Neurol. 2019;26:566–74.
109. Hodel J, Outteryck O, Dubron C, et al. Asymptomatic progressive multifocal leukoencephalopathy associated with natalizumab: diagnostic precision with MR imaging. Radiology. 2016;278:863–72.
110. Wijburg MT, Warnke C, Barkhof F, et al. Performance of PML diagnostic criteria in natalizumab-associated PML: data from the Dutch-Belgian cohort. J Neurol Neurosurg Psychiatry. 2019;90:44–6.
111. Sinnecker T, Hadisurya J, Schneider-Hohendorf T, et al. Extensive immune reconstitution inflammatory syndrome in Fingolimod-associated PML: a case report with 7 tesla MRI data. BMC Neurol. 2019;19:190.
112. Gheuens S, Buggy BP, Tlomak W, et al. A game of viral hide and seek: miliary PML masquerading as EBV encephalitis in an HIVþ patient. Clin Neurol Neurosurg. 2013;115:1861–3.
113. Ishii J, Shishido-Hara Y, Kawamoto M, et al. A punctate magnetic resonance imaging pattern in a patient with systemic lupus erythematosus is an early sign of progressive multifocal leukoencephalopathy: a clinicopathological study. Intern Med. 2018;57:2727–34.
114. Wijburg MT, Kleerekooper I, Lissenberg-Witte BI, et al. Association of progressive multifocal leukoencephalopathy lesion volume with JC virus polymerase chain reaction results in cerebrospinal fluid of natalizumab-treated patients with multiple sclerosis. JAMA Neurol. 2018;75:827–33.
115. Zeller D, Markulin F, Monoranu CM, et al. Spreading along white matter tracts? A case of progressive multifocal leukoencephalopathy with unusual MRI presentation. Clin Neurol Neurosurg. 2013;115:638–40.
116. Ruiz Romagnoli E, Akly MP, Miquelini LA, Funes J, Gillanders T, Besada C. Understanding progressive multifocal leukoencephalopathy: links between milky-way appearance and mismatch T2/FLAIR. Neuroradiol J. 2021;34(6):646–55. https://doi.org/10.1177/19714009211019374.
117. Von Einsiedei RW, Fife TD, Aksamit AJ, et al. Progressive multifocal leukoencephalopathy in AIDS: a clinicopathologic study and review of the literature. J Neurol. 1993;240:391–406.
118. Gagne F, Bouchard JP, Bernier JP. Progressive multifocal leukoencephalopathy: observation with predominant pontocerebellar lesions and association with congenital immune deficiency. Acta Neuropathol. 1977;38:167–9.
119. Jones HR Jr, Hedley-Whyte ET, Freidberg SR, et al. Primary cerebellopontine progressive multifocal

leukoencephalopathy diagnosed premortem by cerebellar biopsy. Ann Neurol. 1982;11:199–202.
120. Yadav R, Ramdas M, Karthik N, et al. "Hot cross bun" sign in HIV-related progressive multifocal leukoencephalopathy. Neurol India. 2011;59:293–4.
121. Padmanabhan S, Cherian A, Iype T, et al. Hot cross bun sign in HIV-related progressive multifocal leukoencephalopathy. Ann Indian Acad Neurol. 2013;16:672–3.
122. Lee YC, Liu CS, Wu HM, et al. The "hot cross bun" sign in the patients with spinocerebellar ataxia. Eur J Neurol. 2009;16:513–6.
123. Soares-Fernandes JP, Ribeiro M, Machado A. "Hot cross bun" sign in variant Creutzfeldt-Jakob disease. AJNR Am J Neuroradiol. 2009;30:E37.
124. Muqit MM, Mort D, Miskiel KA, et al. "Hot cross bun" sign in a patient with parkinsonism secondary to presumed vasculitis. J Neurol Neurosurg Psychiatry. 2001;71:565–6.
125. Adra N, Goodheart AE, Rapalino O, Caruso P, Mukerji SS, González RG, Venna N, Schmahmann JD. MRI shrimp sign in cerebellar progressive multifocal leukoencephalopathy: description and validation of a novel observation. AJNR Am J Neuroradiol. 2021;42(6):1073–9. https://doi.org/10.3174/ajnr.A7145.
126. Thurnher MM, Boban J, Rieger A, Gelpi E. Susceptibility-weighted MR imaging Hypointense rim in progressive multifocal leukoencephalopathy: the end point of Neuroinflammation and a potential outcome predictor. AJNR Am J Neuroradiol. 2019;40(6):994–1000. https://doi.org/10.3174/ajnr.A6072.
127. Carra-Dalliere C, Menjot de Champfleur N, Ayrignac X, et al. Quantitative susceptibility mapping suggests a paramagnetic effect in PML. Neurology. 2015;84:1501–2.
128. Umino M, Maeda M, Ii Y, et al. Low-signal-intensity rim on susceptibility-weighted imaging is not a specific finding to progressive multifocal leukoencephalopathy. J Neurol Sci. 2016;362:155–9.
129. Kwan JY, Jeong SY, Van Gelderen P, et al. Iron accumulation in deep cortical layers accounts for MRI signal abnormalities in ALS: correlating 7 tesla MRI and pathology. PLoS One. 2012;7:e35241.
130. van Duijn S, Bulk M, van Duinen SG, et al. Cortical iron reflects severity of Alzheimer's disease. J Alzheimer's Dis. 2017;60:1533–45.
131. Bulk M, Abelmoula WM, Nabuurs RJA, et al. Post-mortem MRI and histology demonstrate differential iron accumulation and cortical myelin organization in early and late onset Alzheimer's disease. Neurobiol Aging. 2018;62:231–42.
132. Birkl C, Carassiti D, Hussain F, et al. Assessment of ferritin content in multiple sclerosis brains using temperature-induced R*2 changes. Magn Reson Med. 2018;79:1609–15.
133. Konijn AM, Carmel N, Levy R, et al. Ferritin synthesis in inflammation, II: mechanism of increased ferritin synthesis. Br J Haematol. 1981;49:361–70.
134. Khoury MN, Alsop DC, Agnihotri SP, et al. Hyperintense cortical signal on magnetic resonance imaging reflects focal leukocortical encephalitis and seizure risk in progressive multifocal leukoencephalopathy. Ann Neurol. 2014;75:659–69.
135. Takeda S, et al. Progressive multifocal leukoencephalopathy showing extensive spinal cord involvement in a patient with lymphocytopenia. Neuropathology. 2009;29:485–93.
136. Miskin DP, Herman ST, Ngo LH, Koralnik IJ. Predictors and characteristics of seizures in survivors of progressive multifocal leukoencephalopathy. J Neurovirol. 2016;22:464–71.
137. Brooks BR, Walker DL. Progressive multifocal leukoencephalopathy. Neurol Clin. 1984;2:299–313.
138. Carson KR, et al. Progressive multifocal leukoencephalopathy associated with brentuximab vedotin therapy: a report of 5 cases from the southern network on adverse reactions (SONAR) project. Cancer. 2014;120:2464–71.
139. Pavlovic D, Patera AC, Nyberg F, Gerber M, Liu M. Progressive multifocal leukoencephalopathy consortium. Progressive multifocal leukoencephalopathy: current treatment options and future perspectives. Ther Adv Neurol Disord. 2015;8:255–73.
140. Sano Y, et al. Rituximab-associated progressive multifocal leukoencephalopathy derived from non-Hodgkin lymphoma: neuropathological findings and results of mefloquine treatment. Intern Med. 2015;54:965–70.
141. Miller JR, et al. Progressive multifocal leukoencephalopathy in a male homosexual with T-cell immune deficiency. N Engl J Med. 1982;307:1436–8.
142. Christensen KLY, Holman RC, Hammett TA, Belay ED, Schonberger LB. Progressive multifocal leukoencephalopathy deaths in the USA, 1979–2005. Neuroepidemiology. 2010;35:178–84.
143. Wuthrich C, Koralnik IJ. Frequent infection of cortical neurons by JC virus in patients with progressive multifocal leukoencephalopathy. J Neuropathol Exp Neurol. 2012;71:54–65.
144. Miyagawa M, et al. Low signal intensity in U-fiber identified by susceptibility-weighted imaging in two cases of progressive multifocal leukoencephalopathy. J Neurol Sci. 2014;344:198–202.
145. Fournier A, et al. Immune reconstitution inflammatory syndrome unmasking or worsening AIDS-related progressive multifocal leukoencephalopathy: a literature review. Front Immunol. 2017;8:577.
146. Tan CS, et al. JC virus latency in the brain and extraneural organs of patients with and without progressive multifocal leukoencephalopathy. J Virol. 2010;84:9200–9.
147. Warnke C, et al. Cerebrospinal fluid JC virus antibody index for diagnosis of natalizumab-associated progressive multifocal leukoencephalopathy. Ann Neurol. 2014;76:792–801.
148. Behrens GM, Meyer D, Stoll M, Schmidt RE. Immune reconstitution syndromes in human immunodeficiency virus infection following

effective antiretroviral therapy. Immunobiology. 2000;202:186–93.
149. Shelburne SA, et al. Immune reconstitution inflammatory syndrome: emergence of a unique syndrome during highly active antiretroviral therapy. Medicine. 2002;81:213–27. https://doi.org/10.1097/00005792-200205000-00005.
150. Engsig FN, et al. Incidence, clinical presentation, and outcome of progressive multifocal leukoencephalopathy in HIV-infected patients during the highly active antiretroviral therapy era: a nationwide cohort study. J Infect Dis. 2009;199:77–83. https://doi.org/10.1086/595299.
151. Falcó V, et al. Influence of HAART on the clinical course of HIV-1-infected patients with progressive multifocal leukoencephalopathy: results of an observational multicenter study. J Acquir Immune Defic Syndr. 2008;49:26–31. https://doi.org/10.1097/QAI.0b013e31817bec64.
152. Summers NA, Kelley CF, Armstrong W, Marconi VC, Nguyen ML. Not a disease of the past: a case series of progressive multifocal leukoencephalopathy in the established antiretroviral era. AIDS Res Hum Retrovir. 2019;35:544–52. https://doi.org/10.1089/AID.2018.0232.
153. Müller M, et al. Immune reconstitution inflammatory syndrome in patients starting antiretroviral therapy for HIV infection: a systematic review and meta-analysis. Lancet Infect Dis. 2010;10:251–61. https://doi.org/10.1016/S1473-3099(10)70026-8.
154. Vendrely A, et al. Fulminant inflammatory leukoencephalopathy associated with HAART-induced immune restoration in AIDS-related progressive multifocal leukoencephalopathy. Acta Neuropathol. 2005;109:449–55. https://doi.org/10.1007/s00401-005-0983-y.
155. Post MJD, et al. CNS-immune reconstitution inflammatory syndrome in the setting of HIV infection, part 1: overview and discussion of progressive multifocal leukoencephalopathy-immune reconstitution inflammatory syndrome and cryptococcal-immune reconstitution inflammatory syndrome. Am J Neuroradiol. 2013;34:1297–307. https://doi.org/10.3174/ajnr.A3183.
156. Sainz-de-la-Maza S, et al. Incidence and prognosis of immune reconstitution inflammatory syndrome in HIV-associated progressive multifocal leucoencephalopathy. Eur J Neurol. 2016;23:919–25. https://doi.org/10.1111/ene.12963.
157. Berger JR, Levy RM, Flomenhoft D, Dobbs M. Predictive factors for prolonged survival in acquired immunodeficiency syndrome-associated progressive multifocal leukoencephalopathy. Ann Neurol. 1998;44:341–9. https://doi.org/10.1002/ana.410440309.
158. Tan K, Roda R, Ostrow L, McArthur J, Nath A. PML-IRIS in patients with HIV infection: clinical manifestations and treatment with steroids. Neurology. 2009;72:1458–64. https://doi.org/10.1212/01.wnl.0000343510.08643.74.
159. Huang D, et al. Inflammatory progressive multifocal leukoencephalopathy in human immunodeficiency virus-negative patients. Ann Neurol. 2007;62:34–9. https://doi.org/10.1002/ana.21085.
160. Gheuens S, et al. Metabolic profile of PML lesions in patients with and without IRIS: an observational study. Neurology. 2012;79:1041–8. https://doi.org/10.1212/WNL.0b013e318268465b.
161. Khoury MS, et al. Hyperperfusion in progressive multifocal leukoencephalopathy is associated with disease progression and absence of immune reconstitution inflammatory syndrome. Brain. 2013;136:3441–50. https://doi.org/10.1093/brain/awt268.
162. Baheerathan A, et al. The utility of FDG-PET imaging in distinguishing PML-IRIS from PML in a patient treated with natalizumab. Neurology. 2018;91:572–3. https://doi.org/10.1212/WNL.0000000000006213.
163. Bauer J, Gold R, Adams O, Lassmann H. Progressive multifocal leukoencephalopathy and immune reconstitution inflammatory syndrome (IRIS). Acta Neuropathol. 2015;130:751–64. https://doi.org/10.1007/s00401-015-1471-7.
164. Martin-Blondel G, et al. In situ evidence of JC virus control by CD8T cells in PML-IRIS during HIV infection. Neurology. 2013;81:964–70. https://doi.org/10.1212/WNL.0b013e3182a43e6d.
165. Berger JR, Malik V, Lacey S, Brunetta P, Lehane PB. Progressive multifocal leukoencephalopathy in rituximab-treated rheumatic diseases: a rare event. J Neurovirol. 2018;24:323–31. https://doi.org/10.1007/s13365-018-0615-7.
166. Raisch DW, Rafi JA, Chen C, Bennett CL. Detection of cases of progressive multifocal leukoencephalopathy associated with new biologicals and targeted cancer therapies from the FDA'S adverse event reporting system. Expert Opin Drug Saf. 2016;15:1003–11. https://doi.org/10.1080/14740338.2016.1198775.
167. Boren EJ, Cheema GS, Naguwa SM, Ansari AA, Gershwin ME. The emergence of progressive multifocal leukoencephalopathy (PML) in rheumatic diseases. J Autoimmun. 2008;30:90–8. https://doi.org/10.1016/j.jaut.2007.11.013.
168. Bloomgren G, et al. Risk of natalizumab-associated progressive multifocal leukoencephalopathy. N Engl J Med. 2012;366:1870–80. https://doi.org/10.1056/NEJMoa1107829.
169. Campagnolo D, et al. Statistical analysis of PML incidences of natalizumab-treated patients from 2009 to 2016: outcomes after introduction of the stratify JCV® DxSelect™ antibody assay. J Neurovirol. 2016;22:880–1. https://doi.org/10.1007/s13365-016-0482-z.
170. Plavina T, et al. Anti-JC virus antibody levels in serum or plasma further define risk of natalizumab-associated progressive multifocal leukoencephalopathy. Ann Neurol. 2014;76:802–12. https://doi.org/10.1002/ana.24286.

171. Ryerson LZ, et al. Risk of natalizumab-associated PML in patients with MS is reduced with extended interval dosing. Neurology. 2019;93:e1452–62. https://doi.org/10.1212/WNL.0000000000008243.
172. Phan-Ba R, et al. The earlier, the smaller, the better for natalizumab-associated PML: in MRI vigilance veritas? Neurology. 2012;79:1067–9. https://doi.org/10.1212/WNL.0b013e31826846b4.
173. Havla J, Hohlfeld R, Kümpfel T. Unusual natalizumab-associated progressive multifocal leukoencephalopathy starting in the brainstem. J Neurol. 2014;261:232–4. https://doi.org/10.1212/WNL.0b013e31826846b4.
174. Blair NF, Brew BJ, Halpern J-P. Natalizumab-associated PML identified in the presymptomatic phase using MRI surveillance. Neurology. 2012;78:507–8. https://doi.org/10.1212/WNL.0b013e318246d6d8.
175. Vennegoor A, et al. Indolent course of progressive multifocal leukoencephalopathy during natalizumab treatment in MS. Neurology. 2011;76:574–6. https://doi.org/10.1212/WNL.0b013e31820b7644.
176. Bayliss J, Karasoulos T, McLean CA. Immunosuppression increases JC polyomavirus large T antigen DNA load in the brains of patients without progressive multifocal leukoencephalopathy. J Infect Dis. 2013;207:133–6. https://doi.org/10.1093/infdis/jis668.
177. Wattjes MP, et al. MRI pattern in asymptomatic natalizumab-associated PML. J Neurol Neurosurg Psychiatry. 2015;86:793–8.
178. Dong-Si T, et al. Outcome and survival of asymptomatic PML in natalizumab-treated MS patients. Ann Clin Transl Neurol. 2014;1:755–64.
179. Wijburg MT, et al. Association of progressive multifocal leukoencephalopathy lesion volume with JC virus polymerase chain reaction results in cerebrospinal fluid of natalizumab-treated patients with multiple sclerosis. JAMA Neurol. 2018;75:827–33.
180. Wattjes MP, et al. Diagnosis of asymptomatic natalizumab-associated PML: are we between a rock and a hard place? J Neurol. 2014;261:1139–43.
181. McGuigan C, et al. Stratification and monitoring of natalizumab-associated progressive multifocal leukoencephalopathy risk: recommendations from an expert group. J Neurol Neurosurg Psychiatry. 2016;87:117–25.
182. Hall CD, et al. Failure of cytarabine in progressive multifocal leukoencephalopathy associated with human immunodeficiency virus infection. N Engl J Med. 1998;338:1345–51.
183. Royal W, et al. Topotecan in the treatment of acquired immunodeficiency syndrome-related progressive multifocal leukoencephalopathy. J Neurovirol. 2003;9:411–9.
184. Gasnault J, et al. Improved survival of HIV-1-infected patients with progressive multifocal leukoencephalopathy receiving early 5-drug combination antiretroviral therapy. PLoS One. 2011;6:e20967.
185. Clifford DB, et al. A study of mefloquine treatment for progressive multifocal leukoencephalopathy: results and exploration of predictors of PML outcomes. J Neurovirol. 2013;19:351–8.
186. Landi D, et al. No evidence of beneficial effects of plasmapheresis in natalizumab-associated PML. Neurology. 2017;88:1144–52.
187. Scarpazza C, et al. To do or not to do? Plasma exchange and timing of steroid administration in progressive multifocal leukoencephalopathy. Ann Neurol. 2017;82:697–705.
188. Cortese I, et al. Pembrolizumab treatment for progressive multifocal leukoencephalopathy. N Engl J Med. 2019;380:1597–605.
189. Pawlitzki M, et al. Ineffective treatment of PML with pembrolizumab: exhausted memory T-cell subsets as a clue? Neurol Neuroimmunol Neuroinflamm. 2019;6:e627.
190. Boumaza X, Bonneau B, Roos-Weil D, Pinnetti C, Rauer S, Nitsch L, Del Bello A, Jelcic I, Sühs KW, Gasnault J, Goreci Y, Grauer O, Gnanapavan S, Wicklein R, Lambert N, Perpoint T, Beudel M, Clifford D, Sommet A, Cortese I, Martin-Blondel G, Immunotherapy for PML Study Group. Progressive multifocal leukoencephalopathy treated by immune checkpoint inhibitors. Ann Neurol. 2023;93(2):257–70. https://doi.org/10.1002/ana.26512.
191. Balduzzi A, et al. Polyomavirus JC-targeted T-cell therapy for progressive multiple leukoencephalopathy in a hematopoietic cell transplantation recipient. Bone Marrow Transpl. 2011;46:987–92.
192. Muftuoglu M, et al. Allogeneic BK virus-specific T cells for progressive multifocal leukoencephalopathy. N Engl J Med. 2018;379:1443–51.
193. Möhn N, Grote-Levi L, Wattjes MP, Bonifacius A, Holzwart D, Hopfner F, Nay S, Tischer-Zimmermann S, Saßmann ML, Schwenkenbecher P, Sühs KW, Mahmoudi N, Warnke C, Zimmermann J, Hagin D, Goudeva L, Blasczyk R, Koch A, Maecker-Kolhoff B, Eiz-Vesper B, Höglinger G, Skripuletz T. Directly isolated allogeneic virus-specific T cells in progressive multifocal leukoencephalopathy. JAMA Neurol. 2024;81(11):1187–98. https://doi.org/10.1001/jamaneurol.2024.3324.
194. Lambert N, El Moussaoui M, Maquet P. Immune checkpoint inhibitors for progressive multifocal leukoencephalopathy: identifying relevant outcome factors. Eur J Neurol. 2021;28(11):3814–9. https://doi.org/10.1111/ene.15021.
195. Lajaunie R, Mainardi I, Gasnault J, Rousseau V, Tarantino AG, Sommet A, Cinque P, Martin-Blondel G, PML study group. Outcome of progressive multifocal leukoencephalopathy treated by Interleukin-7. Ann Neurol. 2022;91(4):496–505. https://doi.org/10.1002/ana.26307.

7 Spontaneous and Iatrogenic Amyloid-Related Imaging Abnormalities (ARIA): Clues for Immunotherapy in Alzheimer's Disease

Marialuisa Zedde, Giampaolo Basso, Fabrizio Piazza, and Rosario Pascarella

7.1 Introduction

Age-related cognitive impairment is now understood to result from both neurodegenerative and cerebrovascular diseases [1]. Studies like the Religious Orders Study and the Memory and Aging Project [2] found that while Alzheimer's disease (AD) was the most common pathology (in ~65% of brains), vascular issues like ischemic infarcts, cerebral amyloid angiopathy (CAA), atherosclerosis, and arteriolosclerosis were also significant, each present in over 30% of brains and contributing 20–30% to cognitive decline. This overlap informs prevention strategies, as improvements in blood pressure control and vascular health in developed countries over recent decades have coincided with a decline in age-specific dementia incidence [3]. The interaction between neurodegenerative and vascular diseases likely stems from cumulative brain injuries and potential crosstalk between neurodegenerative pathways and blood vessels [4]. A clear example of this interaction is between CAA and AD, both involving amyloid-β (Aβ) deposition. CAA may exacerbate AD by impairing perivascular drainage, a key route for clearing Aβ from the brain [5, 6]. Given the high overlap between CAA and AD, treatments for one condition may also impact the other, emphasizing the need to

M. Zedde (✉)
Neurology Unit, Stroke Unit, Azienda Unità Sanitaria Locale-IRCCS di Reggio Emilia, Reggio Emilia, Italy

ICAβ International Network, Monza, Italy

The Inflammatory Amyloid Angiopathy Study Group of SINdem (Italian neurological society on dementia), Reggio Emilia, Italy
e-mail: zedde.marialuisa@ausl.re.it

G. Basso · F. Piazza
ICAβ International Network, Monza, Italy

CAA and AD Translational Research and Biomarkers Laboratory, School of Medicine and Surgery, University of Milano-Bicocca, Monza, Italy

The Inflammatory Amyloid Angiopathy Study Group of SINdem (Italian neurological society on dementia), Reggio Emilia, Italy

R. Pascarella
ICAβ International Network, Monza, Italy

Neuroradiology Unit, Ospedale Santa Maria della Misericordia, AULSS 5 Polesana, Rovigo, Rovigo, Italy
e-mail: rosario.pascarella@aulss5.veneto.it

M. Zedde, R. Pascarella (eds.), *Neuroimaging of Treatment-Related Conditions in the Brain*,
https://doi.org/10.1007/978-3-032-23618-0_7

understand their interaction in disease development [4].

The mechanisms by which AD and CAA lead to brain injury largely do not overlap. AD-related brain injury mechanisms [7] remain unclear but are believed to involve Aβ-triggered loss of synapses and neurons, resulting in cortical tissue loss and hyperphosphorylated tau-containing neurofibrillary lesions detectable by PET scans. These measures correlate with cognitive performance in Aβ-positive individuals [8]. In contrast, CAA-related brain injuries stem from blood vessel dysfunction, either through vessel integrity loss and hemorrhage or disrupted blood supply and ischemia. CAA-related hemorrhages include large symptomatic intracerebral hemorrhages, small asymptomatic cerebral microbleeds, and bleeding into cortical sulci, detectable by T2*-weighted MRI and forming the basis of the Boston criteria for CAA. Non-hemorrhagic (ischemic) injuries in CAA appear as white matter hyperintensities on T2-weighted MRI, structural disconnection measured with diffusion-tensor MRI, and cerebral microinfarcts [9, 10].

Both AD and CAA might show clinical and neuroimaging correlates of inflammatory pattern, which is the topic of this chapter.

7.2 Definitions and Epidemiology

Amyloid-related imaging abnormalities (ARIA), detectable via MRI, arise from Aβ-targeted immunotherapy seen in AD trials and are the description of an imaging pattern [11, 12]. ARIA has two subtypes [11]:

1. ARIA-E: Characterized by white matter hyperintensities on FLAIR MRI indicating vasogenic edema and sulcal effusions with occasional gyral swelling.
2. ARIA-H: Marked by parenchymal microbleeds and superficial hemosiderin deposition in the leptomeninges, visible on T2*-weighted MRI, and generally persists on subsequent MRIs.

The mechanisms behind ARIA are not fully understood but are thought to involve antibody-mediated breakdown of neuritic plaques, releasing Aβ, which deposits in vessels leading to increased CAA, perivascular inflammation, and impaired clearance.

ARIA has been observed in several passive immunotherapy trials for AD, especially those targeting N-terminal or conformational forms of Aβ, which clear neuritic plaques [12, 13]. The incidence of ARIA-E is dose-dependent and influenced by the APOEε4 allele. For instance, in the bapineuzumab trial, ARIA-E incidence was 14.2% at the highest dose for non-APOEε4 carriers and 15.3% at the lowest dose for APOEε4 carriers [12]. A higher incidence (~40%) was found with aducanumab [14], particularly among APOEε4 carriers. Lower rates of ARIA-E were associated with antibodies targeting mid-peptide and C-terminal regions of Aβ, likely because they bind to monomeric or specific oligomeric Aβ, mobilizing less Aβ from neuritic plaques [15–19]. Placebo-treated participants and those in observational studies with autosomal-dominant and sporadic AD showed a low incidence (<1%) of ARIA-E, primarily in APOEε4 carriers [19, 20]. Anti-amyloid immunotherapy is also linked to ARIA-H, although the increase compared to placebo is less pronounced than for ARIA-E. ARIA-H can occur after ARIA-E, and higher rates of co-occurring ARIA-H and ARIA-E were observed in APOEε4 carriers treated with aducanumab (35% at the highest dose) [21–23].

A meta-analysis revealed that immunotherapy increases the risk of any ARIA and ARIA-E, but not ARIA-H, possibly because participants with more than four microbleeds are usually excluded from trials, and spontaneous microbleeds are common in observational studies [24].

The profile of risk factors for ARIA provides valuable insights into its underlying pathophysiology. The risk of ARIA-E is linked to the antibody dose; however, it remains unclear whether this risk is driven more by the peak antibody concentration or the rate of dose escalation. Limited evidence suggests that dose titration can reduce the risk of ARIA-E. Several studies have shown that a higher dose of the APOE ε4 allele correlates with an increased risk of both ARIA-E and ARIA-H [21, 25, 26]. Moreover, carriers of the APOE ε4 allele face a significantly higher risk of symptomatic ARIA, which can present as headaches, lethargy, confusion, neuropsychiatric symptoms, and, in rare cases, seizures. Symptomatic ARIA is observed in 1–20% of patients with ARIA-E, with variability depending on the antibody used, dosage, and prevalence of the APOE ε4 allele [13, 14, 25, 27].

Interestingly, hypertension, hyperlipidemia, and diabetes do not appear to be risk factors for ARIA-E in AD patients. No associations have been found between ARIA and baseline biomarkers of brain amyloid on PET scans, volumetric MRI measures, or most CSF biomarkers [26–28]. However, lower baseline CSF levels of Aβ42 in individuals without the APOE ε4 allele are associated with a higher risk of ARIA.

A plausible explanation for ARIA, initially proposed based on post-mortem studies of individuals who received the original active immunotherapy AN1792 is that the solubilization of Aβ may overwhelm the capacity for Aβ clearance through perivascular CSF bulk flow pathways [29, 30]. This could lead to amyloid deposition in arterial walls and accelerated development of CAA. The correlation between baseline microbleeds and the APOE*ìε4 allele as risk factors for both ARIA and CAA supports this hypothesis. Microbleeds suggest Aβ presence in vessel walls, while the APOEε4 allele indicates a high Aβ burden. Autopsy studies have shown that individuals who received immunotherapy developed more extensive CAA in cortical and leptomeningeal vessels (common sites for ARIA) compared to untreated individuals [30, 31]. These studies also revealed treatment-associated concentric vessel wall splitting, a key feature of CAA-associated vasculopathy. Therapeutic antibodies against Aβ might not only accelerate vascular deposition but also bind to accessible vascular Aβ, potentially disrupting vessel integrity further and contributing to ARIA-E (proteinaceous fluid leakage) and ARIA-H (red blood cell leakage).

Additionally, ARIA's resemblance to CAA-related inflammation (CAA-ri) provides further evidence of a link between ARIA and CAA. CAA-ri occurs in a subset of CAA patients and shares similar clinical presentations, neuroimaging features, and associations with ARIA [32–34].

CAA-ri involves infiltration of microglia, T cells, and Aβ-containing multinucleated giant cells around CAA-positive vessel segments, suggesting a spontaneous anti-Aβ autoimmune response [34, 35]. During the active phase of CAA-ri, CSF concentrations of autoantibodies against Aβ increase, supporting the hypothesis that ARIA-E is an iatrogenic version of CAA-ri. Typically, CAA-ri is treated with immunosuppression, which improves clinical symptoms, reduces vasogenic edema, and normalizes CSF anti-Aβ antibody concentrations [36–38].

The analogy between ARIA and CAA-ri suggests that repeated or prolonged immunotherapy would increase the inflammatory response. However, ARIA seems to decrease with longer treatment, indicating a more complex relationship. Prolonged immunotherapy might lower plaque burden, reducing amyloid mobilization and subsequent deposition in vessel walls, potentially decreasing vascular inflammation and the risk of ARIA.

Limited evidence suggests that vessels affected by ARIA can recover. Post-mortem examinations of brains from individuals treated long-term with AN1792 did not reveal vascular smooth muscle cell loss or vessel wall thinning [30]. Similarly, in transgenic mice exposed to a bapineuzumab analog for a prolonged period, the thickness of vascular smooth muscle cells and collagen IV extracellular matrix returned to wild-type levels after treatment cessation [39]. These findings suggest that vascular morphology and perivascular clearance can recover. Additionally, in most individuals diagnosed with CAA-ri and treated with immunosuppressive drugs, clinical symptoms improve, and MRI signs of vasogenic edema resolve, supporting the possibility of vessel recovery following an anti-Aβ immune response [40–44]. A detailed description of CAA-ri and ARIA similarities and differences is available in recently published reviews [45, 46].

Since the early 2000s, a multitude of clinical trials have been conducted for disease-modifying

Table 7.1 Incidence of ARIA in clinical trials

Drug	Amyloid binding site	ARIA-E incidence (%)	ARIA-H incidence (%)
Bapineuzumab [12]	Aβ monomers, oligomers, and fibrils (N-terminus)	4.2 in APOE ε4 noncarriers, 15.3 in APOE ε4 carriers	NR
Solanezumab [47]	Aβ monomers (mid-domain)	0.9	4.9
Gantenerumab [13]	Aβ oligomers, fibrils, and plaques (N-terminus and central amino acids)	13.5	16.2
Crenezumab [48]	Aβ oligomers, fibrils, and plaques (aβ peptides)	0.0	4.9
Ponezumab [49]	Soluble Aβ40 (C-terminus)	0.7	16.4
Lecanemab [50]	Aβ protofibrils (aβ protofibril)	9.9	10.7
Donanemab [51]	Aβ plaques (pyroglutamate form of aβ)	27.5	30.5
Aducanumab [52]	Aβ oligomers, fibrils, and plaques (N-terminus conformational epitope)	35–36	19–20

Alzheimer's disease medications, as outlined in Table 7.1.

Variations in patient demographics might also contribute to the observed differences. Individuals who do not carry the ApoE ε4 gene or who have a lower initial amyloid load tend to have a reduced risk of ARIA compared to ApoE ε4 carriers or those with a positive amyloid status. Nonetheless, previous clinical trials may not have evaluated patients for ApoE ε4 presence or confirmed amyloid build-up. Additionally, the inconsistent frequency of MRI monitoring across different clinical studies might partially account for the observed discrepancies [53].

Bapineuzumab was the first monoclonal antibody trialed in humans, revealing a significantly higher incidence of ARIA-E in APOE ε4 carriers (15.3%) compared to noncarriers (4.2%). Due to a high rate of symptomatic ARIA-E, doses over 2 mg/kg were discontinued early [12]. Most ARIA-E cases occurred after the initial infusion, with a 25.6% recurrence rate upon reinitiation of treatment. ARIA-H was observed with treatment but did not show a dose-dependent effect and was associated with baseline microhemorrhages and antithrombotic use. In combined phase 3 trial data involving 2052 participants with Solanezumab [47], only 0.9% developed ARIA-E, while 4.9% exhibited ARIA-H. Using gantenerumab subcutaneously every 4 weeks [13], among those receiving 225 mg, 15% of APOE ε4 carriers developed ARIA-E, compared to 11% of noncarriers, with an overall incidence of 13.5%. Over 80% of ARIA-E cases were asymptomatic. Additionally, ARIA-H was observed in 19.4% of APOE ε4 carriers versus 11% of noncarriers. In patients receiving crenezumab at doses of 45 or 60 mg/kg [48], no ARIA-E cases were reported, while 4.9% developed ARIA-H. Even at a higher dose of 120 mg/kg, no ARIA-E or ARIA-H cases occurred. Ponezumab has a lower potential for activating the complement system. The reported incidence of ARIA-E was 0.7%, while ARIA-H was 16.4% [49]. In a phase 2b study with Lecanemab enrolling 854 patients [50], ARIA-E was reported in 14.3% of APOE ε4 carriers and 8.0% of noncarriers, with an overall incidence of 9.9%. The incidence of ARIA-H was 13.1% for carriers and 4.6% for noncarriers. Donanemab was evaluated in the TRAILBLAZER-ALZ phase 2 trial [51], which included 257 patients with prodromal to mild AD. ARIA-E and ARIA-H were observed in 27.5% and 30.5% of patients, respectively. Aducanumab [52] was evaluated in the EMERGE [54] and ENGAGE [55] phase 3 trials involving 1647 and 1638 patients, respectively. In EMERGE, ARIA-E incidence was 2%, 26%, and 35% for placebo, low-dose, and high-dose groups, respectively. In ENGAGE, the rates were 3%, 26%, and 36%. The incidence of ARIA-E was significantly higher in APOE ε4 carriers compared to noncarriers in both trials. In terms of ARIA-H, incidence rates in EMERGE were 7%, 16%, and 20%, while in

ENGAGE, they were 6%, 16%, and 19%. Notably, ARIA-H was more prevalent among those with ARIA-E. A recent Genome-Wide Association Studies of ARIA from the Aducanumab Phase 3 ENGAGE and EMERGE studies [56], on 1691/3285 European patients with available genotyping array and at least one post-enrolling MRI, showed a significant association between the APOE status and the risk of ARIA ($p < 5.0 \times 10^{-8}$). In this cohort, 31% had ARIA-E, 19% had ARIA-H microhemorrhage, and 14% had ARIA-H superficial siderosis. The APOE association with ARIA was stronger in e4/e4 homozygotes (OR = 4.28, 4.58, 7.84; $p < 2.9 \times 10–14$ for ARIA-E, ARIA-H microhemorrhage, and ARIA-H superficial siderosis, respectively) than in e3/e4 heterozygotes (OR = 1.74, 1.46, 3.14; $p \leq 0.03$). Moreover, e4/e4 homozygotes had greater odds of radiographically severe ARIA (OR = 7.04–24.64, $p \leq 2.72 \times 10^{-5}$) than radiographically mild ARIA (OR = 3.19–5.00, $p \leq 1.37 \times 10^{-5}$).

In a recent metanalysis of all immunotherapy trials [57], the overall incidences of ARIA-E and ARIA-H were 6.5% and 7.8%, respectively, and the pooled proportion of asymptomatic ARIA was 80.4%. The cohorts treated with aducanumab showed a significantly higher incidence of ARIA-E and ARIA-H (30.7% and 30.0%) compared with other drugs.

Notably, MRI-based exclusion criteria of CLARITY AD study [58] (lecanemab phase 3) are the presence of any CNS macrobleed >10 mm in diameter, more than 4 microbleeds (<10 mm in diameter), evidence of superficial siderosis, evidence of brain vasogenic edema, significant white matter hyperintensities, multiple lacunar strokes, and any cerebral strokes involving a major vascular territory. These same restrictions should apply when considering patients for treatment with lecanemab [59], and MRI evidence of underlying CAA-ri or other conditions placing patients at risk for ARIA as well as more serious forms of ARIA should exclude patients as treatment candidates. The diagnostic criteria for probable CAA-ri [34] are illustrated in Table 7.2.

Table 7.2 Criteria for probable CAA-ri

Clinical issues
Age ≥ 40 years of age
Clinical features (at least one): Headache, decrease in consciousness, behavioral change, or focal neurological signs and seizures[a]
MRI findings
Unifocal or multifocal WMH lesions (cortico--subcortical or deep) that are asymmetric and extend to the immediately subcortical white matter[b]
≥1 Cortico-subcortical hemorrhagic lesion: Cerebral macrobleed, cerebral microbleed, or cortical superficial siderosis
Absence of neoplastic, infectious, or other cause

[a]The presentation is not directly attributable to an acute ICH

[b]The asymmetry is not due to past ICH

7.3 Neuroimaging Findings

Neuroimaging findings of ARIA have been extensively described [11, 44, 53, 59–62] in clinical trials of immunotherapy for AD, and their standardization was recently updated.

7.3.1 ARIA-E and CAA-Related Inflammation

ARIA-E is identifiable on MRI, particularly on T2-weighted or FLAIR sequences, by the presence of increased signal intensity. This increased signal indicates edema, effusion, or exudate without signs of cytotoxic edema, such as diffusion restriction [11, 53]. The vasogenic edema in ARIA-E is believed to result from increased extracellular fluid due to the heightened permeability of endothelial cells to serum proteins

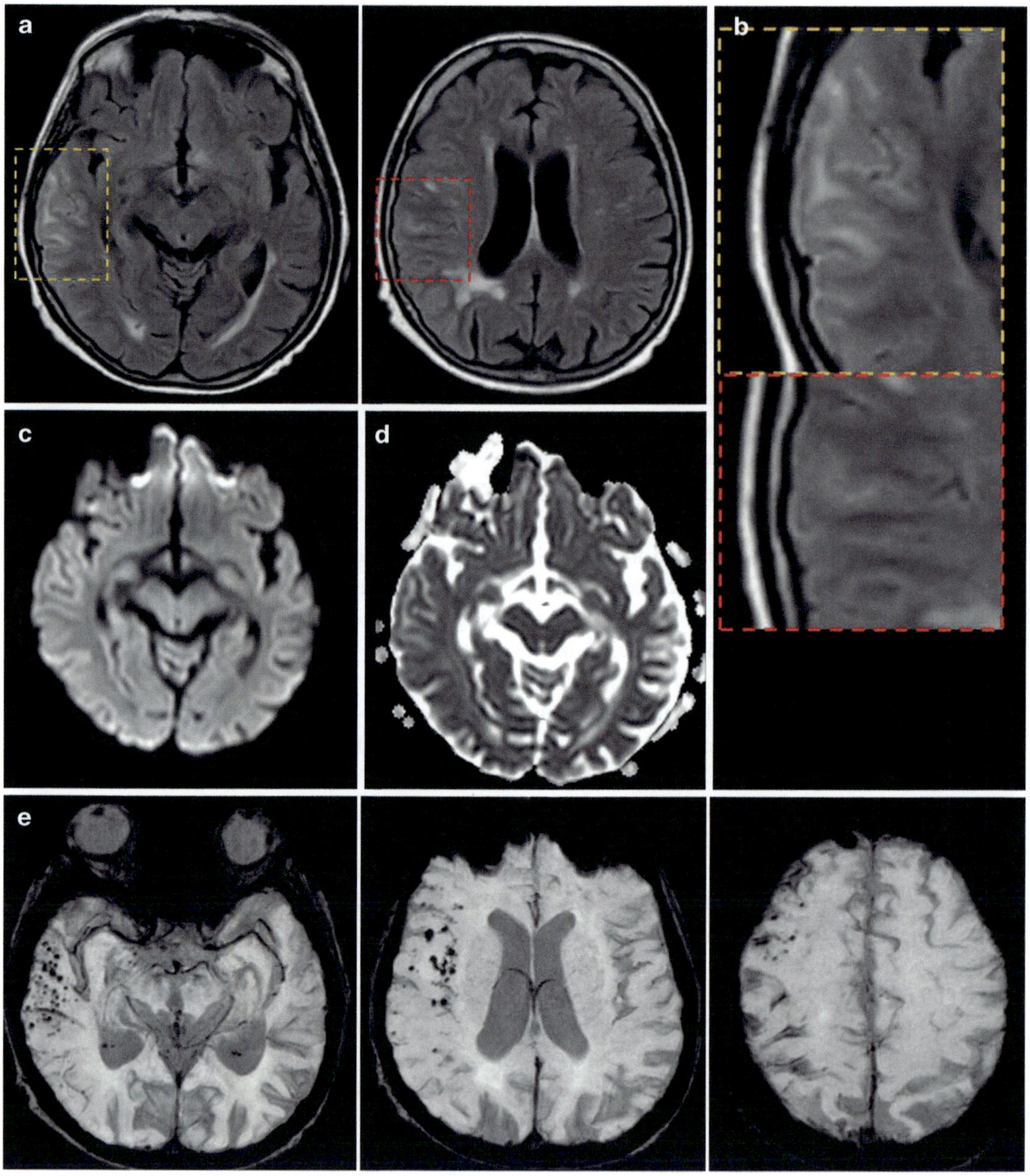

Fig. 7.1 Brain MRI of a patient showing both ARIA-E and ARIA-H. In panel **a**, the axial FLAIR slices show with matter hyperintensities and cortical effacement with sulcal hyperintensities in the right temporal and parietal lobes (magnified details in panel **b**). Panels **c** and **d** show DWI and ADC maps, respectively, with signal features suggestive for vasogenic edema. Panel e shows axial MinIP SWI slices with multiple microbleeds clustered in the regions interested by ARIA-E

[53]. This increased signal can also be observed in the sulci or leptomeningeal spaces, likely due to the leakage of protein-rich fluid from meningeal vessels. Sometimes, the leptomeningeal component is prominent or isolated (Figs. 7.1 and 7.2).

Moreover, ARIA-E can be associated with locoregional mass effect or gyral swelling

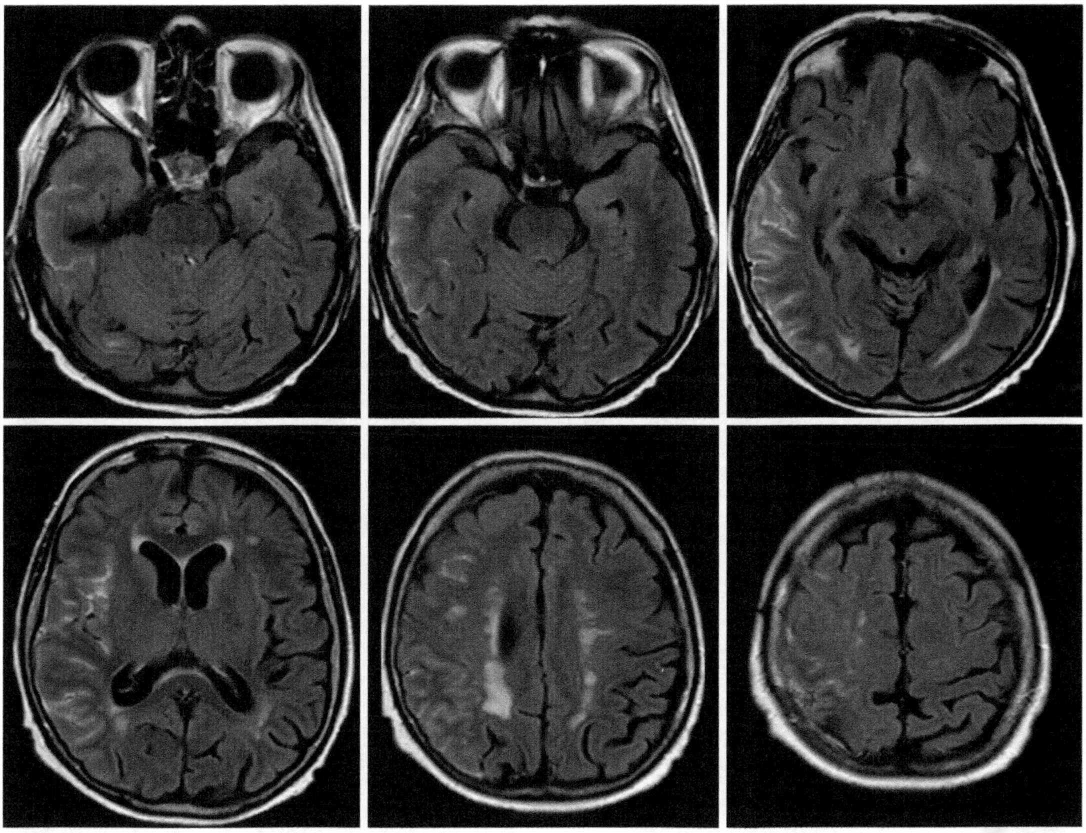

Fig. 7.2 Post-contrast FLAIR MRI of the same patient as in Fig. 7.1 showing diffuse leptomeningeal enhancement in the right hemisphere

(Figs. 7.1, 7.2, and 7.3). It most commonly affects the occipital lobes, followed by the parietal, frontal, and temporal lobes, with cerebellar involvement being rare. Importantly, the MRI findings of ARIA-E are usually transient and tend to resolve upon the interruption or discontinuation of therapy. In some cases, these abnormalities may even resolve spontaneously despite the continuation of treatment.

Proper MRI interpretation of ARIA-E requires awareness of potential mimics, such as incomplete CSF suppression and susceptibility artifacts. A 3D FLAIR sequence is preferred over a 2D FLAIR sequence due to its superior CSF suppression, achieved through a nonselective inversion pulse [11, 53, 63].

Several conditions can exhibit MRI findings similar to ARIA-E:

1. Posterior Reversible Encephalopathy Syndrome (PRES): Often characterized by vasogenic edema predominantly in the posterior regions of the brain.
2. Evolving Subacute Ischemia: Can show increased signal intensity on T2-weighted or FLAIR sequences, similar to ARIA-E.

Having a pretreatment T2-weighted or FLAIR sequence is crucial, particularly in clinical trials, to facilitate the detection of ARIA-E during the course of treatment. This is especially important when ARIA-E findings are subtle and may be easily overlooked without a baseline comparison.

This is not usually available for spontaneous ARIA and for CAA-ri, the relative findings being very similar but potentially missing if subtle and asymptomatic or paucisymptomatic cases.

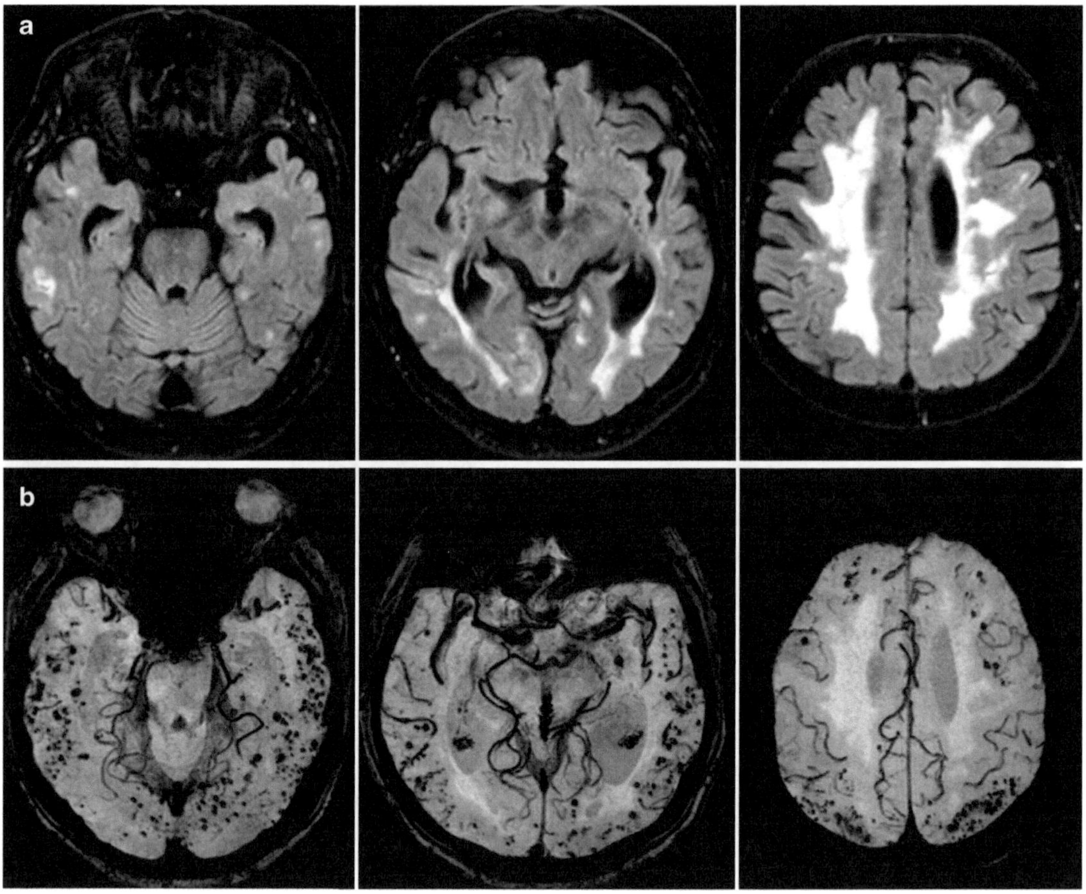

Fig. 7.3 Brain MRI of a patient with mixed CAA/AD showing both spontaneous ARIA-E (panel **a**) and ARIA-H (panel **b**). In panel a axial FLAIR shows extensive, confluent symmetrical white matter hyperintensities on both hemispheres with involvement of the cortical-subcortical junction in the right temporal and occipital lobes. In panel b SWI shows multiple lobar microbleeds

Indeed, the radiological prevalence of CAA-ri is at least three times the prevalence of diagnosed cases in a retrospective MRI study [64].

7.3.2 ARIA-H

ARIA-H is identified by the presence of hemosiderin, a blood degradation product that appears as parenchymal microhemorrhages or leptomeningeal superficial siderosis on MRI. These findings mirror those seen in CAA [65], typically exhibiting a lobar or peripheral distribution at the gray matter-white matter junction or cortex. This distribution contrasts with hypertensive microhemorrhages, which are usually found in deep gray matter, cerebellar hemispheres, and brainstem [26, 66, 67], but mixed patterns are possible outside clinical trials, where the presence of microbleeds (with variable thresholds) and/or siderosis were exclusion criteria.

ARIA-H is best detected using long-TE (T2*-weighted) gradient-recalled echo (GRE) or other susceptibility-weighted sequences [67–72]. On these sequences, ARIA-H appears as markedly hypointense signals in the parenchyma or sulci, and is typically not visible on CT, T1-weighted,

T2-weighted, FLAIR, or diffusion-weighted sequences.

T2*-Weighted GRE Sequences:

- These sequences enhance the effects of local magnetic field variations and spin dephasing caused by microhemorrhages, resulting in a susceptibility-related signal loss known as blooming.
- Compared to conventional T2-weighted spin-echo sequences, T2*-weighted GRE sequences are more effective at highlighting microhemorrhages [53, 69, 70].

Susceptibility-Weighted Imaging (SWI):

- SWI employs a high-resolution 3D spoiled GRE acquisition, offering higher spatial resolution and increased sensitivity to hemosiderin, calcification, and iron deposits.
- It generates both magnitude and phase images, which are multiplied to increase sensitivity [71, 72].
- SWI can be used with quantitative susceptibility mapping to distinguish between paramagnetic substances (e.g., hemosiderin or deoxygenated blood) and diamagnetic substances (e.g., calcium) [70–72].

Microhemorrhage detection is improved by using longer TE, higher field strength (3 T versus 1.5 T), or lower readout bandwidth. Consistent scanning techniques are essential for reliable temporal comparisons, as variations in these parameters can alter the appearance of microhemorrhages [70–72]. Microhemorrhages are small, hypointense, rounded foci within the brain parenchyma, generally measuring less than 5 mm or 10 mm in diameter, depending on the study. Superficial siderosis appears as curvilinear hypointensity within sulci adjacent to the brain parenchyma. The differentiation between these two features is critical for diagnosing ARIA-H [11, 59].

The differences between T2*-weighted GRE and SWI can complicate the use of size criteria for defining ARIA-H if MRI protocols are not standardized. T2*-weighted GRE sequences enhance the effects of local magnetic field variations and spin dephasing caused by microhemorrhages, resulting in susceptibility-related signal loss known as blooming [11, 53, 66]. In contrast, SWI provides higher spatial resolution and increased sensitivity to hemosiderin, calcification, and iron deposits, and generates both magnitude and phase images for increased sensitivity.

Given the increased risk of developing additional microhemorrhages if they are present at baseline, it is essential to performing a baseline screening MRI examination that includes T2*-weighted GRE or SWI sequences before clinical trial entry or treatment initiation (Figs. 7.1 and 7.3). All microhemorrhages, regardless of their location or suspected cause (e.g., even those typical of a hypertensive cause in the deep gray nuclei), affect trial eligibility and treatment management. To ensure proper comparison, all subsequent surveillance MRI examinations should use the same type of blood-sensitive sequence as that used at screening, whether T2*-weighted GRE or SWI. Since patients may be scanned at different facilities with varying protocols during their course of care, it may be prudent to acquire both sequence types at baseline [11, 13, 25, 59, 73].

Most clinical trials to date have utilized T2*-weighted GRE sequences for detecting ARIA-H. This consistency helps maintain the reliability of comparisons and ensures accurate monitoring of microhemorrhage progression or resolution. However, incorporating SWI sequences at baseline can enhance detection sensitivity and provide a more comprehensive assessment of microhemorrhage burden.

In summary, standardized MRI protocols, including both T2*-weighted GRE and SWI sequences, are crucial for the accurate detection and monitoring of ARIA-H, facilitating better patient management in clinical trials and treatment settings.

A recent study aiming to assess the sensitivity of AI software supporting radiologists in identifying and reporting ARIA [74] showed that sensitivity was significantly higher in assisted reading compared with unassisted reading (87% versus 71% for ARIA-E detection; 79% versus 69% for

ARIA-H detection), while specificity remained above 80% for the detection of both ARIA types. This finding highlights the need for a better knowledge, training, and standardization of MRI execution and reading in both clinical trials and routine clinical practice for detecting ARIA.

7.3.3 Grading

Several ARIA severity grading schemes have been proposed [53, 59, 75, 76], including a specific scheme outlined in the FDA guidance [77] for the clinical use of aducanumab. This guidance categorizes ARIA-E and ARIA-H into mild, moderate, and severe grades; it has been used for aducanumab trials and includes a detailed grading scheme for ARIA-E and ARIA-H, which is summarized in Table 7.3.

This 3-point rating scale [78] is easier to apply than Barkhof's rating scale [75, 76], proposed in 2013 for ARIA-E and including three items (parenchymal hyperintensity, sulcal hyperintensity, and brain swelling) with a composite score attributed according to the anatomical location (lobe and side) for six regions bilaterally (frontal, parietal, temporal and occipital lobes, central region, and infratentorial region), depending on the spatial extent and multifocality of the abnormality.

Table 7.3 FDA guidance on ARIA severity grading

Severity	ARIA-E	ARIA-H
Mild	Minimal vasogenic edema or sulcal effusion without mass effect	1–2 focal areas of hemosiderin deposition (microhemorrhages)
Moderate	Localized vasogenic edema or sulcal effusion with mild mass effect	3–10 focal areas of hemosiderin deposition or superficial siderosis
Severe	Extensive vasogenic edema or sulcal effusion with significant mass effect	>10 focal areas of hemosiderin deposition or extensive superficial siderosis

Standardized grading schemes, such as the one provided by the FDA, are essential for consistent assessment and management of ARIA in clinical settings. They help guide treatment decisions and ensure patient safety by categorizing the severity of ARIA and tailoring interventions accordingly (Figs. 7.4, 7.5, 7.6, and 7.7).

7.4 Management

Iatrogenic ARIA is often asymptomatic and detected incidentally during routine MRI surveillance [11, 53]. When symptomatic, ARIA-E can present with nonspecific symptoms such as headache, confusion, visual disturbances, visuospatial impairment, and praxis difficulties. Clinical symptoms, similar to MRI findings, usually resolve spontaneously upon pausing or withdrawing the treatment. Intravenous methylprednisolone has been anecdotally reported to alleviate symptoms [77]. This is a huge difference between ARIA and CAA-ri, the latter one being usually symptomatic from mild encephalopathy symptoms to seizures and coma and usually being treated by immunosuppressive therapy (steroids with or without long-term immunosuppression) [32].

Upon detecting ARIA, a prompt evaluation is crucial to determining whether dose adjustment or discontinuation of therapy is necessary. The presence of a new microhemorrhage or edema after starting anti-Aβ immunotherapy typically suggests ARIA, but other causes must be considered. Decisions on adjusting treatment should factor in the patient's symptoms and overall clinical context [43, 44].

Patients in clinical trials often receive follow-up MRI examinations at 4-week intervals. If ARIA is identified, an additional short-term follow-up MRI may be performed to monitor temporal evolution. A suggested management

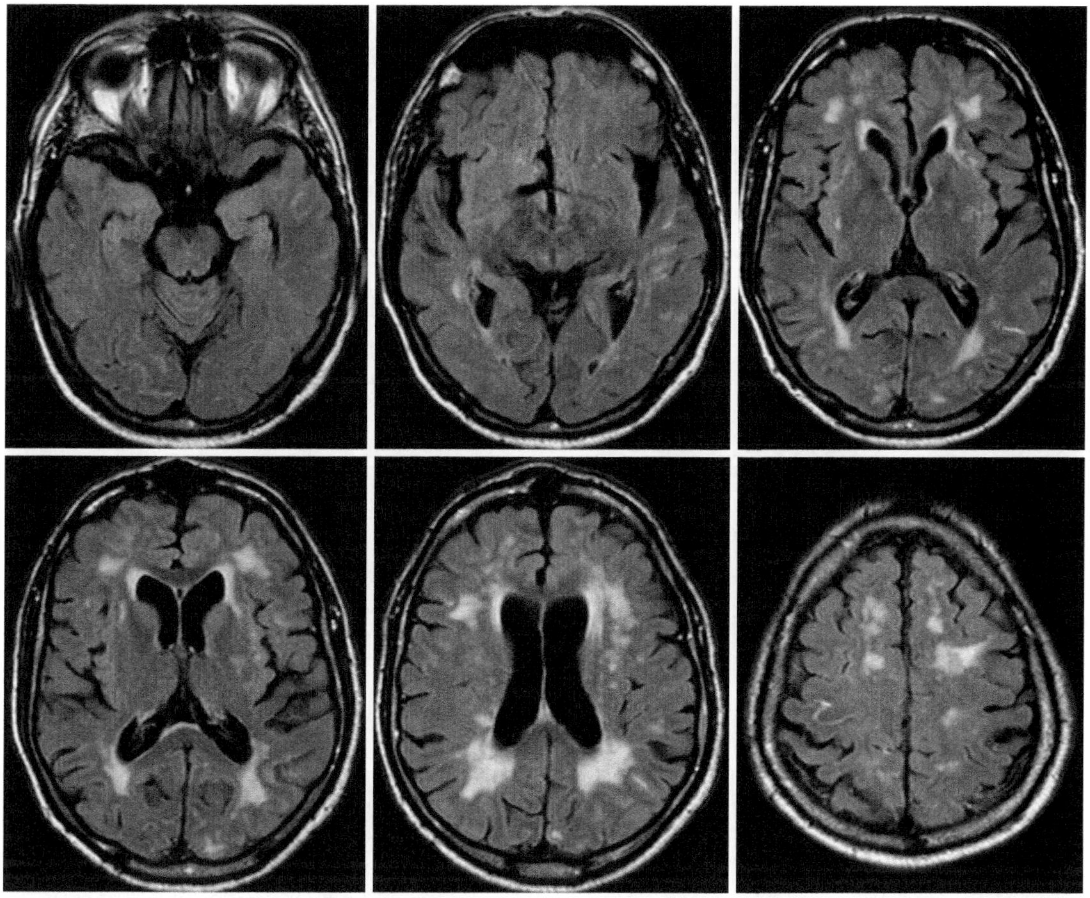

Fig. 7.4 In a patient with mixed CAA/AD, axial FLAIR slices show multifocal leptomeningeal hyperintensities in the right occipital, left temporal, and right frontal lobes, and white matter hyperintensities in the left parietal lobe, as for ARIA-E

scheme for ARIA in patients receiving Aβ-targeting therapy includes

1. Initial Detection:
   - Conduct a thorough clinical evaluation.
   - Assess MRI findings to confirm ARIA and rule out other potential causes.
2. Symptomatic versus Asymptomatic ARIA:
   - Asymptomatic ARIA:
     - Monitor with regular follow-up MRIs.
     - Consider pausing treatment if multiple or severe lesions are detected.
   - Symptomatic ARIA:
     - Temporarily discontinue treatment.
     - Consider corticosteroid therapy (e.g., IV methylprednisolone) if symptoms are severe or persistent.
3. Long-Term Management:
   - Resume treatment cautiously after symptoms and MRI findings resolve.
   - Adjust the dosage or switch to an alternative therapy if recurrent ARIA occurs.
   - Ensure consistent MRI protocols to facilitate reliable temporal comparisons and accurate assessment of ARIA progression or resolution.

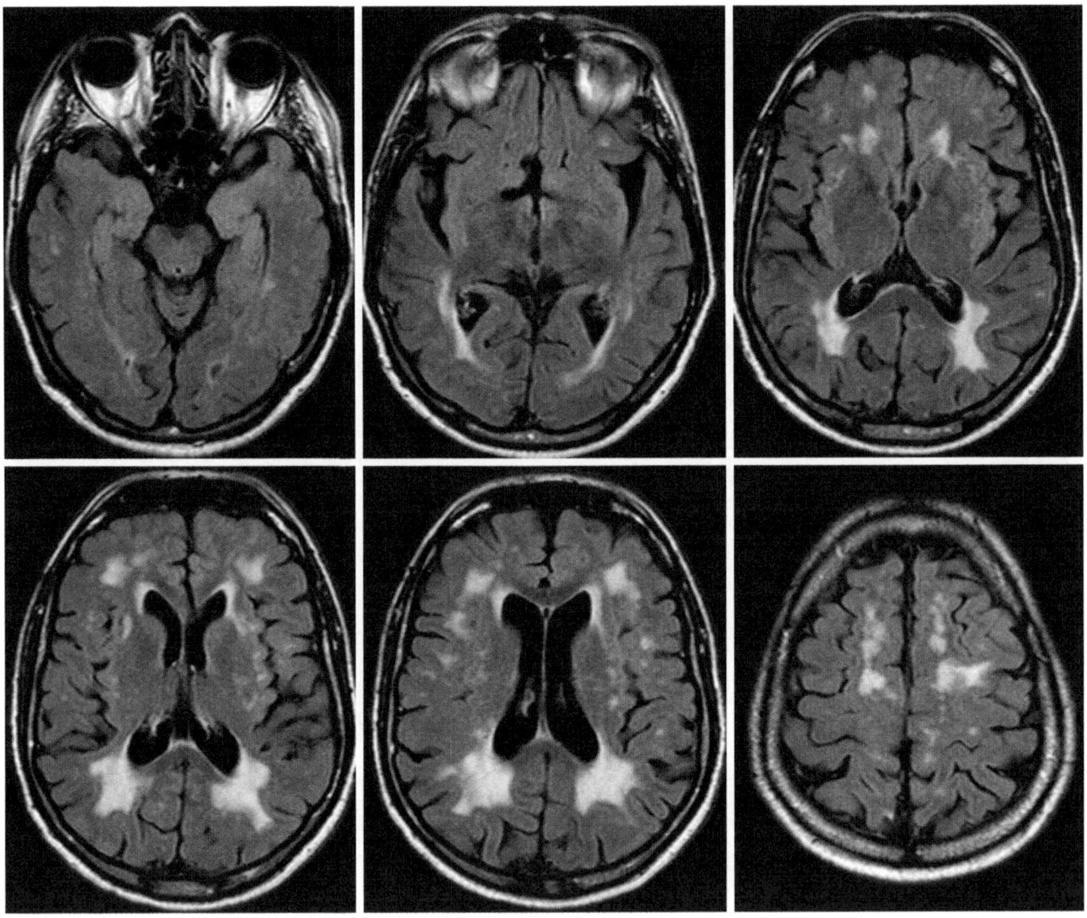

Fig. 7.5 In the same patients as in Fig. 7.4, the three-month control MRI shows resolution of the previously documented leptomeningeal hyperintensities

Managing ARIA requires careful monitoring, prompt evaluation, and appropriate treatment adjustments based on both imaging findings and clinical symptoms. Standardized follow-up protocols and a clear management strategy are essential to ensuring patient safety and optimizing therapeutic outcomes for those undergoing Aβ-targeting therapy.

In the EMERGE (ClinicalTrials.gov NCT02484547) [54] and ENGAGE (ClinicalTrials.gov NCT02477800) [55] phase 3 trials of aducanumab, treatment continued for patients with ARIA if they were asymptomatic and exhibited mild MRI findings of ARIA-E or ARIA-H. In cases of moderate ARIA-E or ARIA-H, therapy was paused and could only resume once there was either resolution of ARIA-E or stabilization of ARIA-H. For patients with severe ARIA-H, treatment was permanently discontinued. Conversely, the FDA's prescribing guidelines for aducanumab state that treatment can cautiously continue for patients with any

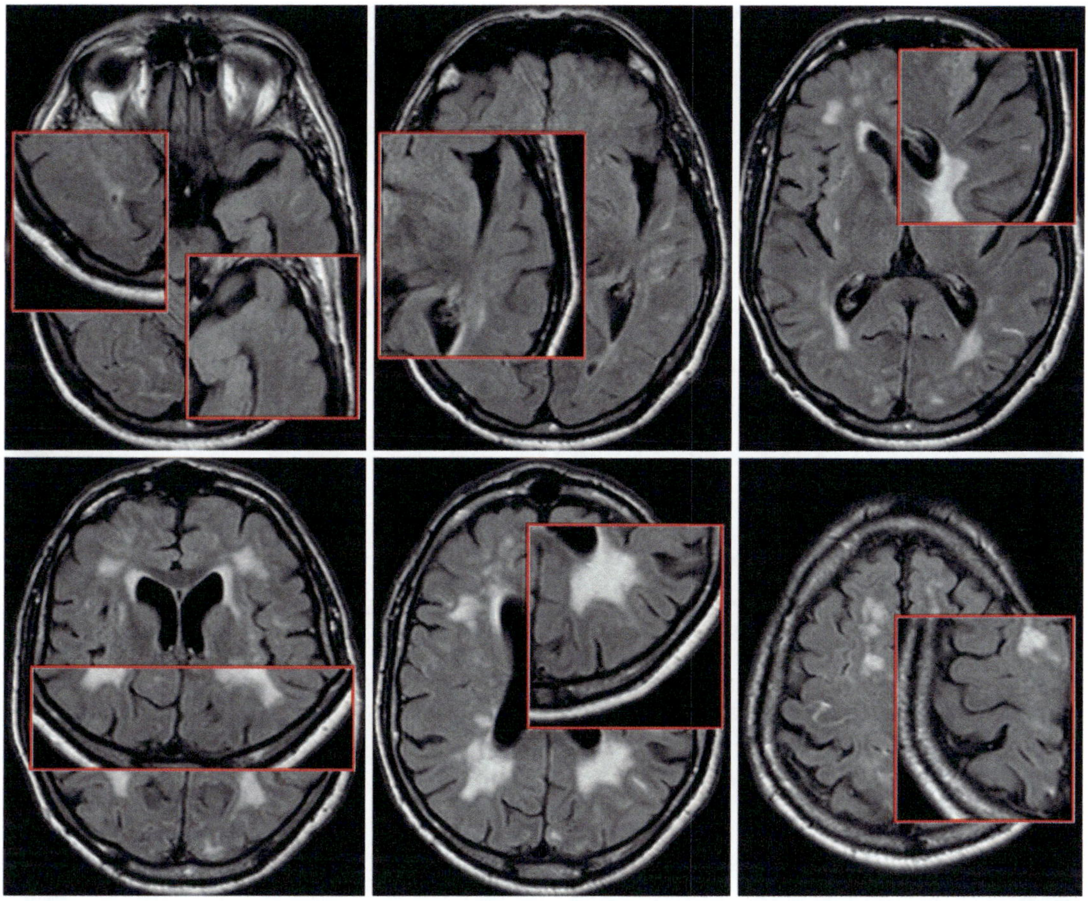

Fig. 7.6 In the same patient as in Figs. 7.4 and 7.5, basal con control (red squares) FLAIR MRI summarized the acute phase of ARIA-E, and its resolution in several brain sites

severity of ARIA-E and for those with mild or moderate ARIA-H. Additionally, if a follow-up MRI shows stable findings in patients with severe ARIA-H, treatment may also continue [77].

The FDA's prescribing information outlines management protocols for aducanumab, emphasizing patient selection and monitoring for ARIA [77]. An expert panel [79, 80] has also provided recommendations for optimal use. As aducanumab was approved via the accelerated approval pathway, a phase 4 post-approval study demonstrating real-world efficacy is required by August 2029, with data submission due by February 2030. In the meanwhile, Aducanumab had been retired and FDA approved both lecanemab and donanemab [79–82].

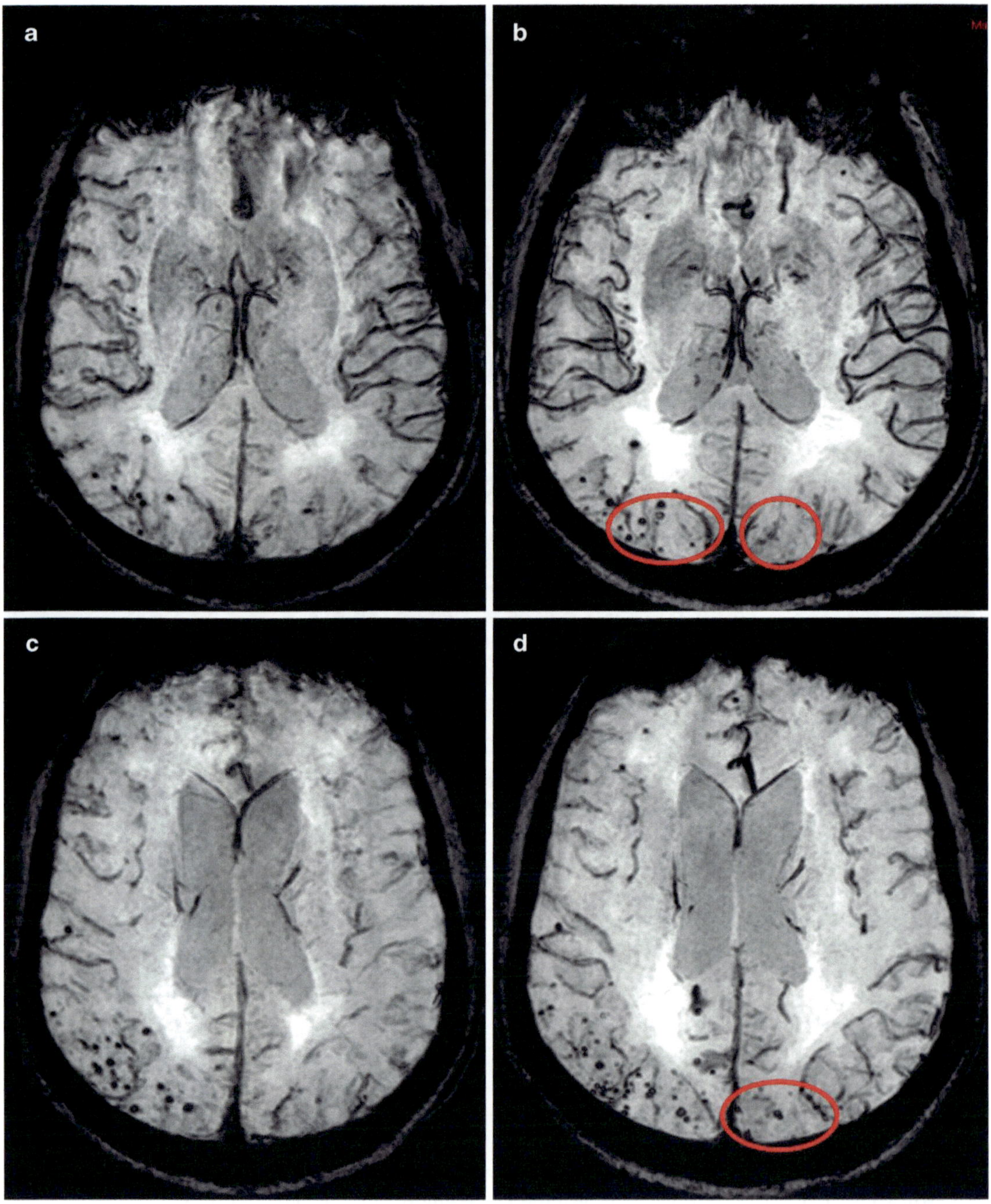

Fig. 7.7 In the same patient as in Figs. 7.4, 7.5, and 7.6, basal (panel **a**) and control (panel **b**) SWI show the increase in ARIA-H in the left parietal lobe (red circle) after ARIA-E resolution

7.5 Conclusions

The increasing implementation of disease-modifying Alzheimer's therapies will result in a larger patient population affected by this condition. Them, it is essential for both neuroradiologists and neurologists to be aware of clinical and imaging features of ARIA, CAA, and CAA-ri and the classification systems for ARIA-E and ARIA-H.

References

1. Corriveau RA, et al. The science of vascular contributions to cognitive impairment and dementia (VCID): a framework for advancing research priorities in the cerebrovascular biology of cognitive decline. Cell Mol Neurobiol. 2016;36:281–8. https://doi.org/10.1007/s10571-016-0334-7.
2. Boyle PA, et al. Person-specific contribution of neuropathologies to cognitive loss in old age. Ann Neurol. 2018;83:74–83. https://doi.org/10.1002/ana.25123.
3. Satizabal CL, et al. Incidence of dementia over three decades in the Framingham heart study. N Engl J Med. 2016;374:523–32. https://doi.org/10.1056/NEJMoa1504327.
4. Greenberg SM, Bacskai BJ, Hernandez-Guillamon M, Pruzin J, Sperling R, van Veluw SJ. Cerebral amyloid angiopathy and Alzheimer disease – one peptide, two pathways. Nat Rev Neurol. 2020;16:30–42. https://doi.org/10.1038/s41582-019-0281-2.
5. Arvanitakis Z, et al. Cerebral amyloid angiopathy pathology and cognitive domains in older persons. Ann Neurol. 2011;69:320–7. https://doi.org/10.1002/ana.22112.
6. Brenowitz WD, Nelson PT, Besser LM, Heller KB, Kukull WA. Cerebral amyloid angiopathy and its co-occurrence with Alzheimer's disease and other cerebrovascular neuropathologic changes. Neurobiol Ageing. 2015;36:2702–8. https://doi.org/10.1016/j.neurobiolaging.2015.06.028.
7. De Strooper B, Karran E. The cellular phase of Alzheimer's disease. Cell. 2016;164:603–15. https://doi.org/10.1016/j.cell.2015.12.056.
8. Sperling RA, et al. The impact of amyloid- beta and tau on prospective cognitive decline in older individuals. Ann Neurol. 2019;85:181–93. https://doi.org/10.1002/ana.25395.
9. van Veluw SJ, et al. Histopathology of diffusion imaging abnormalities in cerebral amyloid angiopathy. Neurology. 2019;92:e933–43. https://doi.org/10.1212/WNL.0000000000007005.
10. van Veluw SJ, et al. Detection, risk factors, and functional consequences of cerebral microinfarcts. Lancet Neurol. 2017;16:730–40. https://doi.org/10.1016/S1474-4422(17)30196-5.
11. Sperling RA, et al. Amyloid- related imaging abnormalities in amyloid- modifying therapeutic trials: recommendations from the Alzheimer's association research roundtable workgroup. Alzheimers Dement. 2011;7:367–85. https://doi.org/10.1016/j.jalz.2011.05.2351.
12. Salloway S, et al. Two phase 3 trials of bapineuzumab in mild- to-moderate Alzheimer's disease. New Engl J Med. 2014;370:322–33. https://doi.org/10.1056/NEJMoa1304839.
13. Ostrowitzki S, et al. A phase III randomized trial of gantenerumab in prodromal Alzheimer's disease. Alzheimer's Res Ther. 2017;9:95. https://doi.org/10.1186/s13195-017-0318-y.
14. Sevigny J, et al. The antibody aducanumab reduces aβ plaques in Alzheimer's disease. Nature. 2016;537:50–6. https://doi.org/10.1038/nature19323.
15. Carlson C, et al. Amyloid-related imaging abnormalities from trials of solanezumab for Alzheimer's disease. Alzheimers Dement (Amst). 2016;2:75–85. https://doi.org/10.1016/j.dadm.2016.02.004.
16. Cummings JL, et al. ABBY: a phase 2 randomized trial of crenezumab in mild to moderate Alzheimer disease. Neurology. 2018;90:e1889–97. https://doi.org/10.1212/WNL.0000000000005550.
17. Leurent C, et al. Immunotherapy with ponezumab for probable cerebral amyloid angiopathy. Ann Clin Transl Neurol. 2019;6:795–806. https://doi.org/10.1002/acn3.761.
18. Ultsch M, et al. Structure of crenezumab complex with aβ shows loss of β-hairpin. Sci Rep. 2016;6:39374. https://doi.org/10.1038/srep39374.
19. Raman MR, et al. Spontaneous amyloid-related imaging abnormalities in a cognitively normal adult. Neurology. 2014;83:1771–2. https://doi.org/10.1212/WNL.0000000000000957.
20. Ryan NS, et al. Spontaneous ARIA (amyloid-related imaging abnormalities) and cerebral amyloid angiopathy related inflammation in presenilin 1-associated familial Alzheimer's disease. J Alzheimer's Dis. 2015;44:1069–74. https://doi.org/10.3233/JAD-142325.
21. Ketter N, et al. Central review of amyloid-related imaging abnormalities in two phase III clinical trials of bapineuzumab in mild-to-moderate Alzheimer's disease patients. J Alzheimer's Dis. 2017;57:557–73. https://doi.org/10.3233/JAD-160216.
22. Penninkilampi R, Brothers HM, Eslick GD. Safety and efficacy of anti-amyloid-β immunotherapy in Alzheimer's disease: a systematic review and meta-analysis. J Neuroimmune Pharmacol. 2017;12:194–203. https://doi.org/10.1007/s11481-016-9722-5.
23. Haeberlein SB, et al. 24-month analysis of change from baseline in clinical dementia rating scale cognitive and functional domains in PRIME: a randomized phase 1b study of the anti-amyloid beta monoclonal antibody aducanumab [abstract O1-09-06]. Alzheimers Dement. 2018;14(Suppl. 7):P242.
24. Goos JD, et al. Incidence of cerebral microbleeds: a longitudinal study in a memory clinic popula-

tion. Neurology. 2010;74:1954–60. https://doi.org/10.1212/WNL.0b013e3181e396ea.
25. Sperling R, et al. Amyloid-related imaging abnormalities in patients with Alzheimer disease treated with bapineuzumab: a retrospective analysis. Lancet Neurol. 2012;11:241–9. https://doi.org/10.1016/S1474-4422(12)70015-7.
26. Arrighi HM, et al. Amyloid-related imaging abnormalities-haemosiderin (ARIA-H) in patients with Alzheimer's disease treated with bapineuzumab: a historical, prospective secondary analysis. J Neurol Neurosurg Psychiatry. 2016;87:106–12. https://doi.org/10.1136/jnnp-2014-309493.
27. Liu E, et al. Biomarker pattern of ARIA-E participants in phase 3 randomized clinical trials with bapineuzumab. Neurology. 2018;90:e877–86. https://doi.org/10.1212/WNL.0000000000005060.
28. Brashear HR, et al. Clinical evaluation of amyloid-related imaging abnormalities in bapineuzumab phase III studies. J Alzheimer's Dis. 2018;66:1409–24. https://doi.org/10.3233/JAD-180675.
29. Boche D, Denham N, Holmes C, Nicoll JA. Neuropathology after active Abeta42 immunotherapy: implications for Alzheimer's disease pathogenesis. Acta Neuropathol. 2010;120:369–84. https://doi.org/10.1007/s00401-010-0719-5.
30. Sakai K, et al. Aβ immunotherapy for Alzheimer's disease: effects on apoE and cerebral vasculopathy. Acta Neuropathol. 2014;128:777–89. https://doi.org/10.1007/s00401-014-1340-9.
31. Mandybur TI. Cerebral amyloid angiopathy: the vascular pathology and complications. J Neuropathol Exp Neurol. 1986;45:79–90.
32. Antolini L, DiFrancesco JC, Zedde M, Basso G, Arighi A, Shima A, Cagnin A, Caulo M, Carare RO, Charidimou A, Cirillo M, Di Lazzaro V, Ferrarese C, Giossi A, Inzitari D, Marcon M, Marconi R, Ihara M, Nitrini R, Orlandi B, Padovani A, Pascarella R, Perini F, Perini G, Sessa M, Scarpini E, Tagliavini F, Valenti R, Vázquez-Costa JF, Villarejo-Galende A, Hagiwara Y, Ziliotto N, Piazza F. Spontaneous ARIA-like events in cerebral amyloid Angiopathy-related inflammation: a multicenter prospective longitudinal cohort study. Neurology. 2021;97(18):e1809–22. https://doi.org/10.1212/WNL.0000000000012778.
33. Zedde M, Napoli M, Moratti C, Pavone C, Bonacini L, Di Cecco G, D'Aniello S, Grisendi I, Assenza F, Boulouis G, Nguyen TN, Valzania F, Pascarella R. Tumor-like lesions in primary Angiitis of the central nervous system: the role of magnetic resonance imaging in differential diagnosis. Diagnostics (Basel). 2024;14(6):618. https://doi.org/10.3390/diagnostics14060618.
34. Auriel E, Charidimou A, Gurol ME, Ni J, Van Etten ES, Martinez-Ramirez S, Boulouis G, Piazza F, DiFrancesco JC, Frosch MP, Pontes-Neto OV, Shoamanesh A, Reijmer Y, Vashkevich A, Ayres AM, Schwab KM, Viswanathan A, Greenberg SM. Validation of Clinicoradiological criteria for the diagnosis of cerebral amyloid Angiopathy-related inflammation. JAMA Neurol. 2016 Feb;73(2):197–202. https://doi.org/10.1001/jamaneurol.2015.4078.
35. Piazza F, Caminiti SP, Zedde M, Presotto L, DiFrancesco JC, Pascarella R, Giossi A, Sessa M, Poli L, Basso G, Perani D. Association of microglial activation with spontaneous ARIA-E and CSF levels of anti-aβ autoantibodies. Neurology. 2022;99(12):e1265–77. https://doi.org/10.1212/WNL.0000000000200892.
36. Piazza F, Greenberg SM, Savoiardo M, Gardinetti M, Chiapparini L, Raicher I, Nitrini R, Sakaguchi H, Brioschi M, Billo G, Colombo A, Lanzani F, Piscosquito G, Carriero MR, Giaccone G, Tagliavini F, Ferrarese C, DiFrancesco JC. Anti-amyloid β autoantibodies in cerebral amyloid angiopathy-related inflammation: implications for amyloid-modifying therapies. Ann Neurol. 2013 Apr;73(4):449–58. https://doi.org/10.1002/ana.23857.
37. DiFrancesco JC, Longoni M, Piazza F. Anti-aβ autoantibodies in amyloid related imaging abnormalities (ARIA): candidate biomarker for immunotherapy in Alzheimer's disease and cerebral amyloid angiopathy. Front Neurol. 2015 Sep;25(6):207. https://doi.org/10.3389/fneur.2015.00207.
38. Carmona-Iragui M, Fernández-Arcos A, Alcolea D, Piazza F, Morenas-Rodriguez E, Antón-Aguirre S, Sala I, Clarimon J, Dols-Icardo O, Camacho V, Sampedro F, Munuera J, Nuñez-Marin F, Lleó A, Fortea J, Gómez-Ansón B, Blesa R. Cerebrospinal fluid anti-amyloid-β autoantibodies and amyloid PET in cerebral amyloid Angiopathy-related inflammation. J Alzheimer's Dis. 2016;50(1):1–7. https://doi.org/10.3233/JAD-150614.
39. Zago W, et al. Vascular alterations in PDAPP mice after anti-aβ immunotherapy: implications for amyloid-related imaging abnormalities. Alzheimers Dement. 2013;9:S105–15. https://doi.org/10.1016/j.jalz.2012.11.010.
40. van Dyck CH. Anti-amyloid-β monoclonal antibodies for Alzheimer's disease: pitfalls and promise. Biol Psychiatry. 2018;83:311–9. https://doi.org/10.1016/j.biopsych.2017.08.010.
41. Cummings J, Lee G, Zhong K, Fonseca J, Taghva K. Alzheimer's disease drug development pipeline: 2021. Alzheimers Dement (N Y). 2021;7:e12179. https://doi.org/10.1002/trc2.12179.
42. Jeremic D, Jiménez-Díaz L, Navarro-López JD. Past, present and future of therapeutic strategies against amyloid-β peptides in Alzheimer's disease: a systematic review. Ageing Res Rev. 2021;72:101496. https://doi.org/10.1016/j.arr.2021.101496.
43. Tolar M, Abushakra S, Hey JA, Porsteinsson AM. Aducanumab, gantenerumab, BAN2401, and ALZ-801-the first wave of amyloid-targeting drugs for Alzheimer's disease with potential for near term approval. Alzheimer's Res Ther. 2020;12:95. https://doi.org/10.1186/s13195-020-00663-w.
44. Cogswell PM, Barakos JA, Barkhof F, et al. Amyloid-related imaging abnormalities with emerging

Alzheimer disease therapeutics: detection and reporting recommendations for clinical practice. AJNR. 2022;43:E19–35. https://doi.org/10.3174/ajnr.A7586.
45. Zedde M, Losa M, Donniaquio A, Gandoglia I, Sette, MD, Roccatagliata L, Piazza F, Pardini M, Pascarella R. Drug-Induced Amyloid-Related Imaging Abnormalities: A Neurovascular Perspective on Risk Assessment. Pharmaceuticals 2026;19:579. https://doi.org/10.3390/ph19040579
46. Zedde M, Losa M, Grisafi E, Lucia DD, Gandoglia I, Del Sette M, Pardini M, Roccatagliata L, Pascarella R, Piazza F. Spontaneous and Drug-Induced Amyloid-Related Imaging Abnormalities: Overlaps, Divergences, and Clinical Implications Across a Continuum Between Alzheimer's Disease and Cerebral Amyloid Angiopathy. Biomolecules. 2026;5:16(1):89. https://doi.org/10.3390/biom16010089
47. Doody RS, Thomas RG, Farlow M, et al. Phase 3 trials of solanezumab for mild-to-moderate Alzheimer's disease. N Engl J Med. 2014;370:311–21. https://doi.org/10.1056/NEJMoa1312889.
48. Guthrie H, Honig LS, Lin H, et al. Safety, tolerability, and pharmacokinetics of crenezumab in patients with mild-to-moderate Alzheimer's disease treated with escalating doses for up to 133 weeks. J Alzheimer's Dis. 2020;76:967–79. https://doi.org/10.3233/JAD-200134.
49. Landen JW, Cohen S, Billing CB Jr, et al. Multiple-dose ponezumab for mild-to-moderate Alzheimer's disease: safety and efficacy. Alzheimers Dement (N Y). 2017;3:339–47. https://doi.org/10.1016/j.trci.2017.04.003.
50. Swanson CJ, Zhang Y, Dhadda S, et al. A randomized, double-blind, phase 2b proof-of-concept clinical trial in early Alzheimer's disease with lecanemab, an anti-aβ protofibril antibody. Alzheimer's Res Ther. 2021;13:80. https://doi.org/10.1186/s13195-021-00813-8.
51. Mintun MA, Lo AC, Duggan Evans C, et al. Donanemab in early Alzheimer's disease. N Engl J Med. 2021;384:1691–704. https://doi.org/10.1056/NEJMoa2100708.
52. Haeberlein SB, Aisen PS, Barkhof F, et al. Two randomized phase 3 studies of aducanumab in early Alzheimer's disease. J Prev Alzheimers Dis. 2022;9:197–210. https://doi.org/10.14283/jpad.2022.30.
53. Barakos J, Purcell D, Suhy J, Chalkias S, Burkett P, Marsica Grassi C, Castrillo-Viguera C, Rubino I, Vijverberg E. Detection and management of amyloid-related imaging abnormalities in patients with Alzheimer's disease treated with anti-amyloid Beta therapy. J Prev Alzheimers Dis. 2022;9(2):211–20. https://doi.org/10.14283/jpad.2022.21.
54. ClinicalTrials.gov. Bethesda (MD): National Library of Medicine (US). February 29, 2000. Identifier NCT02484547, 221AD302 Phase 3 study of aducanumab (BIIB037) in early Alzheimer's disease (EMERGE). https://clinicaltrials.gov/study/NCT02484547?term=EMERGE&intr=Aducanumab. Accessed 1 June 2023.
55. ClinicalTrials.gov. Bethesda (MD): National Library of Medicine (US). February 29, 2000. Identifier NCT02477800, 221AD301 Phase 3 study of aducanumab (BIIB037) in early Alzheimer's disease (ENGAGE). https://clinicaltrials.gov/study/NCT02477800?term=ENGAGE&intr=Aducanumab. Accessed 1 June 2023.
56. Loomis SJ, Miller R, Castrillo-Viguera C, Umans K, Cheng W, O'Gorman J, Hughes R, Budd Haeberlein S, Whelan CD. Genome-wide association studies of ARIA from the Aducanumab phase 3 ENGAGE and EMERGE studies. Neurology. 2024;102(3):e207919. https://doi.org/10.1212/WNL.0000000000207919.
57. Jeong SY, Suh CH, Shim WH, Lim JS, Lee JH, Kim SJ. Incidence of amyloid-related imaging abnormalities in patients with Alzheimer disease treated with anti-β-amyloid immunotherapy: a meta-analysis. Neurology. 2022;99(19):e2092–101. https://doi.org/10.1212/WNL.0000000000201019.
58. Honig LS, Barakos J, Dhadda S, Kanekiyo M, Reyderman L, Irizarry M, Kramer LD, Swanson CJ, Sabbagh M. ARIA in patients treated with lecanemab (BAN2401) in a phase 2 study in early Alzheimer's disease. Alzheimers Dement (N Y). 2023;9(1):e12377. https://doi.org/10.1002/trc2.12377.
59. Barakos J, Sperling R, Salloway S, Jack C, Gass A, Fiebach JB, Tampieri D, Melançon D, Miaux Y, Rippon G, Black R, Lu Y, Brashear HR, Arrighi HM, Morris KA, Grundman M. MR imaging features of amyloid-related imaging abnormalities. AJNR Am J Neuroradiol. 2013;34(10):1958–65. https://doi.org/10.3174/ajnr.A3500.
60. Roytman M, Mashriqi F, Al-Tawil K, Schulz PE, Zaharchuk G, Benzinger TLS, Franceschi AM. Amyloid-related imaging abnormalities: an update. AJR Am J Roentgenol. 2023;220(4):562–74. https://doi.org/10.2214/AJR.22.28461.
61. Salloway S, Chalkias S, Barkhof F, Burkett P, Barakos J, Purcell D, Suhy J, Forrestal F, Tian Y, Umans K, Wang G, Singhal P, Budd Haeberlein S, Smirnakis K. Amyloid-related imaging abnormalities in 2 phase 3 studies evaluating Aducanumab in patients with early Alzheimer disease. JAMA Neurol. 2022;79(1):13–21. https://doi.org/10.1001/jamaneurol.2021.4161.
62. Sotoudeh H, Alizadeh M, Shahidi R, Shobeiri P, Saadatpour Z, Wheeler CA, Natelson Love M, Tanwar M. Imaging spectrum of amyloid-related imaging abnormalities associated with aducanumab immunotherapy. Front Radiol. 2024;3:1305390. https://doi.org/10.3389/fradi.2023.1305390.
63. Kallmes DF, Hui FK, Mugler JP 3rd. Suppression of cerebrospinal fluid and blood flow artifacts in FLAIR MR imaging with a single-slab three-dimensional pulse sequence: initial experience. Radiology. 2001;221:251–5. https://doi.org/10.1148/radiol.2211001712.

64. Amin M, Aboseif A, Southard K, Uchino K, Kiczek M, Hajj-Ali R, Kharal GA. The prevalence of radiological cerebral amyloid angiopathy-related inflammation in patients with cerebral amyloid angiopathy. J Stroke Cerebrovasc Dis. 2023;32(12):107436. https://doi.org/10.1016/j.jstrokecerebrovasdis.2023.107436.
65. Charidimou A, Boulouis G, Frosch MP, Baron JC, Pasi M, Albucher JF, Banerjee G, Barbato C, Bonneville F, Brandner S, Calviere L, Caparros F, Casolla B, Cordonnier C, Delisle MB, Deramecourt V, Dichgans M, Gokcal E, Herms J, Hernandez-Guillamon M, Jäger HR, Jaunmuktane Z, Linn J, Martinez-Ramirez S, Martínez-Sáez E, Mawrin C, Montaner J, Moulin S, Olivot JM, Piazza F, Puy L, Raposo N, Rodrigues MA, Roeber S, Romero JR, Samarasekera N, Schneider JA, Schreiber S, Schreiber F, Schwall C, Smith C, Szalardy L, Varlet P, Viguier A, Wardlaw JM, Warren A, Wollenweber FA, Zedde M, van Buchem MA, Gurol ME, Viswanathan A, Al-Shahi Salman R, Smith EE, Werring DJ, Greenberg SM. The Boston criteria version 2.0 for cerebral amyloid angiopathy: a multicentre, retrospective, MRI-neuropathology diagnostic accuracy study. Lancet Neurol. 2022;21(8):714–25. https://doi.org/10.1016/S1474-4422(22)00208-3.
66. Gregoire SM, Brown MM, Kallis C, Jäger HR, Yousry TA, Werring DJ. MRI detection of new microbleeds in patients with ischemic stroke: five-year cohort follow-up study. Stroke. 2010;41:184–6. https://doi.org/10.1161/STROKEAHA.109.568469.
67. Haller S, Vernooij MW, Kuijer JPA, Larsson E-M, Jäger HR, Barkhof F. Cerebral microbleeds: imaging and clinical significance. Radiology. 2018;287:11–28. https://doi.org/10.1148/radiol.2018170803.
68. Hodel J, Rodallec M, Gerber S, et al. Susceptibility weighted magnetic resonance sequences "SWAN, SWI and VenoBOLD": technical aspects and clinical applications [in French]. J Neuroradiol. 2012;39:71–86. https://doi.org/10.1016/j.neurad.2011.11.006.
69. Docampo J, Gonzalez N, Bravo F, Sarroca D, Morales C, Bruno C. Susceptibility-weighted angiography of intracranial blood products and calcifications compared to gradient echo sequence. Neuroradiol J. 2013;26:493–500. https://doi.org/10.1177/197140091302600501.
70. Haller S, Haacke EM, Thurnher MM, Barkhof F. Susceptibility-weighted imaging: technical essentials and clinical neurologic applications. Radiology. 2021;299:3–26. https://doi.org/10.1148/radiol.2021203071.
71. Haacke EM, Liu S, Buch S, Zheng W, Wu D, Ye Y. Quantitative susceptibility mapping: current status and future directions. Magn Reson Imaging. 2015;33:1–25. https://doi.org/10.1016/j.mri.2014.09.004.
72. Ruetten PPR, Gillard JH, Graves MJ. Introduction to quantitative susceptibility mapping and susceptibility weighted imaging. Br J Radiol. 2019;92:20181016. https://doi.org/10.1259/bjr.20181016.
73. Ferrero J, Williams L, Stella H, et al. First-in-human, double-blind, placebo-controlled, single-dose escalation study of aducanumab (BIIB037) in mild-to-moderate Alzheimer's disease. Alzheimers Dement (N Y). 2016;2:169–76. https://doi.org/10.1016/j.trci.2016.06.002.
74. Sima DM, Phan TV, Van Eyndhoven S, Vercruyssen S, Magalhães R, Liseune A, Brys A, Frenyo P, Terzopoulos V, Maes C, Guo J, Hughes R, Gabr RE, Huijbers W, Saha-Chaudhuri P, Curiale GG, Becker A, Belachew S, Van Hecke W, Ribbens A, Smeets D. Artificial intelligence assistive software tool for automated detection and quantification of amyloid-related imaging abnormalities. JAMA Netw Open. 2024;7(2):e2355800. https://doi.org/10.1001/jamanetworkopen.2023.55800.
75. Barkhof F, Daams M, Scheltens P, et al. An MRI rating scale for amyloid-related imaging abnormalities with edema or effusion. AJNR. 2013;34:1550–5. https://doi.org/10.3174/ajnr.A3475.
76. Bechten A, Wattjes MP, Purcell DD, et al. Validation of an MRI rating scale for amyloid-related imaging abnormalities. J Neuroimaging. 2017;27:318–25. https://doi.org/10.1111/jon.12422.
77. U.S. FDA website. Highlights of prescribing information ADUHELM (aducanumab-avwa) injection, for intravenous use. www.accessdata.fda.gov/drugsatfda_docs/label/2021/761178s000lbl.pdf.
78. Bracoud L, Klein G, Lyons M, Scelsi MA, Wojtowicz J, Bullain S, Purcell D, Fiebach JB, Barakos J, Suhy J. Validation of 3- and 5-point severity scales to assess ARIA-E. Alzheimers Dement (Amst). 2023;15(4):e12503. https://doi.org/10.1002/dad2.12503. Erratum in: Alzheimers Dement (Amst) 31 Jan 2024;16(1):e12546. doi:10.1002/dad2.12546.
79. Cummings J, Aisen P, Apostolova LG, Atri A, Salloway S, Weiner M. Aducanumab: appropriate use recommendations. J Prev Alzheimers Dis. 2021;8:398–410. https://doi.org/10.14283/jpad.2021.41.
80. Cummings J, Rabinovici GD, Atri A, et al. Aducanumab: appropriate use recommendations update. J Prev Alzheimers Dis. 2022;9:221–30. https://doi.org/10.14283/jpad.2022.34.
81. https://www.accessdata.fda.gov/drugsatfda_docs/label/2023/761269Orig1s001lbl.pdf
82. https://www.accessdata.fda.gov/drugsatfda_docs/label/2025/761248s004lbl.pdf

8 Posterior Reversible Encephalopathy Syndrome: Clinical and Neuroimaging Clues in Drug-Triggered Cases

Sara Botelho Rosa and Diana Aguiar de Sousa

8.1 Definition

Posterior reversible encephalopathy syndrome (PRES) consists of a broad spectrum of clinical and radiological changes [1] caused by endothelial dysfunction leading to disruption of the blood-brain barrier (BBB) and vasogenic edema [2]. Despite its name, although posterior brain lesions are more common, abnormalities are not usually limited to these regions [3, 4]. Also, albeit rare, lesions are not always completely reversible [3]. Thus, the name does not accurately describe the syndrome.

8.2 Etiopathogenesis

In order to maintain normal brain function, it is determinant that cerebral blood flow (CBF) does not fluctuate with changes in arterial blood pressure [5]. In physiological conditions, within the normal range of 60–150 mmHg of mean arterial pressure [6], a complex interplay between cells of the neurovascular unit (neurons, glial cells, endothelial cells, and other vessel wall components) allows for the tight regulation of CBF [7]. This is attained by reactive vasodilation of cerebral arteries when blood pressure decreases and vasoconstriction when the opposite occurs, a mechanism referred to as "cerebral autoregulation" [2]. When these mechanisms fail, regardless of the cause, there is a common final cascade of events that culminates in BBB disruption, vasogenic edema, and paradoxical hypoperfusion [8].

Regarding the mechanisms that lead to this common pathway, two principal theories have been put forward:

- "Vasogenic" or "Hyperperfusion" theory (classic theory), which proposes that a severe and rapid increase in arterial blood pressure (above the physiological threshold for that particular individual) results in mechanical damage to endothelial cells, with vascular leakage and loss of adaptive ability to changes in blood pressure [8, 9]. This hypothesis is supported by the observation that about 70% of patients with PRES initially present with hypertension [3, 10, 11]. Traditionally, it has been suggested that the posterior cerebral circulation has a lower density of sympathetic innervation, which could limit vasoconstriction in response to increases in blood pressure and therefore increase this region's susceptibility to damage in this context [2]. Additionally, this mechanism could help explain why PRES occurs in 9–38% of reversible cerebral vasoconstriction syndrome (RCVS)

S. Botelho Rosa
Neuroradiology Department, Lisbon Central University Hospital—ULS S José, Lisbon, Portugal
e-mail: sararosa@campus.ul.pt

D. Aguiar de Sousa (✉)
Stroke Center, Lisbon Central University Hospital—ULS S José, Lisbon, Portugal

Faculdade de Medicina, Universidade de Lisboa, Lisbon, Portugal
e-mail: dianasousa@campus.ul.pt

M. Zedde, R. Pascarella (eds.), *Neuroimaging of Treatment-Related Conditions in the Brain*,
https://doi.org/10.1007/978-3-032-23618-0_8

cases [12–15]. The focal vasoconstriction of cerebral arteries seen in RCVS may lead to a local increase in hydrostatic pressure and subsequent endothelial damage, similar to what is seen globally in cases of hypertension. However, given that common triggers are shared between the two diseases, it is difficult to pinpoint whether one causes the other or if they occur simultaneously in the presence of the same trigger [16].
- "Cytotoxic" theory proposes that the triggers of endothelial dysfunction are endogenous or exogenous toxins that damage the endothelial lining [8, 17]. This would justify the variety of conditions and medications that have been associated with the syndrome [18]. A derivation of this hypothesis that elucidates cases of PRES in patients with sepsis or autoimmune diseases is that excessive release of inflammatory cytokines triggers endothelial activation [9, 19, 20]. This activation subsequently leads to release of vasoactive substances, thus resulting in BBB disruption [9, 19, 20].

In most cases, there probably are concurring factors leading to the common pathway of BBB disruption, and a combination of pathophysiological mechanisms likely better explains the disease [18, 20] (Fig. 8.1).

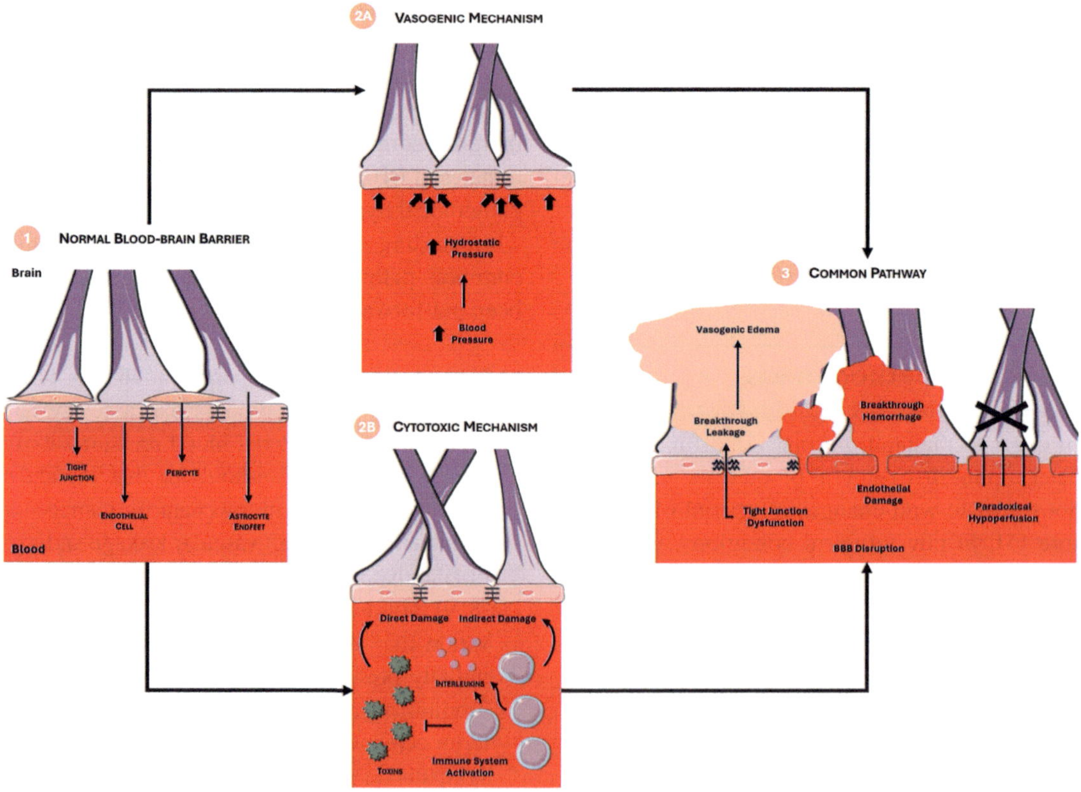

Fig. 8.1 PRES Etiopathogenesis. (1) In physiologic conditions, the BBB protects brain tissue from endogenous and exogenous insults [7]. The BBB is composed of endothelial cells (ECs), pericytes, and astrocyte endfeet [7]. (2A) The "vasogenic" hypothesis states that rapid increases in blood pressure above the physiological threshold for cerebral autoregulation result in increased capillary hydrostatic pressure and subsequent damage to endothelial tight junctions, as well as endothelial cells [8, 9]. (2B) An alternative theory, the "cytotoxic" hypothesis, proposes that endogenous or exogenous toxins may cause direct and indirect damage to the endothelial lining [8, 17]. In some cases, immune system activation seems to play an important role, mainly due to endothelial activation in response to cytokine release [9, 19, 20]. (3) Regardless of the trigger, these changes result in a common pathway of BBB disruption with consequent breakthrough leakage and vasogenic edema [18, 20]. With disease progression, brain hemorrhage and paradoxical hypoperfusion may ensue [18, 20]

8.3 Etiology

The etiopathogenesis and etiologies of PRES are not well established, but a wide variety of conditions and medications have been associated with disease onset [10, 18, 20, 21].

The most recognized etiology is hypertension [18, 20, 22]. However, about 30% of patients are normotensive or even hypotensive [3, 10, 11]. Other etiologies can be grouped in the following categories: cytotoxic and immunosuppressive medications, hematopoietic growth factors, toxins, other medications, systemic conditions, and autoimmune disorders [22–24]. Table 8.1 details a comprehensive list of possible etiologies.

Table 8.1 Etiologies associated with development of PRES

Cytotoxic and immunosuppressive medications
Adriamycin
Azathioprine
Bevacizumab
Bortezomib
Carboplatin
Cisplatin
Corticosteroids
Cyclophosphamide
Cyclosporine
Cytarabine
Etoposide
Gemcitabine
Interferon
L-asparaginase
Methotrexate
Mycophenolate mofetil
Rituximab
Sirolimus
Tacrolimus
Tumor necrosis factor antagonist
Ustekinumab
Vincristine
Hematopoietic growth factors
Erythropoietin
Granulocyte colony stimulating factor (G-CSF)
Toxins
Alcohol
Amide of lysergic acid
Amphetamines
Cocaine
Ephedra
Licorice
LSD
Mephedrone
Mushrooms
Organophosphates
Scorpion venom
Snake venom
Wasp venom
Other medications
Acetaminophen
Antiretroviral therapy for human immunodeficiency virus infection
Bismuth
Butal-bital-acetaminophen-caffeine therapy
Dextroamphetamine
Digitoxin
Ephedrine
Intravenous immunoglobulin
Linezolid
Lithium
Phenylpropanolamine
Pseudoephedrine
Tyrosine kinase inhibitors
Voriconazole
Systemic conditions
Hypertension
Eclampsia/pre-eclampsia
Renal failure
Thrombotic microangiopathies
Sickle cell disease
Tumor lysis syndrome
Sepsis/shock
COVID-19
Solid organ transplantation
Bone marrow transplantation
Stem cell transplantation
Hypomagnesemia
Hypercalcemia
Autoimmune disorders
Chron's disease
Neuromyelitis spectrum disorder
Rheumatoid arthritis
Scleroderma
Systemic lupus erythematosus
Vasculitis

Etiologies can be divided into two main groups: general conditions and drug toxicity. These groups can be further subdivided into systemic conditions and autoimmune diseases; cytotoxic and immunosuppressive medications, hematopoietic growth factors, toxins, and other medications, respectively [22–24]

8.4 Epidemiology

There are no studies reporting the incidence of PRES in the general population. It occurs in all age groups, with peak incidence among 20–40-year-olds [25–27]. It is slightly more frequent in females, even after excluding cases of eclampsia [3, 4, 28].

8.5 Diagnosis

There are no validated diagnostic criteria. Diagnosis is proposed when in the presence of (1) a possible trigger, (2) at least one acute neurological symptom (headache, visual disturbance, seizure, or altered mental status), (3) radiological features compatible with the disease, and when (4) no alternative diagnosis is more likely [2].

8.6 Clinical Presentation

Patients usually present with acute-onset non-specific neurological symptoms [3, 9, 10, 12, 20, 22–24, 28, 29] (Fig. 8.2), specifically:

- Encephalopathy seems to be the most frequent symptom (28–94%), ranging from mild confusion to coma [25, 28, 29].
- Seizures are present in 74–87% of patients [28, 29], with a subgroup (3–18%) presenting with or evolving to status epilepticus [29–32].
- Symptoms of raised intracranial pressure, namely headache (50%), nausea, and vomiting, may also occur [26]. Headache is typically of low intensity and progressive onset [2, 25]. Diagnosis of RCVS should be considered in cases where the patient presents with thunderclap headache [2, 25, 33].
- Focal neurological symptoms are less frequent and depend on which brain regions are affected. Among these, visual disturbances are the most common (20–39%) [1, 3, 29]. These may include decreased visual acuity, diplopia, visual field deficits, cortical blindness, visual neglect, and visual hallucinations [1, 3, 29]. Other focal deficits, such as paresis, aphasia, and ataxia, are rarer (4–19%) [2, 28, 34, 35].

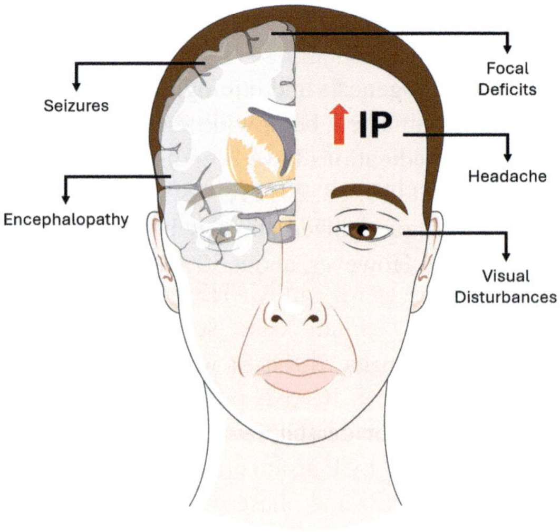

Fig. 8.2 Clinical presentation of PRES. PRES presents with acute-onset neurological symptoms [3, 9, 10, 12, 20, 22–24, 28, 29]: encephalopathy (mild confusion, stupor, coma) [25, 28, 29], seizures (partial or complex; status epilepticus is less frequent) [28, 29], intracranial hypertension syndrome (headache, vomiting; papilledema can be seen) [26], and focal neurological deficits, with visual disturbances being the most common [1, 3, 29]. IP: Intracranial Pressure

8.7 Neuroimaging

Magnetic Resonance Imaging (MRI) is the most appropriate exam to support the diagnosis of PRES and determine its extension. Nevertheless, in an emergency setting, computed tomography (CT) is usually the first modality of imaging performed and it is frequently able to show changes compatible with the syndrome [36].

The hallmark imaging feature is bilateral symmetric vasogenic edema involving the subcortical white matter, often extending into the cortex [4, 8, 36]. These changes can be appreciated as hypointense on T1-weighted sequences and hyperintense on T2-weighted imaging, including T2 fluid-attenuation inversion recovery (FLAIR) sequences. Signal on diffusion-weighted imaging (DWI) ranges from hypointense to slightly hyperintense, whereas apparent diffusion coefficient (ADC) is usually increased, reflecting the spectrum of changes from facilitated diffusion to T2 shine-through effect, respectively [4, 8, 36, 37]. Small foci of restricted diffusion may be seen within larger areas of vasogenic edema in cases where hypoperfusion and cytotoxic edema have ensued (15–30%) [38, 39]. Also, these may be related to hemorrhagic foci. Post-contrast enhancement is also common (38–50% of cases) and may be leptomeningeal, cortical, or cortico-subcortical with patchy enhancement in areas of vasogenic edema [4, 32]. Imaging reveals intracranial hemorrhage in 10–25% of cases, which can be better appreciated on T2* or susceptibility-weighted imaging (SWI) [3, 11, 28, 40, 41]. Hemorrhage may be subarachnoid or intraparenchymal (lobar or dispersed microbleeds) [3, 11, 28, 40, 41].

There are four main patterns regarding lesion location, particularly:

- Classic PRES (50%), which is a pattern limited to the parieto-occipital lobes [4, 39] (Fig. 8.3).
- Superior frontal sulcus pattern (27%), which presents as edema predominantly of the watershed territory between the anterior cerebral artery (ACA) and middle cerebral artery (MCA) [4] (Fig. 8.4).
- Holohemispheric watershed pattern (23%), with involvement of all watershed areas, i.e., ACA-MCA, ACA-posterior cerebral artery (PCA), and MCA-PCA [4] (Fig. 8.5).
- Central pattern (13%), with edema of subcortical structures, namely the deep white matter, basal ganglia, thalami, and brainstem [4, 39] (Fig. 8.4).

Although less frequent, cerebellar involvement is also possible (34–53%) [4, 39]. Additionally, medullary edema has also been described, but cases reporting it are scarce [42].

These patterns may manifest as combinations in 28% of cases [4] (Fig. 8.4). Also, patients may present with lesions that do not follow the enumerated patterns [4, 39]. Figure 8.6 specifies percentage of patients that exhibit abnormalities in each topography.

Another relevant concept is that patterns and lesion extension are not related to symptom severity [11, 28]. Additionally, there seems to be no relation between etiology and imaging pattern. Table 8.2 summarizes the main neuroimaging features of PRES.

With regard to other imaging exams, CT and MR angiography, as well as digital subtraction angiography, may be useful to clarify the differential diagnosis between PRES and RCVS [43]. Overlap is common, with 9–38% of RCVS cases presenting simultaneously with PRES [12–15, 44] and 87% of PRES cases presenting with angiographic changes compatible with RCVS [8]. If PRES is complicated with RCVS, angiographic examination will reveal a diffuse or focal pattern of vasoconstriction and vasodilation resembling a "string of beads" [38, 45].

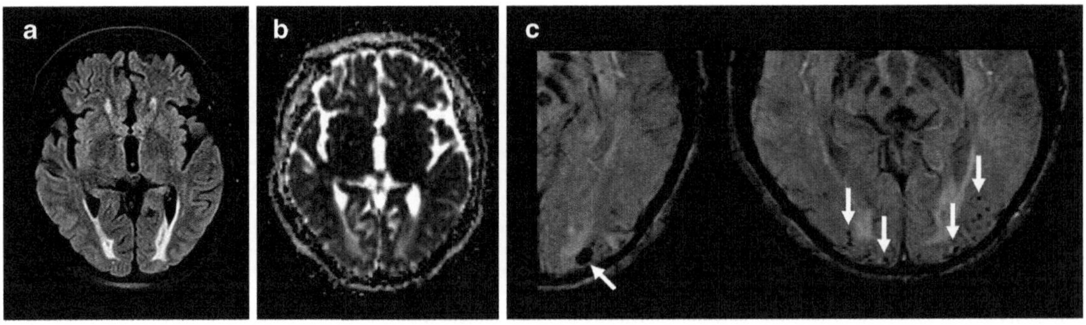

Fig. 8.3 Parieto-occipital pattern with micro-hemorrhages. Case of a 59-year-old female patient who presented with new-onset generalized tonic-clonic seizures two months after being submitted to lung transplantation. The patient was on corticosteroids and a tyrosine kinase inhibitor. MR revealed (**a**) subcortical vasogenic edema in the parieto-occipital regions, (**b**) with facilitated diffusion on ADC map. (**c**) On SWI, cortico-subcortical micro-hemorrhages, as well as a larger hemorrhage could be seen (arrows). Hemorrhage in PRES may also be subarachnoid (not depicted)

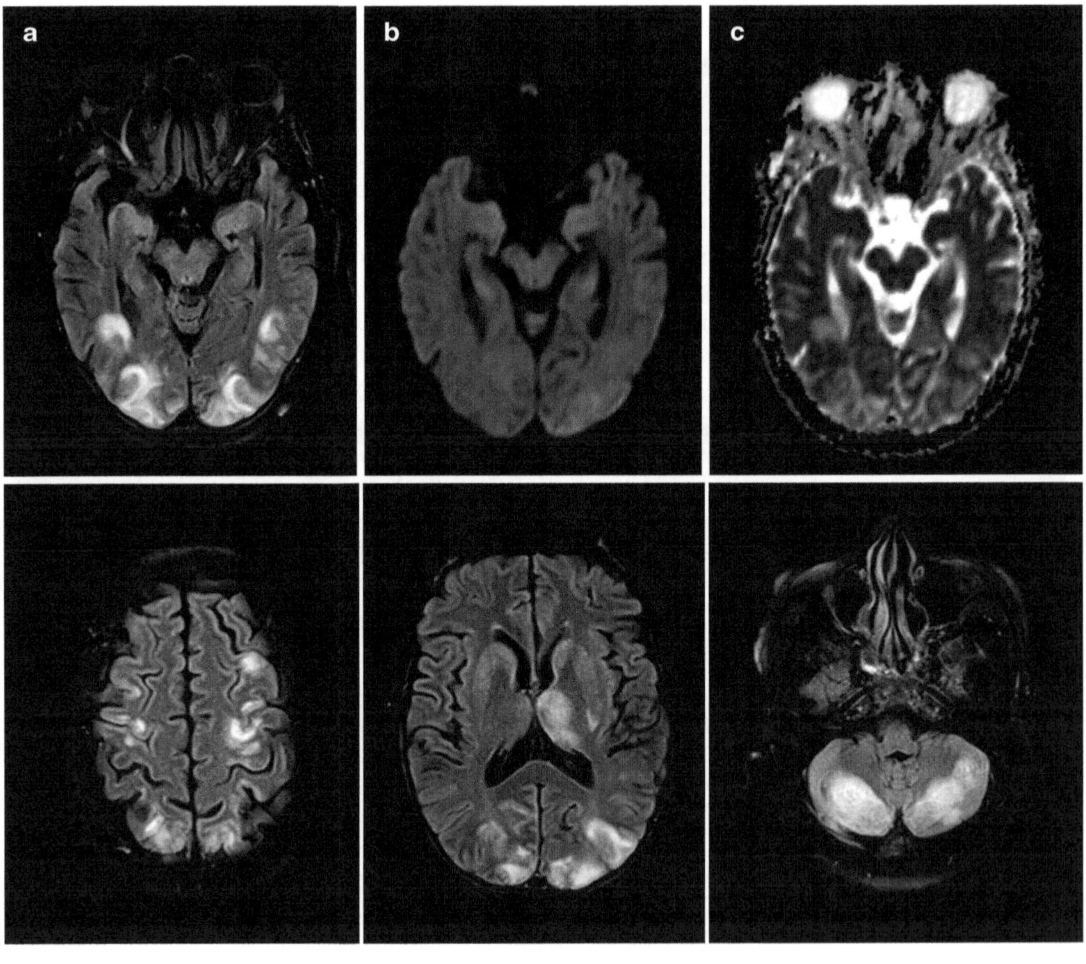

Fig. 8.4 Parieto-occipital, superior frontal sulcus and central (atypical, asymmetrical) patterns displayed simultaneously in the same patient. Case of a 44-year-old male patient under interferon-alfa for treatment of chronic hepatitis B who presented to the emergency room with acute-onset confusion, headache, and decreased visual acuity. MR showed (**a**) areas of vasogenic edema on T2 FLAIR predominantly in the parieto-occipital regions, around the superior frontal sulci, left thalamus, posterior segment of left lenticular nucleus, pons (not depicted), and in the cerebellar hemispheres. The areas of edema displayed (**b**) isointense to slightly hyperintense signal on DWI and (**c**) increased ADC

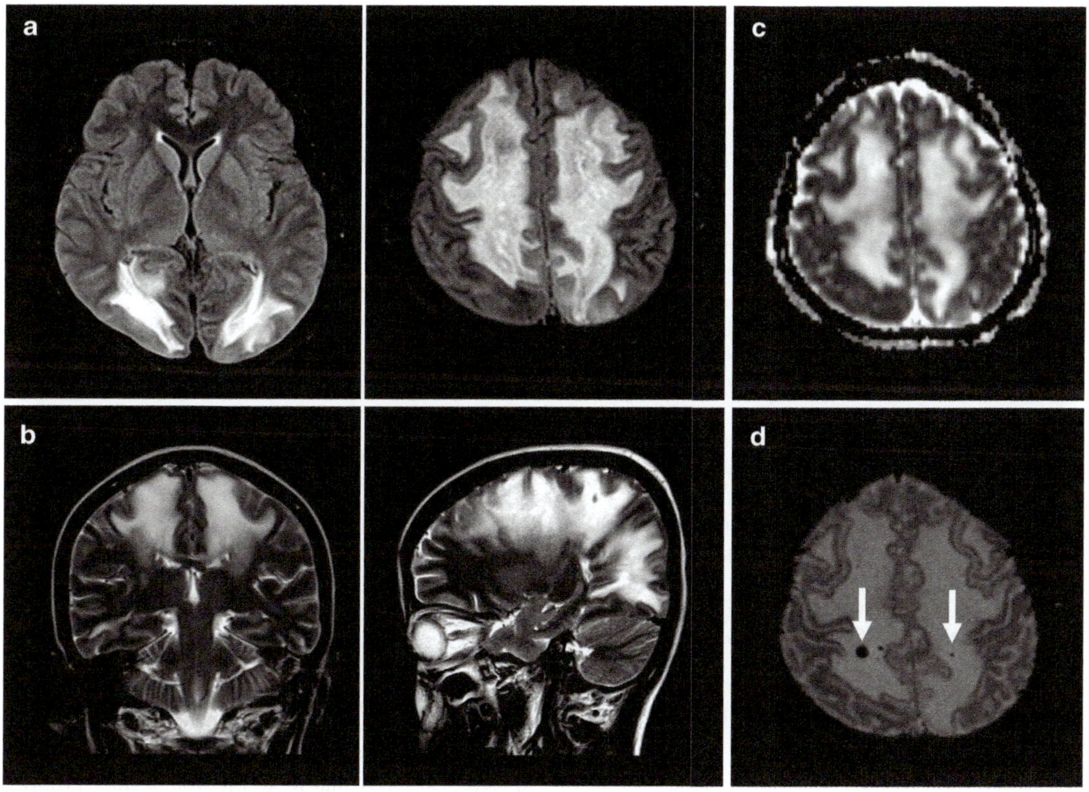

Fig. 8.5 Holohemispheric watershed pattern. Case of a 27-year-old male patient with systemic lupus erythematosus and lupus nephritis, under treatment with corticosteroids and mycophenolate mofetil, who presented with new-onset encephalopathy and status epilepticus. MR showed (**a** and **b**) a holohemispheric pattern of vasogenic edema, involving the ACA-MCA, ACA-PCA, and MCA--PCA, as well as deep-superficial watershed areas, (**c**) with facilitated diffusion on ADC map. (**d**) SWI revealed subcortical micro-hemorrhages within the areas of vasogenic edema (arrows)

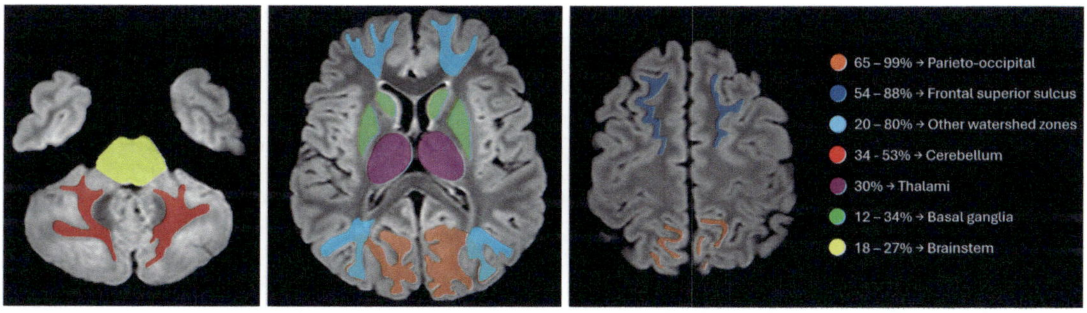

Fig. 8.6 Percentage of cases that exhibit abnormalities in each topography. Vasogenic edema is more often present in the parieto-occipital regions (65–99% of cases), followed by the areas around the superior frontal sulcus (54–88%), other watershed zones (20–80%), cerebellum (34–53%), thalami (30%), basal ganglia (12–34%), and the brainstem (18–27%) [4, 37]

Table 8.2 Main neuroimaging features of PRES

Location	Parieto-occipital lesions involving subcortical white matter
	Frequently associated with watershed territory lesions
	Occasionally, there is involvement of thalami, basal ganglia, and posterior fossa
Pattern	Bilateral and relatively symmetric
Signal	T2 and T2 FLAIR hyperintensities
	Usually, there is facilitated diffusion (high ADC), but foci of restricted diffusion are sometimes present (low ADC)
	Subarachnoid or intraparenchymal hemorrhage (hematoma or microbleeds) are possible
	Contrast enhancement is common and may be leptomeningeal, cortical, or cortico-subcortical

PRES is characterized by subcortical white matter edema, which is usually bilateral and symmetric and involves the parieto-occipital regions. Involvement of the watershed territories is also frequent. These changes can be appreciated as hyperintense on T2/T2 FLAIR sequences and usually show facilitated diffusion (increased ADC values). Foci of cytotoxic edema are possible. Subarachnoid and parenchymal hemorrhages may also be seen. Adapted from Lamy et al. (2014) [37]

8.8 Other Complementary Diagnostic Exams

There are no serum or cerebrospinal fluid biomarkers specifically associated with PRES [18]. Laboratory analyses may be helpful in identifying potential etiologies.

EEG can be useful in ruling out non-convulsive status epilepticus, but there are no specific EEG patterns that are characteristic of the syndrome [46–48].

8.9 Differential Diagnosis

Depending on clinical features and imaging patterns, different diagnoses should be considered. The more common differential diagnoses include ischemic stroke involving the posterior circulation, watershed infarcts, cerebral venous thrombosis (CVT), RCVS, and hypoglycemia [2, 20, 22, 49].

Concerning the vascular group, in the case of ischemic stroke (PCA or watershed territories), patients will present with cytotoxic, instead of vasogenic edema. Furthermore, large vessel occlusion/stenosis or clinical context of hypoperfusion, respectively, will be apparent [50, 51]. If CVT is suspected, CT or MR venogram should be performed to rule out the diagnosis [52].

Hypoglycemic encephalopathy may present with similar symptoms to PRES. Usually, MRI will reveal T2 hyperintensity involving the posterior limb of the internal capsule, cerebral cortex (particularly the parieto-occipital regions), hippocampus, and basal ganglia, with diffusion restriction [53]. Some cases may present with atypical changes, which complicates the differential diagnosis.

Table 8.3 summarizes the different diagnoses that may be considered. A detailed analysis of clinical history and complementary diagnostic exams should help shedding light on the correct diagnosis.

Table 8.3 Differential diagnoses of PRES

Vascular
Acute cerebral ischemia (mainly PCA stroke and ischemia of the watershed territory)
Cerebral venous thrombosis
Hemorrhagic stroke
Vasculitis
Thrombotic microangiopathies
RCVS
Hypoxic-ischemic encephalopathy
Inflammatory cerebral amyloid angiopathy
Metabolic
Hypoglycemia
Other metabolic encephalopathies
Toxic leukoencephalopathy
Osmotic demyelinating syndrome
Inflammatory
Acute disseminated encephalomyelitis (ADEM)
Autoimmune encephalitis
Infectious
Infectious encephalitis
Progressive multifocal leukoencephalopathy
Tumoral
Malignancy (lymphoma, gliomatosis cerebri, metastasis)
Paraneoplastic encephalitis
Radiation necrosis
Stroke-like migraine attacks after radiation therapy (SMART) syndrome
Genetic
Cerebral autosomal dominant arteriopathy with subcortical infarcts and leukoencephalopathy (CADASIL)
Mitochondrial encephalomyopathy with lactic acidosis and stroke-like episodes (MELAS)
Others
Status epilepticus

There is a wide range of diseases that can be included in the differential diagnosis for PRES, from vascular to inflammatory conditions [2, 20, 22, 49]. Clinical history, as well as neuroimaging features, are determinant to reach the most likely diagnosis

8.10 Management

Supportive care and elimination of the trigger are the mainstay of treatment.

Patients with severe hypertension should undergo treatment with antihypertensors, aiming at a reduction in blood pressure (BP) of less than 25% of the systolic pressure within the first hour, followed by progressive lowering to normal values over 24 to 48 hours [54]. Continuous monitoring of BP by intra-arterial line is recommended [55]. Admission to an intensive care unit should be considered [56]. Intravenous antiepileptic drugs are indicated for treatment of seizures [57]. Brain edema and raised intracranial pressure should be managed, with some patients requiring surgical intervention [58].

It is not clear yet if in drug-triggered cases the drug should be discontinued permanently or if reintroduction does not imply a risk of recurrence [59]. Also, it is still not known if switching the drug to a similar agent is safe [60]. Treatment recommendations are based on small retrospective studies or case series, so more evidence is still required.

8.11 Prognosis

When treated appropriately, PRES patients usually have a favorable prognosis, with symptoms and neuroimaging findings being reversible within hours to days [48, 57, 61–63]. Nonetheless, 8–17% of patients die and 26–36% experience poor functional outcomes [48, 57, 61–63]. Furthermore, follow-up imaging may reveal residual lesions, such as foci of gliosis and focal atrophy, in 40% of cases [3].

Older age, presence of subarachnoid hemorrhage, and altered mental state as initial symptoms are predictors of inpatient mortality [39]. Severe brain edema, cytotoxic edema, and brain hemorrhage are associated with poor functional outcomes [39]. Meanwhile, PRES due to eclampsia/pre-eclampsia is related to a favorable prognosis [64].

Recurrence seems to occur in 4–10% of patients, particularly in patients with persistent risk factors [65].

8.12 Summary (Table 8.4)

Table 8.4 Summary of key features of PRES

Definition
Clinicoradiological syndrome caused by endothelial dysfunction leading to BBB disruption and vasogenic edema
Etiology
Hypertension is the most recognized etiology (present in 70% of patients).
Other possible etiologies are cytotoxic and immunosuppressive medications, hematopoietic growth factors, toxins, autoimmune disorders, and other systemic conditions, such as eclampsia, renal failure, and sepsis
Diagnosis
Diagnosis is based on four key features: (1) presence of an identifiable trigger, (2) at least one acute neurological symptom, (3) compatible neuroimaging findings, and (4) absence of a better alternate diagnosis
Clinical presentation
Acute-onset neurological symptoms:
Encephalopathy
Seizures
Headache
Focal neurological symptoms, the most common being visual disturbances
Imaging findings
Vasogenic edema in typical patterns: Classic PRES (parieto-occipital), superior frontal sulcus pattern, holohemispheric watershed pattern, and central pattern.
Hemorrhages may be present as micro-hemorrhages, lobar hemorrhage, and subarachnoid hemorrhage.
Areas of restricted diffusion are less common
Management
Supportive care + elimination of precipitant factor are the mainstay of treatment
Prognosis
Prognosis is usually favorable under appropriate treatment. Recurrence is very rare

Acknowledgements Figures 8.1 and 8.2 were drawn in part using images from Servier Medical Art. Servier Medical Art by Servier is licensed under a Creative Commons Attribution 3.0 Unported License (https://creativecommons.org/licenses/by/3.0/).

References

1. Hinchey J, Chaves C, Appignani B, et al. A reversible posterior leukoencephalopathy syndrome. N Engl J Med. 1996;334:494–500. https://doi.org/10.1056/NEJM199602223340803.
2. Fugate JE, Rabinstein AA. Posterior reversible encephalopathy syndrome: clinical and radiological manifestations, pathophysiology, and outstanding questions. Lancet Neurol. 2015;14(9):914–25. https://doi.org/10.1016/S1474-4422(15)00111-8.
3. Liman TG, Bohner G, Heuschmann PU, et al. The clinical and radiological spectrum of posterior reversible encephalopathy syndrome: the retrospective Berlin PRES study. J Neurol. 2012;259:155–64. https://doi.org/10.1007/s00415-011-6152-4.
4. Bartynski WS, Boardman JF. Distinct imaging patterns and lesion distribution in posterior reversible encephalopathy syndrome. AJNR Am J Neuroradiol. 2007;28:1320–7. https://doi.org/10.3174/ajnr.A0549.
5. Lassen NA. Regulation of cerebral circulation. Acta Anaesthesiol Scand Suppl. 1971;45:78–80. https://doi.org/10.1111/j.1399-6576.1971.tb00661.x.
6. Cipolla MJ. Control of cerebral blood flow. San Rafael: Morgan & Claypool Publishers; 2009. ISBN:9781615047222
7. Muoio V, Persson PB, Sendeski MM. The neurovascular unit—concept review. Acta Physiol. 2014;210:790–8. https://doi.org/10.1111/apha.12250.
8. Bartynski WS. Posterior reversible encephalopathy syndrome, part 2: controversies surrounding pathophysiology of vasogenic edema. AJNR Am J Neuroradiol. 2008;29(6):1043–9. https://doi.org/10.3174/ajnr.A0929.
9. Granata G, Greco A, Iannella G, et al. Posterior reversible encephalopathy syndrome—insight into pathogenesis, clinical variants and treatment approaches. Autoimmun Rev. 2015;14:830–6. https://doi.org/10.1016/j.autrev.2015.05.006.
10. Feske SK. Posterior reversible encephalopathy syndrome: a review. Semin Neurol. 2011;31(2):202–15. https://doi.org/10.1055/s-0031-1277990.
11. Mueller-Mang C, Mang T, Pirker A, et al. Posterior reversible encephalopathy syndrome: do predisposing risk factors make a difference in MRI appearance? Neuroradiology. 2009;51:373–83. https://doi.org/10.1007/s00234-009-0504-0.
12. Ducros A, Boukobza M, Porcher R, et al. The clinical and radiological spectrum of reversible cerebral vasoconstriction syndrome. A prospective series of 67 patients. Brain. 2007;130:3091–101. https://doi.org/10.1093/brain/awm256.

13. Ducros A, Fiedler U, Porcher R, et al. Hemorrhagic manifestations of reversible cerebral vasoconstriction syndrome: frequency, features, and risk factors. Stroke. 2010;41:2505–11. https://doi.org/10.1161/STROKEAHA.109.572313.
14. Singhal AB, Hajj-Ali RA, Topcuoglu MA, et al. Reversible cerebral vasoconstriction syndromes: analysis of 139 cases. Arch Neurol. 2011;68:1005–12. https://doi.org/10.1001/archneurol.2011.68.
15. Chen SP, Fuh JL, Wang SJ, et al. Magnetic resonance angiography in reversible cerebral vasoconstriction syndromes. Ann Neurol. 2010;67:648–56. https://doi.org/10.1002/ana.21951.
16. Cappelen-Smith C, Calic Z, Cordato D. Reversible cerebral vasoconstriction syndrome: recognition and treatment. Curr Treat Options Neurol. 2017;19:21. https://doi.org/10.1007/s11940-017-0460-7.
17. Marra A, Vargas M, Striano P, Del Guercio L, Buonanno P, Servillo G. Posterior reversible encephalopathy syndrome: the endothelial hypotheses. Med Hypotheses. 2014;82(5):619–22. https://doi.org/10.1016/j.mehy.2014.02.022.
18. Fischer M, Schmutzhard E. Posterior reversible encephalopathy syndrome. J Neurol. 2017;264(8):1608–16. https://doi.org/10.1007/s00415-016-8377-8.
19. Pruitt JH, Copeland EM III, Moldawer LL. Interleukin-1 and interleukin-1 antagonism in sepsis, systemic inflammatory response syndrome, and septic shock. Shock. 1995;3(4):235–51. https://doi.org/10.1097/00024382-199504000-00001.
20. Liman TG, Siebert E, Endres M. Posterior reversible encephalopathy syndrome. Curr Opin Neurol. 2019;32(1):25–35. https://doi.org/10.1097/WCO.0000000000000640.
21. Gewirtz AN, Gao V, Parauda SC, Robbins MS. Posterior reversible encephalopathy syndrome. Curr Pain Headache Rep. 2021;25:1–9. https://doi.org/10.1007/s11916-020-00932-1.
22. Triplett JD, Kutlubaev MA, Kermode AG, Hardy T. Posterior reversible encephalopathy syndrome (PRES): diagnosis and management. Pract Neurol. 2022;22(3):183–9. https://doi.org/10.1136/practneurol-2021-003194.
23. Geocadin RG. Posterior reversible encephalopathy syndrome. N Engl J Med. 2023;388(23):2171–8. https://doi.org/10.1056/NEJMra2114482.
24. Parasher A, Jhamb R. Posterior reversible encephalopathy syndrome (PRES): presentation, diagnosis and treatment. Postgrad Med J. 2020;96(1140):623–8. https://doi.org/10.1136/postgradmedj-2020-137706.
25. Legriel S, Schraub O, Azoulay E, Hantson P, Magalhaes E, Coquet I, et al. Determinants of recovery from severe posterior reversible encephalopathy syndrome. PLoS One. 2012;7(9):e44534. https://doi.org/10.1371/journal.pone.0044534.
26. Li K, Yang Y, Guo D, Sun D, Li C. Clinical and MRI features of posterior reversible encephalopathy syndrome with atypical regions: a descriptive study with a large sample size. Front Neurol. 2020;11:194. https://doi.org/10.3389/fneur.2020.00194.
27. Thavamani A, Umapathi KK, Puliyel M, Super D, Allareddy V, Ghori A. Epidemiology, comorbidities, and outcomes of posterior reversible encephalopathy syndrome in children in the United States. Pediatr Neurol. 2020;103:21–6. https://doi.org/10.1016/j.pediatrneurol.2019.07.007.
28. Fugate JE, Claassen DO, Cloft HJ, Kallmes DF, Kozak OS, Rabinstein AA. Posterior reversible encephalopathy syndrome: associated clinical and radiologic findings. Mayo Clin Proc. 2010;85(5):427–32. https://doi.org/10.4065/mcp.2009.0590.
29. Lee VH, Wijdicks EFM, Manno EM, Rabinstein AA. Clinical spectrum of reversible posterior leukoencephalopathy syndrome. Arch Neurol. 2008;65:205–10. https://doi.org/10.1001/archneurol.2007.46.
30. Kozak OS, Wijdicks EF, Manno EM, Miley JT, Rabinstein AA. Status epilepticus as initial manifestation of posterior reversible encephalopathy syndrome. Neurology. 2007;69(9):894–7. https://doi.org/10.1212/01.wnl.0000269780.45472.16.
31. Sha Z, Moran BP, McKinney AM IV, Henry TR. Seizure outcomes of posterior reversible encephalopathy syndrome and correlations with electroencephalographic changes. Epilepsy Behav. 2015;48:70–4. https://doi.org/10.1016/j.yebeh.2015.05.027.
32. Hinduja A, Habetz K, Raina SK, Fitzgerald RT, Sahaya K. Predictors of seizures in patients with posterior reversible encephalopathy syndrome. Epilepsy Behav. 2016;61:97–101. https://doi.org/10.1016/j.yebeh.2016.05.001.
33. Ducros A. Reversible cerebral vasoconstriction syndrome. Lancet Neurol. 2012;11:906–17. https://doi.org/10.1016/S1474-4422(12)70135-7.
34. McKinney AM, Short J, Truwit CL, McKinney ZJ, Kozak OS, SantaCruz KS, Teksam M. Posterior reversible encephalopathy syndrome: incidence of atypical regions of involvement and imaging findings. AJR Am J Roentgenol. 2007;189(4):904–12. https://doi.org/10.2214/AJR.07.2024.
35. Pizon AF, Wolfson AB. Postpartum focal neurologic deficits: posterior leukoencephalopathy syndrome. J Emerg Med. 2005;29:163–6. https://doi.org/10.1016/j.jemermed.2005.02.006.
36. Bartynski WS. Posterior reversible encephalopathy syndrome, part 1: fundamental imaging and clinical features. AJNR Am J Neuroradiol. 2008;29(6):1036–42. https://doi.org/10.3174/ajnr.A0928.
37. Lamy C, Oppenheim C, Mas JL. Posterior reversible encephalopathy syndrome. Handb Clin Neurol. 2014;121:1687–701. https://doi.org/10.1016/B978-0-7020-4088-7.00109-7.
38. Covarrubias DJ, Luetmer PH, Campeau NG. Posterior reversible encephalopathy syndrome: prognostic utility of quantitative diffusion-weighted MR images. AJNR Am J Neuroradiol. 2002;23:1038–48.
39. Siebert E, Bohner G, Liebig T, et al. Factors associated with fatal outcome in posterior reversible encephalopathy syndrome: a retrospective analysis of

the Berlin PRES study. J Neurol. 2017;264:237–42. https://doi.org/10.1007/s00415-016-8328-4.
40. Sharma A, Whitesell RT, Moran KJ. Imaging pattern of intracranial hemorrhage in the setting of posterior reversible encephalopathy syndrome. Neuroradiology. 2010;52:855–63. https://doi.org/10.1007/s00234-009-0632-6.
41. Hefzy HM, Bartynski WS, Boardman JF, Lacomis D. Hemorrhage in posterior reversible encephalopathy syndrome: imaging and clinical features. AJNR Am J Neuroradiol. 2009;30:1371–9. https://doi.org/10.3174/ajnr.A1588.
42. Saad AF, Chaudhari R, Wintermark M. Imaging of atypical and complicated posterior reversible encephalopathy syndrome. Front Neurol. 2019;10:964. https://doi.org/10.3389/fneur.2019.00964.
43. Brady E, Parikh NS, Navi BB, Gupta A, Schweitzer AD. The imaging spectrum of posterior reversible encephalopathy syndrome: a pictorial review. Clin Imaging. 2018;47:80–9. https://doi.org/10.1016/j.clinimag.2017.08.008.
44. Bartynski WS, Boardman JF. Catheter angiography, MR angiography, and MR perfusion in posterior reversible encephalopathy syndrome. AJNR Am J Neuroradiol. 2008;29:447–55. https://doi.org/10.3174/ajnr.A0839.
45. Pilato F, Distefano M, Calandrelli R. Posterior reversible encephalopathy syndrome and reversible cerebral vasoconstriction syndrome: clinical and radiological considerations. Front Neurol. 2020;11:34. https://doi.org/10.3389/fneur.2020.00034.
46. Kastrup O, Gerwig M, Frings M, Diener HC. Posterior reversible encephalopathy syndrome (PRES): electroencephalographic findings and seizure patterns. J Neurol. 2012;259(7):1383–9. https://doi.org/10.1007/s00415-011-6362-9.
47. Bastide L, Legros B, Rampal N, et al. Clinical correlates of periodic discharges and nonconvulsive seizures in posterior reversible encephalopathy syndrome (PRES). Neurocrit Care [Internet]. 2018; https://doi.org/10.1007/s12028-018-0548-2.
48. Hinduja A. Posterior reversible encephalopathy syndrome: clinical features and outcome. Front Neurol. 2020;11:71. https://doi.org/10.3389/fneur.2020.00071.
49. Faille LD, Fieuws S, Van Paesschen W. Clinical predictors and differential diagnosis of posterior reversible encephalopathy syndrome. Acta Neurol Belg. 2017;117:469–75. https://doi.org/10.1007/s13760-017-0750-6.
50. Tedyanto EH, Tini K, Pramana NA. Magnetic resonance imaging in acute ischemic stroke. Cureus. 2022;14(7). https://doi.org/10.7759/cureus.27224.
51. Mangla R, Kolar B, Almast J, Ekholm SE. Border zone infarcts: pathophysiologic and imaging characteristics. Radiographics. 2011;31(5):1201–14. https://doi.org/10.1148/rg.315105014.
52. Aguiar de Sousa D, Lucas NL. Advances in cerebral venous thrombosis. Stroke. 2024; https://doi.org/10.1161/STROKEAHA.123.044266.
53. Kang EG, Jeon SJ, Choi SS, Song CJ, Yu IK. Diffusion MR imaging of hypoglycemic encephalopathy. Am J Neuroradiol. 2010;31(3):559–64. https://doi.org/10.3174/ajnr.A1856.
54. Aronow WS. Treatment of hypertensive emergencies. Ann Transl Med. 2017;5(Suppl 1):S5. https://doi.org/10.21037/atm.2017.03.34.
55. Whelton PK, Carey RM, Aronow WS, et al. ACC/AHA/AAPA/ABC/ACPM/AGS/APhA/ASH/ASPC/NMA/PCNA guideline for the prevention, detection, evaluation, and management of high blood pressure in adults: a report of the American College of Cardiology/American Heart Association task force on clinical practice guidelines. Hypertension. 2018;71(6):e13–e115. https://doi.org/10.1161/HYP.0000000000000065.
56. Hinduja A, Habetz K, Raina SK, et al. Predictors of intensive care unit utilization in patients with posterior reversible encephalopathy syndrome. Acta Neurol Belg. 2017;117:201–6. https://doi.org/10.1007/s13760-016-0703-5.
57. Legriel S, Pico F, Azoulay E. Understanding posterior reversible encephalopathy syndrome. In: Annual Update in Intensive Care and Emergency Medicine; 2011. p. 631–53.
58. Akins PT, Axelrod Y, Silverthorn JW, Guppy K, Banerjee A, Hawk MW. Management and outcomes of malignant posterior reversible encephalopathy syndrome. Clin Neurol Neurosurg. 2014;125:52–7. https://doi.org/10.1016/j.clineuro.2014.06.034.
59. Hammerstrom AE, Howell J, Gulbis A, Rondon G, Champlin RE, Popat U. Tacrolimus-associated posterior reversible encephalopathy syndrome in hematopoietic allogeneic stem cell transplantation. Am J Hematol. 2013;88:301–5. https://doi.org/10.1002/ajh.23402.
60. Singer S, Grommes C, Reiner AS, Rosenblum MK, DeAngelis LM. Posterior reversible encephalopathy syndrome in patients with cancer. Oncologist. 2015;20:806–11. https://doi.org/10.1634/theoncologist.2014-0149.
61. Chen Z, Zhang G, Lerner A, Wang AH, Gao B, Liu J. Risk factors for poor outcome in posterior reversible encephalopathy syndrome: systematic review and meta-analysis. Quant Imaging Med Surg. 2018;8:421–32. https://doi.org/10.21037/qims.2018.05.07.
62. Roth C, Ferbert A. Posterior reversible encephalopathy syndrome: long-term follow-up. J Neurol Neurosurg Psychiatry. 2010;81:773–7. https://doi.org/10.1136/jnnp.2009.189647.
63. Alhilali LM, Reynolds AR, Fakhran S. A multidisciplinary model of risk factors for fatal outcome in posterior reversible encephalopathy syndrome. J Neurol Sci. 2014;347:59–65. https://doi.org/10.1016/j.jns.2014.09.019.
64. Liman TG, Bohner G, Endres M, Siebert E. Discharge status and in-hospital mortality in posterior reversible encephalopathy syndrome. Acta Neurol Scand. 2014;130:34–9. https://doi.org/10.1111/ane.12213.
65. Li R, Mitchell P, Dowling R, Yan B. Is hypertension predictive of clinical recurrence in posterior reversible encephalopathy syndrome? J Clin Neurosci. 2013;20:248–52. https://doi.org/10.1016/j.jocn.2012.02.023.

9 Treatment-Related Reversible Cerebral Vasoconstriction Syndrome

Giulia Avola and Alessandro Pezzini

9.1 Introduction

The reversible cerebral vasoconstriction syndrome (RCVS) is a clinical-radiological entity whose main characteristic is the reversible vasoconstriction of segments of intracranial arterial vessels. Actually, only in the last two decades this disease has been recognized, and the term RCVS was proposed in 2007 to describe a group of pathologies characterized by reversible narrowing and dilation of cerebral arteries [1]. This condition was previously known as "Call–Fleming syndrome," "thunderclap headache with reversible vasospasm," "benign angiopathy of the central nervous system," "postpartum angiopathy," "migrainous vasospasm or migraine angiitis," "drug-induced cerebral arteritis or angiopathy" [2].

RCVS can be idiopathic or drug-related [3]. The pathogenic mechanism is still unclear, but in both cases, endothelial dysfunction and sympathetic hyperactivation are thought to play a crucial role [4].

Imaging plays a critical role in the diagnosis and management of RCVS. Non-invasive techniques such as MR angiography are increasingly being used in clinical practice, although cerebral angiography is the gold standard for the detection of cerebral vasoconstriction [5]. Imaging is also helpful for a differential diagnosis with other disorders of the central nervous system, particularly primary angiitis of the central nervous system (PACNS).

9.2 Epidemiology

The estimated incidence of RCVS is 3 per million in adults [6], but it is likely the most probable form of intracranial arteriopathy and a frequent cause of stroke in young adults [7]. It can affect any age group, but the average age is 40–55 years, with a prevalence in females [2]. Male patients tend to be younger (fourth to fifth decade in women vs. third to fourth decade in men) [8], or adolescents (>85% of affected adolescents are male) [9], but the reason for this disparity is unknown. Additionally, male sex is more often associated with a better outcome [4].

G. Avola
Dipartimento di Medicina e Chirurgia, Università degli Studi di Parma, Parma, Italy

A. Pezzini (✉)
Dipartimento di Medicina e Chirurgia, Università degli Studi di Parma, Parma, Italy

Dipartimento di Emergenza e Urgenza, Programma Stroke Care Azienda Ospedaliero Universitaria, Parma, Italy
e-mail: alessandro.pezzini@unipr.it

M. Zedde, R. Pascarella (eds.), *Neuroimaging of Treatment-Related Conditions in the Brain*,
https://doi.org/10.1007/978-3-032-23618-0_9

9.3 Clinical Presentation

Between 85% and 100% of cases present at onset with a thunderclap headache, which is described as the worst headache of life, reaching its maximum intensity in ≤1 min and often being accompanied by not only crying, photophobia, nausea, and vomiting, but also seizures and hypertensive peaks during the attack [10, 11]. The diagnostic criteria for the diagnosis of primary thunderclap headache are reported in Table 9.1. The headache episodes are often triggered by factors such as coughing [12], bathing [13], physical excerption, sexual activity [14], Valsalva maneuver, and emotional outbursts [2]. Headaches are recurrent and persist for up to 4 weeks; they can arise 2–3 weeks before the overt clinical manifestation of RCVS, characterized by the association of other focal neurological manifestations with the headache [15]. Between episodes, a form of mild to moderate intensity holocranial headache persists [7]. Neurological signs (present in 8–43% of cases) depend on the complications associated with RCVS, involving cerebral ischemia, cerebral hemorrhage, and Posterior Reversible Encephalopathy Syndrome (PRES) [4]. Depending on the affected area, aphasia, hemiparesis, hemianopia, seizures, or Balint's syndrome can be observed [16]. The incidence of seizures, however, is rare (7–17% of cases) [4]. Table 9.2 shows the diagnostic criteria of headache attributed to reversible cerebral vasoconstriction syndrome, according to the Headache Classification Committee of the International Headache Society (IHS) [15].

In the treatment of headache, the first-line treatment is nimodipine, administered orally, or intra-arterially in clinically more severe cases [17]. Vasoconstriction, however, persists even after the resolution of the headache. But the headache itself can also persist: some patients, about half, develop a post-RCVS headache that can last for over a year after the resolution of vasoconstriction [4].

Table 9.1 Diagnostic criteria for primary thunderclap headache, according to Headache Classification Committee of the International Headache Society (IHS)

Primary thunderclap headache criteria
A. Intense headache fulfilling criteria B and C
B. Sudden onset, reaching maximum intensity in less than 1 min
C. Persists for at least 5 min
D. Not attributable to another ICHD-3 diagnosis

9.4 Pathogenesis

RCVS can occur spontaneously, in the absence of a predisposing factor, but in 40–60% of cases it is induced by factors considered as triggers [2]. The spontaneous form appears to be predominant in Asian populations, while the trigger-induced one prevails among Europeans and Americans [2, 18]. Regarding the pathophysiological mechanisms, although there is more evidence related to idiopathic forms to date, they are still unknown. However, the two main pathophysiological hypotheses are the following: (1) alteration of vascular tone and (2) endothelial dysfunction.

9.4.1 Dysregulation of Cerebral Vascular Tone and Sympathetic Over-Reactivity

The pial cerebral vessels receive rich innervation from the superior cervical ganglion, the sphenopalatine ganglion, and the trigeminal nerve, whose nerve endings release vasoactive substances such as neuropeptide Y and norepinephrine, resulting in vasoconstriction [19]. Similarly, the cerebral vessels of the microcirculation receive sympathetic innervation from the locus coeruleus, the raphe nucleus, and the basal forebrain [19]. Vascular tone regulation is possible through various receptor populations. Norepinephrine exerts a vasoconstrictive effect on the walls of the middle cerebral arteries through α-1 adrenergic receptors [20], while it induces vasodilation of parenchymal arterioles through β-adrenergic receptors [21]. An imbalance in vascular tone, driven by heightened sympathetic activity on vessel walls, causes the characteristic vasoconstriction seen in

Table 9.2 Diagnostic criteria of headache attributed to reversible cerebral vasoconstriction syndrome and headache probably attributed to reversible cerebral vasoconstriction syndrome, according to Headache Classification Committee of the HIS

Headache attributed to reversible cerebral vasoconstriction syndrome (RCVS)	Headache probably attributed to reversible cerebral vasoconstriction syndrome (RCVS)
A. Any new headache meeting criterion C	A. Any new headache meeting criterion C
B. Diagnosed reversible cerebral vasoconstriction syndrome (RCVS)	B. Reversible cerebral vasoconstriction syndrome (RCVS) is suspected, but cerebral angiography shows normal findings
C. At least one of the following: 1. Headache, with or without focal deficits and/or seizures, has prompted angiography (showing "strings and beads" appearance) and the diagnosis of RCVS 2. Headache has one or both of the following characteristics: a. recurs within 1 month, with thunderclap onset, b. triggered by sexual activity, exertion, Valsalva maneuver, emotion, bathing, and/or showering 3. No new significant headache occurs more than 1 month after onset	C. Probability of causation supported by all of the following: 1. At least two headaches within 1 month, with each of the following characteristics: (a) Thunderclap onset, peaking in less than 1 min (b) Severe intensity (c) Lasting 5 min or more 2. At least one thunderclap headache has been triggered by one or more of the following: (a) sexual activity (just before or at orgasm), (b) exertion, (c) Valsalva-like maneuver, (d) emotion, (e) bathing and/or showering, and (f) bending 3. No new thunderclap or other significant headache occurs more than 1 month after onset
D. Not better explained by another ICHD-3 diagnosis, and aneurysmal subarachnoid hemorrhage has been ruled out by appropriate investigations	D. Does not fulfill ICHD-3 criteria for any other headache disorder
	E. Not better explained by another ICHD-3 diagnosis, and aneurysmal subarachnoid hemorrhage has been ruled out through appropriate investigations

RCVS. Studies on cerebrovascular vasoreactivity support this hypothesis. Specifically, a retrospective case series revealed significant impairment in the breath holding index during the acute phases of the disease, reflecting compromised vasodilatory capacity in response to hypercapnia [22]. Additionally, more recent studies have suggested the role of a genetic predisposition and identified circulating microRNAs that target genes responsible for vascular tone, such as the gene for endothelin 1, or that are involved in the transforming growth factor beta signaling pathway [23]. A polymorphism (val66Met) in the brain-derived neurotrophic factor (BDNF) gene has also been identified, which could be responsible for the severity of vasoconstriction in RCVS [24], as it upregulates neuropeptide Y. On the other hand, an aberrant response to sympathetic stimulation can make patients more vulnerable to sympathetic stimulation [4]: this could explain why some patients develop RCVS after the intake of sympathomimetics.

9.4.2 Endothelial Dysfunction

The second hypothesized mechanism is endothelial dysfunction. The integrity of the endothelium plays a crucial role as endothelial cells secrete vasoconstrictive and vasodilatory substances that act on the muscular wall of the arterioles, thus contributing to the constant maintenance of cerebral blood flow through vasoconstriction/vasodilation. It has been demonstrated that patients with RCVS also have fewer CD34KDR endothelial progenitor cells compared to controls, especially those with more severe vasoconstriction [25]. Since this cell class is responsible for re-endothelialization [26], it is possible that in the acute phases of the disease, patients who have suffered endothelial damage also have a deficit in the mechanisms of endothelial repair. An endothelial damage could be favored by sympathetic hypertonia (or hyperreactivity to sympathetic stimulation) or by excessive oxidative stress [2]. In fact, in the acute phases of the disease, increased levels of 8-iso prostaglandin F2α have been shown in both urine and plasma [27]. The 8-iso prostaglandin F2α is considered a marker of oxidative stress and has a strong vasoconstrictive effect. The result is the breakdown of the blood–brain barrier (BBB), leading to increased permeability of the vascular wall, which is radiologically observed with contrast-enhanced FLAIR in 50% of cases [28]. Recently, a technique called dynamic contrast-enhanced magnetic resonance imaging (DCE-MRI) has demonstrated increased microscopic permeability in the acute phase, indicating that barrier damage is present even when not microscopically visible [29]. Finally, a study based on high-resolution vascular wall imaging has shown enhancement of the affected vessels in almost half of the patients with RCVS, suggesting that a perivascular inflammatory process might also contribute to endothelial damage [30]. However, evidence supporting this hypothesis is scarce and controversial. The main difficulty lies in obtaining histopathological samples of the affected vessels that could help shed light on the actual pathogenic mechanism of this disease [2].

9.4.3 Pathogenesis of Thunderclap Headache

The pathophysiological mechanism underlying thunderclap headache is unclear, but it is unlikely to depend on the vasoconstriction of large vessels because vasoconstriction occurs approximately 2 weeks after the headache onset. More likely, the involvement of distal cerebral and pain-sensitive pial vessels leads to the activation of the trigeminovascular nociceptive pathway [31], resulting in the release of vasodilatory substances such as CGRP. Physiologically, the trigeminovascular reflex restores vascular tone after a vasoconstrictive stimulus [32]; in patients with RCVS, this mechanism seems to be altered. Trigeminal nociceptors could also be activated by leaked intravascular components when the BBB permeability is altered [4].

9.4.4 Trigger Factors in RCVS

The same factors that can trigger thunderclap headache are also precipitating factors for RCVS, where intense headache is associated with other focal neurological signs and neuroradiological findings. However, the two most common risk factors (approximately 31% of cases) are the intake of vasoactive drugs and the postpartum period [2, 10, 32]. The pathogenic mechanism might be slightly different in these two subcategories. Table 9.3 summarizes the possible precipitating factors [4]. Vasoactive drugs act through specific receptors located in the smooth muscle and cause overstimulation of the sympathetic system on the vessel wall. In 1962, a study involving the direct injection of serotonin into the carotid arteries of monkeys showed a significant increase in cerebral perfusion pressure and a 50% narrowing of the internal carotid artery [33]. This explains the association of RCVS with the intake of selective serotonin reuptake inhibitors (SSRIs) and serotonin-norepinephrine reuptake inhibitors (SNRIs). Other case reports suggested drugs that act as agonists of serotonergic receptors, such as

Table 9.3 Precipitating factors/triggers causing RCVS

Various precipitating factors/conditions and triggers causing RCVS
Drugs: selective serotonin (and noradrenaline) reuptake inhibitors, cyclophosphamide, fingolimod, tacrolimus, erythropoietin, intravenous immune globulin, red blood cell transfusion triptans, ergotamine, pseudoephedrine, cocaine, amphetamine derivatives, ecstasy, lysergic acid diethylamide, tetrahydrocannabinol, prednisolone, oral contraceptive pills
Tumors: pheochromocytoma, neuroendocrine tumor (e.g., bronchial carcinoid)
Traumatic brain injury, neurosurgical procedures
Porphyria
Early and late pregnancy, pre-eclampsia, (postpartum) eclampsia
Vascular conditions: post-carotid endarterectomy, unruptured cerebral aneurysm, spinal subdural hematoma COVID-19
Triggers: laughing, coughing, bathing, Valsalva maneuver, exertion, emotion, sexual activity

triptans [34, 35], and benzodiazepines (e.g., clonazepam), can cause vasoconstriction of cerebral arteries through the activation of serotonin receptors, thus precipitating RCVS [36]. For the same reason, some authors have hypothesized a possible association with sympathomimetics that have serotonergic effects [4].

Another class of drugs associated with RCVS is immunosuppressants. Several case reports discuss the association with Fingolimod, approved for the treatment of multiple sclerosis. Fingolimod acts as an inhibitor of the sphingosine 1-phosphate receptor, thus inhibiting lymphocyte migration to sites of inflammation; additionally, since sphingolipids have a vasoactive effect, their inhibition can explain the vasospasm. Specifically, the inhibition of ceramide, which is a vasodilator, causes vasoconstriction [37]. The cases described in the literature are few; during the phase three Fingolimod trial, a case of peripheral vasoconstriction was also described in patients taking a higher dose of 1.25 mg daily [38]. Interferon is also a possible trigger. Raynaud's phenomenon and livedo reticularis have been described as possible side effects, both characterized by vasoconstriction of small arteries and peripheral arterioles [39, 40]. It is therefore hypothesized that interferon may have a vasoactive effect on cerebral vessels as well. In some case reports, certain anticancer and other immunosuppressive drugs have been reported as possible RCVS triggers. In the case of Methotrexate, an immunosuppressant used in hematological cancers that acts as a dihydrofolate reductase inhibitor, neurotoxic effects have been observed primarily at high doses, typically after intravenous administration of at least 1000 mg/m^2 or after intrathecal administration [41].

Among immunosuppressive drugs, a possible trigger can be the anti-calcitonin gene-related peptide (CGRP) monoclonal antibody. This association is actually dubious since there are only a few case reports and the patients had also concurrently taken triptans for headaches [42]. CGRP is a potent vasodilator that acts on the cardiovascular and cerebrovascular systems, so its sustained inhibition could justify cerebral vasospasm. However, it is unclear whether the administration of the antibody alone is sufficient to trigger the condition. Additionally, CGRP receptors are located in the smooth muscle, so the luminal administration of these antibodies does not allow them to reach muscle cells and trigger vasospasm unless there is a barrier disruption [43]. Therefore, the monoclonal antibody alone, in the absence of preexisting barrier damage, might not be sufficient to induce RCVS.

The association of RCVS with immunosuppressive treatments (steroids, mycophenolate mofetil, hydroxychloroquine) also explains the association of RCVS with conditions such as systemic lupus erythematosus (SLE), antiphospholipid antibody syndrome (APS), and systemic sclerosis (SS) [44, 45]. In these cases, RCVS is not only treatment-related, as endothelial damage is also present in these diseases, as in RCVS. In particular, in APS, autoantibodies affect the coagulation cascade and activate endothelial cells that release vasoactive agents such as Endothelin-1 (ET1) [46]. ET1 regulates the intracellular influx of calcium and thus modulates the muscular tone of the vessel. Indeed, a decrease in plasma ET1 levels has been demonstrated after the resolution of vasospasm in patients with RCVS [45]. Another noteworthy discovery is that cilostazol, by inhibiting ET1's effect on vascular walls, may potentially alleviate vasospasm, making it a reasonable treatment option for RCVS associated with antiphospholipid syndrome (APS) [47].

The role of immunosuppressants as triggers also explains the association of RCVS with transplantation. In the literature, only four cases of RCVS after heart transplantation have been described [48]. The leading cause of heart transplantation-related RCVS could be the administration of tacrolimus. In this case, the neurological symptoms caused by RCVS appear within 2 weeks of the transplant and could be irreversible due to the neurotoxicity of the drug. Therefore, the administration of tacrolimus should be gradual and closely monitored with plasma-level measurements. It has also been observed that its discontinuation, rather than dosage reduction, reduces long-term neurological sequelae.

Other possible triggers identified in the literature include ergot derivatives, erythropoietin, intravenous immunoglobulins, anesthetic drugs, and antimuscarinic drugs. In particular, some case reports described RCVS potentially related to therapy with oxybutynin. This is an antimuscarinic drug that acts selectively on the M3 receptor, which is one of the most expressed receptors in the brain parenchyma, as well as M1 and M5 receptors. When M3 receptors are bound, they mediate vasoconstriction through the activation of pericytes or vasodilation through the release of endothelial nitric oxide. As a result, by blocking M3, oxybutynin could modify the balance between vasoconstriction and vasodilation [49].

According to some sources, RCVS can also occur after a red blood cell transfusion. In fact, the brain is not commonly an organ exposed to blood transfusion reactions; however, it has been hypothesized that the autoregulatory response of vessels to changes in blood volume and oxygenation could be the main pathogenic mechanism [50]. Chronic anemia leads to hypoxemia and thus vasodilation [51]; a rapid correction of hemoglobin, with an increase in its value ≥5 g/dL, causes the loss of vasodilation [52]. Additionally, the increase in hematocrit and thus blood viscosity can cause endothelial damage and hence vasospasm [53]. The timing of these mechanisms varies: cases where RCVS develops immediately after the transfusion and cases where it develops about a week later have been described [50].

Other triggers include illicit drugs such as 3,4-methylenedioxymethamphetamine (ecstasy), cocaine, amphetamines, lysergic acid diethylamide (LSD), and tetrahydrocannabinol [54]. Even more commonly used drugs, such as non-steroidal anti-inflammatory drugs (NSAIDs) and contraceptive pills, are trigger factors. NSAIDs are not commonly associated with RCVS, but a few case reports have highlighted a possible association between the administration of indomethacin and RCVS. The mechanism by which they induce RCVS is not known, but their effect is likely mediated by the inhibition of cyclooxygenases [55]. Indomethacin, in particular, inhibits prostacyclin, which has a vasodilatory effect, and, unlike other NSAIDs, it counteracts nitric oxide-induced vasodilation, thereby favoring vasoconstriction [56].

Some case reports also support that RCVS can be triggered by hypercalcemia following calcium supplementation [57]. Animal models have shown that calcium acts to initiate actin–myosin binding within cerebrovascular smooth muscle cells to promote contractility and causes inflammation and endothelial damage, leading to the permeability and breakdown of the blood–brain barrier [58]. The serum calcium value above which this alteration is observed is not known; several cases have noted a critical value >13 mg/dL [57].

Finally, contraceptive pills may play a role as a trigger factor due to their estrogen content. Estrogens act as modulators of vascular tone and consequently of cerebral blood flow. Specifically, they reduce the effects of the sympathetic system, stimulate the production of nitric oxide synthase by the endothelium and its phosphorylation, promoting vasodilation, and favor the production of prostacyclins with consequent vasodilatory effect [59]. However, the role of estrogens in the pathogenesis of RCVS remains currently unclear. An association of the disease with contraceptive pills has been proposed [60], as well as with hormonal stimulation for intrauterine insemination [61], and intrauterine devices releasing levonorgestrel [62]. Of note, also a sudden reduction in estrogen levels may favor the onset of RCVS; as mentioned previously, the postpartum period (2 weeks after delivery) is a predisposing condition, more often associated with PRES (>25% of cases), which in 7–38% of cases is associated with RCVS [4]. The abrupt reduction in estrogens in the postpartum period could therefore explain the recurrence of RCVS during this time frame. For the same reasons, treatments such as bilateral salpingo-oophorectomy have been proposed as trigger, since they induce a sudden reduction in estrogen production [63].

However, the major risk factor in postpartum-related RCVS is thought to be eclampsia. The placenta plays a crucial role in the development of eclampsia. The placenta secretes pro-inflammatory cytokines, pro-angiogenic proteins such as placental growth factor, its soluble receptor, and soluble endoglin into the maternal circulation, leading to an immune response and subsequent endothelial dysfunction, which likely causes vasoconstriction [64].

Unfortunately, treatment-related forms of RCVS are mainly described in case reports, so further research is necessary to fully understand the role of drugs or estrogens. Additionally, only limited experience suggests that re-exposure to these trigger factors does not lead to relapse, so if clinically indicated, vasoactive drugs can be re-prescribed to the patient.

9.5 Pathophysiological Models

A pathophysiological model of RCVS is illustrated in Fig. 9.1. In patients with a genetic predisposition and therefore greater vulnerability to triggering factors, when the sympathetic system is overstimulated, there is a more likely release of vasoactive substances such as neuropeptide Y, endothelin 1, and catecholamines, leading to vasoconstriction. Arterioles respond with initial vasodilation, partially due to trigeminovascular reflex activation, resulting in perivascular nociceptor activation and thunderclap headache. Conversely, in response to peripheral vasodilation, larger proximal vessels vasoconstriction. The alteration in vascular tone contributes, alongside blood–brain barrier breakdown, to the onset of clinical and radiological complications of RCVS.

9.6 Imaging Findings

Imaging findings at onset are often normal. Shortly thereafter, changes in neuroradiological findings are a hallmark of RCVS [7].

9.6.1 Brain Magnetic Resonance Imaging (MRI) and Magnetic Resonance Angiography (MRA)

As previously said, vasospasm initially involves only small distal cerebral vessels not depicted by MRA, and then centripetally spreads to larger vessels over days or weeks. As a consequence, initial brain MRI is normal in 30–55% of cases, while initial MRA is normal in 22% of cases [4]. Nevertheless, investigators describe vascular FLAIR hyperintensities as early signs that can be visible on T2/FLAIR sequences, even before vasospasm becomes visible on MRA [65]. They described well-circumscribed dot or tubular-like appearances of hyperintense lesions running through the sulci, correlating with slow flow on the cortical surface. These hyperintense vessels (HVs) are often bilateral, involving the territories of the middle cerebral artery (MCA) and posterior cerebral artery (PCA) (Fig. 9.2). More frequently, HVs are observed in patients with PRES and ischemic stroke, suggesting that they may not only serve as a useful marker of RCVS but also indicate clinical severity. HVs are distinct from subarachnoid hemorrhage, as they do not appear hypointense on SWI sequences [65]. Vasospasm, on the other hand, can be visualized with magnetic resonance angiography (MRA) or through computed tomography angiography (CTA) (as shown on Fig. 9.3), when it starts involving larger cerebral vessels. As a result, the diagnosis could be challenging in the acute phase, and often delayed. In cases of treatment-related RCVS, cerebral edema is more frequently observed and vasoconstriction is more widespread and severe compared to the idiopathic form where vasoconstriction is usually segmental. The addition of contrast medium in T2/FLAIR + gadolinium sequences is useful as it reflects blood–brain barrier breakdown. It has also been shown that breakdown of the blood–brain barrier can be an independent risk factor for neurological complications such as subarachnoid hemorrhage and PRES [66].

The radiological findings of RCVS are distinct from other vascular pathologies (such as

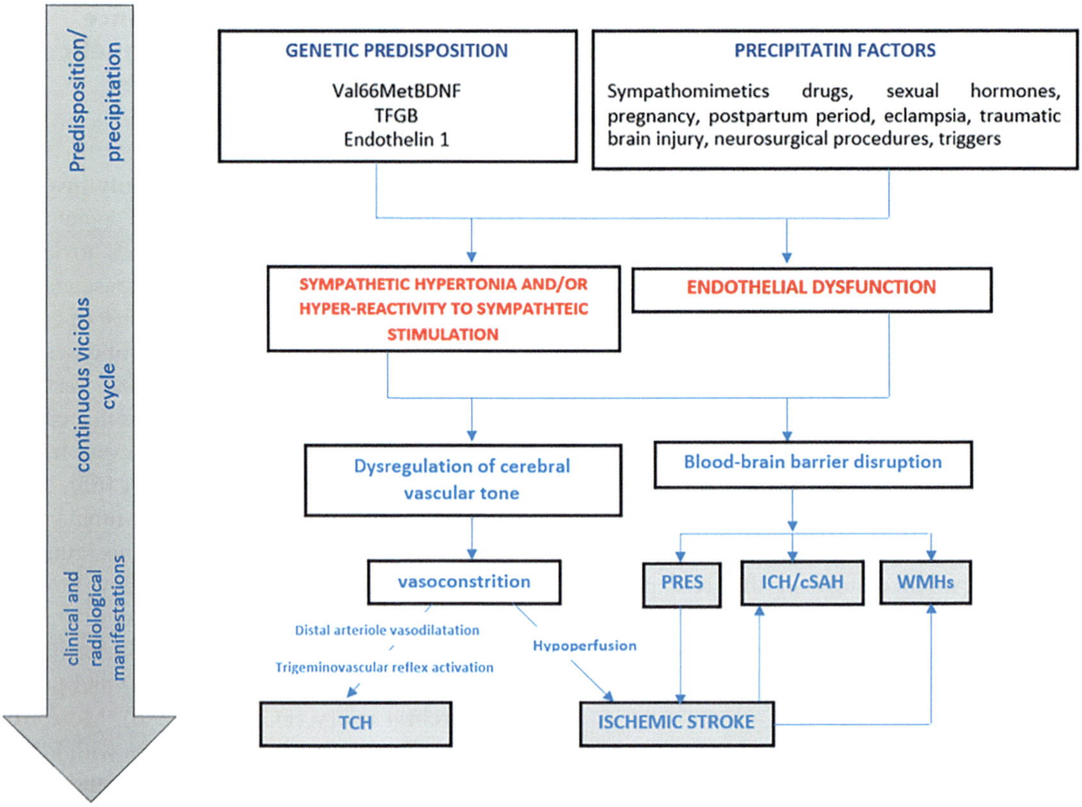

Fig. 9.1 Proposed model of the pathophysiology of RCVS. Development of RCVS is sequential (as indicated by the gradient arrow on the left of the figure). Predisposition and precipitating factors are both required to initiate and perpetuate a vicious cycle of pathogenic mechanisms that result in the clinical and radiological manifestations of RCVS. Dysregulation of cerebral vascular tone and disruption of blood–brain barrier (BBB) seem to be crucial in the pathophysiology of RCVS. Both of them are a consequence of the endothelial disfunction, the sympathetic overactivity, and the oxidative stress, mediated by mechanical and biochemical stimuli. When autoregulatory mechanisms and BBB integrity are further compromised, and the body's protective responses fail, symptoms such as headaches, vasoconstriction, and other complications may arise. In particular hemorrhagic complications (cSAH and ICH) or PRES are consequences of the breakdown of BBB, while the ischemic stroke is linked to hypoperfusion caused by vasoconstriction of major cerebral arteries. White matter hyperintensity lesions could be explained by either the increased BBB permeability or partial ischemia due to cerebral hypoperfusion. The thunderclap headache could be attributable to the dilatation of distal arterioles or meningeal arteries that activate the trigeminovascular nociceptive fibers

atherosclerosis, dissection, fibromuscular dysplasia, and vasculitis). The main mimics is primary central nervous system vasculitis (PACNS). In PACNS, large-caliber vessels of the circle of Willis and their collateral branches are involved. Additionally, vessel wall MRI sequences (vw-MRI) can be useful in the differential diagnosis, since there is no contrast enhancement of the affected arterial wall in RCVS, whereas enhancement is detectable in vasculitis [5, 67]. Moreover, while in PACNS only cerebral vessels are involved, involvement of extracranial vessels is rare in RCVS.

9.6.2 Catheter Angiography

The diagnostic gold standard remains digital subtraction angiography. During angiography, smooth tapered narrowings followed by abnormal dilated segments can be visualized. This

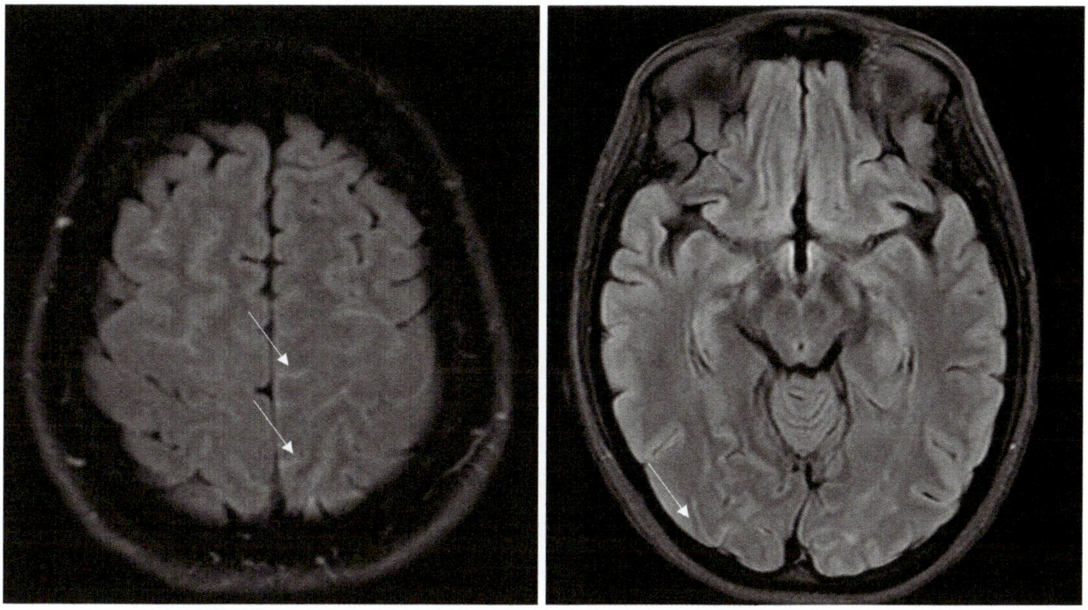

Fig. 9.2 Hyperintense vessels on FLAIR images in two patients affected by RCVS (arrows)

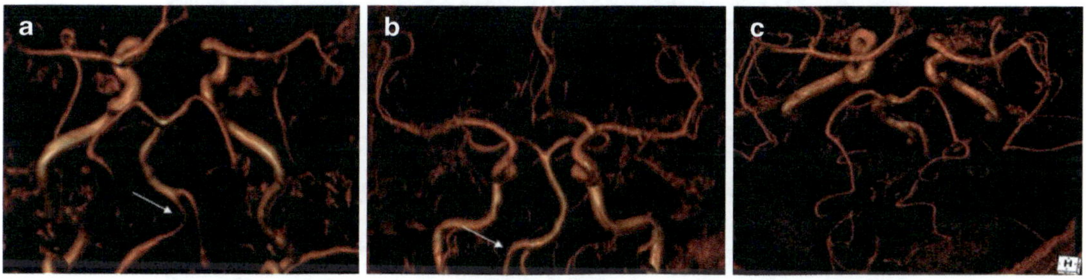

Fig. 9.3 Radiological findings of a 58-year-old female who was admitted to the emergency department due to a thunderclap headache, and diagnosed with RCVS. (**a**) The initial angio CT showed bilateral V4 vasoconstriction (arrow) and narrowing posterior cerebral arteries. (**b**) Three months later, a complete resolution of vertebral arteries vasoconstriction was observed on angio-TC (arrows). (**c**) Also posterior cerebral arteries appeared completely normalized on the follow-up imaging

alternation of narrowings and dilatations is responsible for the typical "sausage on strings" appearance [68]. Angiography also allows for the exclusion of alternative diagnoses and the study of vasospasm reversibility through intra-arterial administration of vasodilators [31]. This is particularly useful because the diagnosis of RCVS is often made retrospectively once the reversible nature of vasospasm is demonstrated. Being able to assert early in the disease process that it is reversible vasospasm significantly advances diagnosis and enables more informed patient monitoring. In fact, in up to a third of cases angiographic evaluation is normal within the first week of symptom onset, due to centripetally proceeding vasospasm [65].

Finally, normalization of angiographic findings is typically observed within 8–12 weeks. However, the evolution of cerebral vasospasm is not uniform, so while some vessels improve, others worsen during the monitoring period [69].

9.6.3 Perfusion Imaging

Lastly, there is limited data on the use of perfusion CT: from clinical experience and a few published case reports, we know that perfusion CT shows multiple areas of hypoperfusion, reflecting the effect of vasospasm that can acutely progress to ischemia [70, 71]. This information could potentially be used in the future to monitor response to treatment with vasodilators [70].

Alternatively, arterial spin-labeling perfusion is a completely non-invasive MRI technique that does not require the administration of gadolinium contrast. Instead, it utilizes electromagnetic spin inversion to label water molecules, which then act as freely diffusible flow tracers [5] (Fig. 9.4).

9.6.4 Transcranial Doppler Sonography

Transcranial Doppler ultrasound can play a role in demonstrating increased morpho-velocimetric profiles suggesting vasospasm and reduced caliber of Internal Carotid arteries (ICA), MCAs, and anterior cerebral arteries (ACAs) [7, 72]. Sonographic studies may also be inconclusive in the early stages, while higher peak velocities are typically observed after approximately 3 weeks. Moreover, peak velocities >120 cm/s and a Lindegaard index (maximum velocity in MCA/maximum velocity in ICA) >3 are associated with an increased risk of developing PRES [72]. Patients with hyperintense vessels (HVs) initially exhibited maximum velocities in the middle cerebral artery (MCA) of up to

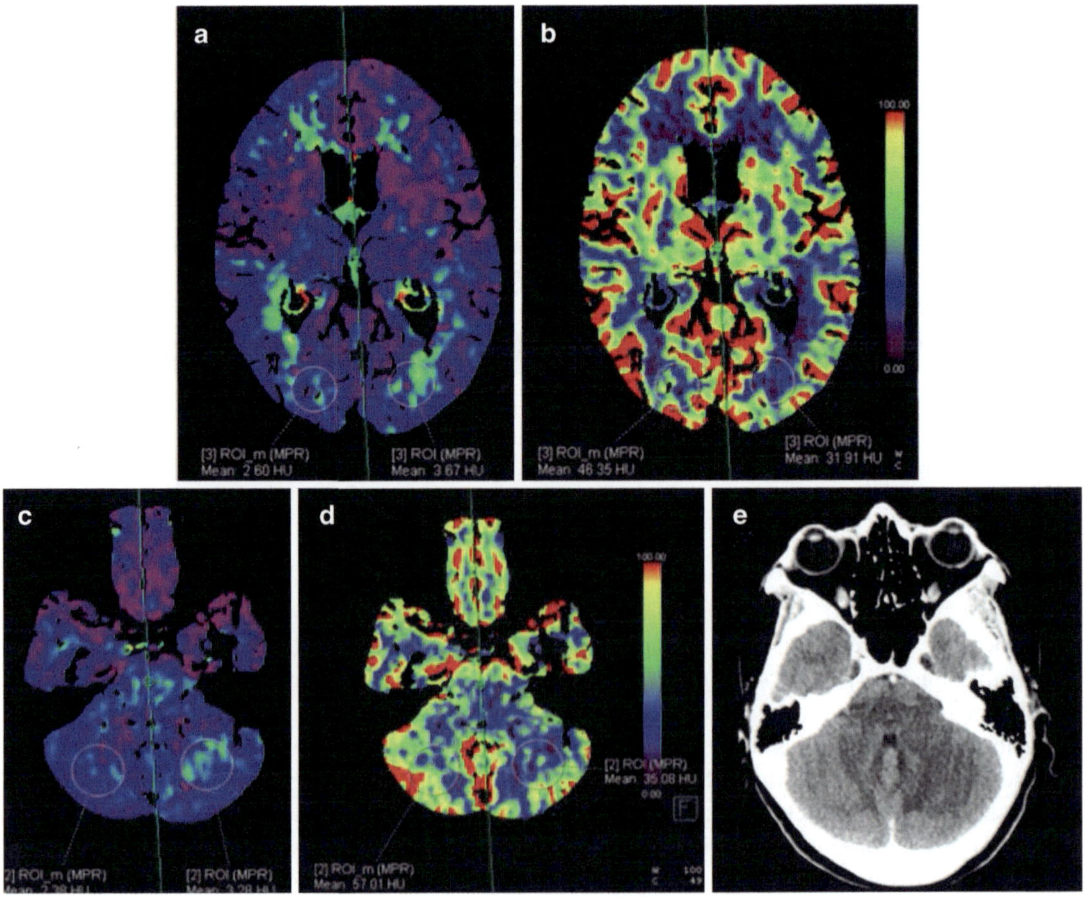

Fig. 9.4 Radiological features of a 37-year-old female with cocaine-induced RCVS, admitted to the emergency department due to headache and bilateral hypovision. Perfusion CT showed an increased TMAX and reduced CBF in the left occipital lobe (**a**, **b**) and in the left cerebellar hemisphere (**c**, **d**). (**e**) CT scan revealed a cerebral infarct in the left cerebellar hemisphere, corresponding to the region identified on the perfusion CT

121.0 ± 39.5 cm/s and a Lindegaard index (LI) up to 2.8 ± 1.2, approaching the cutoff criteria for predicting severe outcomes such as PRES or ischemic stroke (VMCA >120 cm/s and LI >3). This underscores HVs as a severity marker in RCVS. Bedside ultrasound is also useful for follow-up. Normalization of findings in this case is typically achieved within 12 weeks [72].

9.6.5 Clinical-Radiological Complications

Complications from RCVS are more commonly observed in treatment-related forms [73]. Up to 81% of patients exhibit the following radiological abnormalities appearing days to weeks after the onset of thunderclap headache: cerebral ischemia (39%), intraparenchymal hemorrhage typically lobar in 20%, convexity subarachnoid hemorrhage in 34%, and PRES in 38% [4] (Fig. 9.5).

Cerebral vasoconstriction peaks 9–13 days after the initial thunderclap headache [10, 74] and progresses in a disto-proximal direction. This is the reason why ischemic and hemorrhagic complications have a different temporal distribution, occurring at varying times throughout the course of RCVS. Initially, ischemic lesions are due to perfusion deficits caused by altered arteriolar autoregulation and are small, peripheral, and cortical (at the cortico–subcortical junction) [4, 7]. After approximately 2 weeks, vasoconstriction of larger caliber vessels leads to severe hypoperfusion and lesions are larger, wedge-shaped, and watershed [4]. Vasoconstriction of small distal pial vessels may lead to reperfusion injury with subsequent vessel wall rupture and hemorrhagic stroke typically in watershed areas (as shown in Fig. 9.5), which tends to manifest earlier (2–4 days after the headache attack) than ischemic counterparts [75]. RCVS is also the leading cause of convexity subarachnoid hemorrhage in individuals <60 years old [76]. In these patients, thunderclap headache, FLAIR dot sign, and multifocal vasoconstriction are diagnostic of RCVS [7]. Young age, history of severe headache, chronic obstructive pulmonary disease requiring sympathomimetics (e.g., ephedrine), antidepressant use, low Hunt Hess score or Fisher score, and involvement of multiple arteries including bilateral were independent predictors of RCVS-SAH [77].

The type of lesion cannot be reliably predicted based on triggering factors, except for eclampsia, since it is associated with both PRES and RCVS. PRES and RCVS share the same pathophysiological mechanisms: blood–brain barrier disruption and endothelial dysfunction, leading to passive extravasation of fluids and proteins resulting in vasogenic edema, which appears as hyperintensities on apparent diffusion coefficient (ADC) mapping. Impaired cerebral autoregulation in cases of PRES is observed in >85% of cases, leading to vasospasm [4]. Furthermore, also estrogens are supposed to play a role in both pathologies.

Female sex, cocaine use, and a history of hypertension are risk factors for hemorrhagic complications, instead [75].

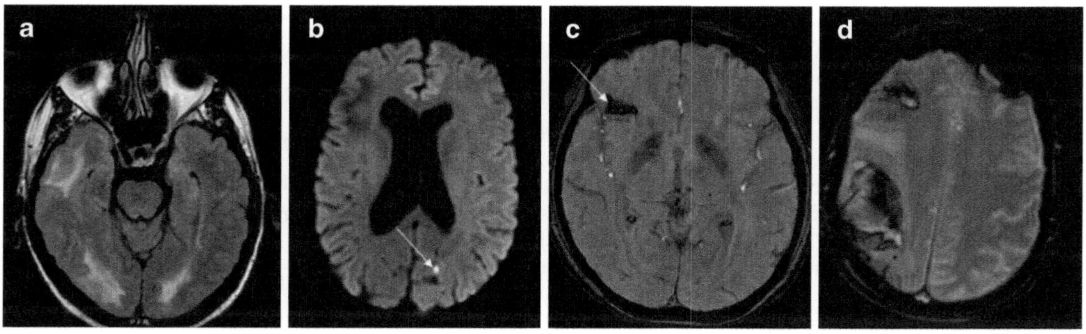

Fig. 9.5 Overview of potential complications of RCVS in four different patients. (**a**) Posterior reversible encephalopathy syndrome appearing as hyperintense lesions on fluid attenuated inversion recovery imaging (FLAIR). (**b**) Ischemic strokes (arrow) appearing as hyperintensities on diffusion weighted imaging (DWI). (**c**) Convexity subarachnoid hemorrhage shown as the hypointensity on gradient echo imaging. (**d**) Parenchymal hemorrhages in temporo-parietal and frontal lobar areas

9.7 Diagnostic Process and Differential Diagnosis

Thunderclap headache, especially if occurring in a single episode, necessitates differential diagnosis with other potentially fatal conditions such as subarachnoid hemorrhage due to aneurysm rupture, parenchymal hemorrhage, posterior or middle cerebral artery embolism, cervical dissection, venous sinus thrombosis, and brain infections. Useful elements for differential diagnosis include medical history focusing particularly on RCVS triggers, imaging, and lumbar puncture [5]. Immediate brain Computerized Tomography (CT) should be performed, and, if possible, Computerized Tomography Angiography (CTA) should be obtained immediately [7]. If subarachnoid hemorrhage is present, the distribution of blood allows for further evaluations: in cases of RCVS, subarachnoid hemorrhage is most often confined to superficial sulci, which differs from aneurysmal subarachnoid hemorrhage where blood is localized in the basal cisterns/circle of Willis [5]. If brain CT does not show acute findings, lumbar puncture should be performed to rule out subarachnoid or parenchymal hemorrhage and inflammatory conditions [78, 79]. Conversely, if lumbar puncture is also normal, brain MRI and MRA are warranted. MRI venography should be considered in order to exclude a cerebral venous thrombosis.

PACNS represents the most important mimic due to overlapping characteristics such as headache, stroke, and vessel wall irregularities [68]. Distinguishing these two entities is particularly important because glucocorticoids administered in cases of vasculitis would worsen outcomes in patients with RCVS [80]. Table 9.4 summarizes the main diagnostic findings helpful for differential diagnosis. Patients with primary angiitis of the central nervous system also present with dull chronic headache, scattered deep infarcts, and involvement of smaller cerebral arteries [7]. Additionally, noncontrast CT scan with multiple ischemic lesions of different ages suggests a form of vasculitis.

Diagnostic criteria have been proposed. The RCVS2 scoring system (Table 9.5) allows confirmation of the diagnostic suspicion with high accuracy, excluding mimics such as primary angiitis of the central nervous system [81].

Table 9.5 $RCVS_2$ score

Criteria	Value
Recurrent or single TCH	Present 5 Absent 0
Involvement of intracranial carotid artery	Affected 2 Not affected 0
Vasoconstrictive trigger	Present 3 Absent 0
Sex	Female 1 Male 0
Subarachnoid hemorrhage	Present 1 Absent 0

Score ≥ 5 had high sensitivity and specificity for diagnosing RCVS, and score ≤ 2 for excluding RCVS. Intermediate scores 3 and 4 had moderate specificity and low sensitivity for RCVS

Table 9.4 Different causes of narrowing of cerebral arteries and thunderclap-like headache

Variable	RCVS	PACNS	SAH-induced vasospasm
CSF findings	Usually normal or mild increase in protein levels and mild pleocytosis	Abnormal up to 90% elevated levels of proteins, moderate pleocytosis, presence of oligoclonal bands and intrathecal IgG synthesis	Xanthochromia, elevated red blood cell count
Parenchymal and vascular brain imaging findings	Normal MRI or presence of watershed ischemic strokes, parieto-occipital vasogenic edema (PRES), parenchymal (lobar and deep) hemorrhages or cSAH. Widespread, symmetrical tapering reversible vasoconstriction and vasodilation of intracranial vessels	Acute/subacute/chronic disseminated ischemic lesions in gray and white matter, hemorrhagic lesions with mass effect and possible white matter lesions. Irregular, eccentric, notched with distal cutoffs, irreversible Multiple, irreversible intracranial stenoses Meningeal and vessel wall enhancement	Blood in the Sylvian fissure and the basal cisterna Possible ruptured aneurysm or arteriovenous malformation. Reversal segmental narrowing occurs after 4–14 days

9.8 Prognosis and Management

Prognosis in RCVS is favorable both in adults and adolescents. More than 90% of patients achieve a good outcome, defined as Modifying Rankin score (mRs) 0–1 [4]. A worse outcome is associated with baseline neurological deficits and the onset of cerebral ischemia in the early phase of the disease [82]. Furthermore, despite the term "reversible," recurrence can occur in 5–10% of cases [83]. Headache may persist beyond vasospasm resolution; follow-up studies show that about 50% of patients continue to experience chronic headaches for more than a year, and 26% develop depression [84]. In these cases, triptan administration is often avoided due to limited data on the effects of re-exposure to triggering factors. Non-pharmacological approaches should be preferred for antidepressant administration for the same reason [7].

Treatment remains symptomatic to date: analgesics or calcium channel blockers for headache relief, removal of vasoconstrictive factors, and avoidance of glucocorticoids, which can significantly worsen outcomes. Actually, calcium channel blockers (verapamil, nimodipine) do not appear to affect vasospasm but rather the intensity of headache [7]. A prospective observational study in 2019 demonstrated that early administration of nimodipine (6–13 days post-onset) was independently linked to a shorter clinical course [17]. Nimodipine effectively prevented recurrent thunderclap headaches (TCHs), with few complications reported. The authors suggested that nimodipine could stabilize vasoconstriction and subsequent vasodilation in distal small arteries, potentially halting the centripetal spread of vasoconstriction and reducing the likelihood of complications.

Some case reports have shown clinical and angiographic benefit with intra-arterial administration of vasodilators. However, this strategy may be reserved for patients with clear clinical deterioration, considering the procedural risks such as reperfusion injury and rebound vasoconstriction, which could be fatal [85].

There is currently no evidence supporting specific treatment or prevention. Despite the high risk of ischemic stroke, there is no indication for antiplatelet agents or anticoagulants [7]. Furthermore, in cases of severe vasoconstriction, hypotension should be avoided. Given the sympathomimetic action of infused drugs in hypotension state, maintaining stable blood pressure through adequate hydration is to be preferred [7].

9.9 Conclusions

RCVS is a unifying term used to describe a group of disorders characterized by thunderclap headaches, which may or may not be associated with neurological complications, and reversible centripetal narrowing and dilatation of cerebral arteries. It exhibits a dynamic course, and despite its reversibility, clinical presentation can be severe and its complications dramatic. The pathophysiology remains unknown, necessitating further studies not only to understand its enigmatic origins but also to identify effective treatments.

References

1. Calabrese LH, Dodick DW, Schwedt TJ, Singhal AB. Narrative review: reversible cerebral vasoconstriction syndromes. Ann Intern Med. 2007;146(1):34–44. https://doi.org/10.7326/0003-4819-146-1-200701020-00007.
2. Chen SP, Wang SJ. Pathophysiology of reversible cerebral vasoconstriction syndrome. J Biomed Sci. 2022;29(1):72. https://doi.org/10.1186/s12929-022-00857-4.
3. Chen SP, Fuh JL, Lirng JF, Chang FC, Wang SJ. Recurrent primary thunderclap headache and benign CNS angiopathy: spectra of the same disorder? Neurology. 2006;67(12):2164–9. https://doi.org/10.1212/01.wnl.0000249115.63436.6d.
4. Erhart DK, Ludolph AC, Althaus K. RCVS: by clinicians for clinicians—a narrative review. J Neurol. 2023;270(2):673–88. https://doi.org/10.1007/s00415-022-11425-z.
5. Miller TR, Shivashankar R, Mossa-Basha M, Gandhi D. Reversible cerebral vasoconstriction syndrome, part 2: diagnostic work-up, imaging evaluation, and differential diagnosis. AJNR Am J Neuroradiol. 2015;36(9):1580–8. https://doi.org/10.3174/ajnr.A4215.
6. Parikh NS, Navi BB, Schneider Y, Jesudian A, Kamel H. Association between cirrhosis and stroke in a nationally representative cohort. JAMA

Neurol. 2017;74(8):927–32. https://doi.org/10.1001/jamaneurol.2017.0923.
7. Singhal AB. Reversible cerebral vasoconstriction syndrome: A review of pathogenesis, clinical presentation, and treatment. Int J Stroke. 2023;18(10):1151–60. https://doi.org/10.1177/17474930231181250.
8. Topcuoglu MA, McKee KE, Singhal AB. Gender and hormonal influences in reversible cerebral vasoconstriction syndrome. Eur Stroke J. 2016;1(3):199–204. https://doi.org/10.1177/2396987316656981.
9. Coffino SW, Fryer RH. Reversible cerebral vasoconstriction syndrome in pediatrics: a case series and review. J Child Neurol. 2017;32(7):614–23. https://doi.org/10.1177/0883073817696817.
10. Ducros A, Boukobza M, Porcher R, Sarov M, Valade D, Bousser MG. The clinical and radiological spectrum of reversible cerebral vasoconstriction syndrome. A prospective series of 67 patients. Brain. 2007;130(Pt 12):3091–101. https://doi.org/10.1093/brain/awm256.
11. Schwedt TJ, Matharu MS, Dodick DW. Thunderclap headache. Lancet Neurol. 2006;5(7):621–31. https://doi.org/10.1016/S1474-4422(06)70497-5.
12. Kato Y, Hayashi T, Sano H, Kato R, Tanahashi N, Takao M. Cough headache presenting with reversible cerebral vasoconstriction syndrome. Intern Med. 2018;57(10):1459–61. https://doi.org/10.2169/internalmedicine.0061-17.
13. Mak W, Tsang KL, Tsoi TH, et al. Bath-related headache. Cephalalgia. 2005;25(3):191–8. https://doi.org/10.1111/j.1468-2982.2004.00832.x.
14. Hu CM, Lin YJ, Fan YK, Chen SP, Lai TH. Isolated thunderclap headache during sex: orgasmic headache or reversible cerebral vasoconstriction syndrome? J Clin Neurosci. 2010;17(10):1349–51. https://doi.org/10.1016/j.jocn.2010.01.052.
15. Headache Classification Committee of the International Headache Society (IHS). The international classification of headache disorders, 3rd ed (beta version). Cephalalgia. 2013;33(9):629–808. https://doi.org/10.1177/0333102413485658.
16. Singhal AB, Hajj-Ali RA, Topcuoglu MA, et al. Reversible cerebral vasoconstriction syndromes: analysis of 139 cases. Arch Neurol. 2011;68(8):1005–12. https://doi.org/10.1001/archneurol.2011.68.
17. Cho S, Lee MJ, Chung CS. Effect of nimodipine treatment on the clinical course of reversible cerebral vasoconstriction syndrome. Front Neurol. 2019;10:644. https://doi.org/10.3389/fneur.2019.00644.
18. Lange KS, Choi SY, Ling YH, Chen SP, Mawet J, Duflos C, Lee MJ, Ducros A, Wang SJ, Pezzini A. Reversible cerebral vasoccostrition syndrome international Collaborative (REVERCE) network: study protocol and rationale of a multicentre research collaboration. Eur Stroke J. 2023;8(4):1107–13. https://doi.org/10.1177/23969873231182207.
19. Hamel E. Perivascular nerves and the regulation of cerebrovascular tone. J Appl Physiol (1985). 2006;100(3):1059–64. https://doi.org/10.1152/japplphysiol.00954.2005.
20. Duckworth JW, Wellman GC, Walters CL, Bevan JA. Aminergic histofluorescence and contractile responses to transmural electrical field stimulation and norepinephrine of human middle cerebral arteries obtained promptly after death. Circ Res. 1989;65(2):316–24. https://doi.org/10.1161/01.res.65.2.316.
21. Mayhan WG. Responses of cerebral arterioles to activation of beta-adrenergic receptors during diabetes mellitus. Stroke. 1994;25(1):141–6. https://doi.org/10.1161/01.str.25.1.141.
22. Topcuoglu MA, Chan ST, Silva GS, Smith EE, Kwong KK, Singhal AB. Cerebral vasomotor reactivity in reversible cerebral vasoconstriction syndrome. Cephalalgia. 2017;37(6):541–7. https://doi.org/10.1177/0333102416650706.
23. Chen SP, Chang YA, Chou CH, Juan CC, Lee HC, Chen LK, Wu PC, Wang YF, Fuh JL, Lirng JF, Ducros A, Huang HD, Wang SJ. Circulating microRNAs Associated With reversible cerebral vasoconstriction syndrome. Ann Neurol. 2021;89(3):459–73. https://doi.org/10.1002/ana.25965.
24. Chen SP, Fuh JL, Wang SJ, Tsai SJ, Hong CJ, Yang AC. Brain-derived neurotrophic factor gene Val66Met polymorphism modulates reversible cerebral vasoconstriction syndromes. PLoS One. 2011;6(3):e18024. https://doi.org/10.1002/ana.25965.
25. Chen SP, Wang YF, Huang PH, Chi CW, Fuh JL, Wang SJ. Reduced circulating endothelial progenitor cells in reversible cerebral vasoconstriction syndrome. J Headache Pain. 2014;15(1):82. https://doi.org/10.1186/1129-2377-15-82.
26. Urbich C, Dimmeler S. Endothelial progenitor cells: characterization and role in vascular biology. Circ Res. 2004;95(4):343–53. https://doi.org/10.1161/01.RES.0000137877.89448.78.
27. Chen SP, Chung YT, Liu TY, Wang YF, Fuh JL, Wang SJ. Oxidative stress and increased formation of vasoconstricting F2-isoprostanes in patients with reversible cerebral vasoconstriction syndrome. Free Radic Biol Med. 2013;61:243–8. https://doi.org/10.1016/j.freeradbiomed.2013.04.022.
28. Pun PB, Lu J, Moochhala S. Involvement of ROS in BBB dysfunction. Free Radic Res. 2009;43(4):348–64. https://doi.org/10.1080/10715760902751902.
29. Wu CH, Lirng JF, Wu HM, et al. Blood-brain barrier permeability in patients with reversible cerebral vasoconstriction syndrome assessed with dynamic contrast-enhanced MRI. Neurology. 2021;97(18):e1847–59. https://doi.org/10.1212/WNL.0000000000012776.
30. Chen CY, Chen SP, Fuh JL, et al. Vascular wall imaging in reversible cerebral vasoconstriction syndrome – a 3-T contrast-enhanced MRI study. J Headache Pain. 2018;19(1):74. https://doi.org/10.1186/s10194-018-0906-7.
31. Elstner M, Linn J, Müller-Schunk S, Straube A. Reversible cerebral vasoconstriction syn-

drome: a complicated clinical course treated with intra-arterial application of nimodipine. Cephalalgia. 2009;29(6):677–82. https://doi.org/10.1111/j.1468-2982.2008.01768.x.
32. Katz BS, Fugate JE, Ameriso SF, et al. Clinical worsening in reversible cerebral vasoconstriction syndrome. JAMA Neurol. 2014;71(1):68–73. https://doi.org/10.1001/jamaneurol.2013.4639.
33. Karlsberg P, Adams JE, Elliot HW. Inhibition and reversal of serotonin-induced cerebral vasospasm. Surg Forum. 1962;13:425–7.
34. Meschia JF, Malkoff MD, Biller J. Reversible segmental cerebral arterial vasospasm and cerebral infarction: possible association with excessive use of sumatriptan and Midrin. Arch Neurol. 1998;55(5):712–4. https://doi.org/10.1001/archneur.55.5.712.
35. Kato Y, Hayashi T, Mizuno S, et al. Triptan-induced reversible cerebral vasoconstriction syndrome: two case reports with a literature review. Intern Med. 2016;55(23):3525–8. https://doi.org/10.2169/internalmedicine.55.7185.
36. Griffin CE 3rd, Kaye AM, Bueno FR, Kaye AD. Benzodiazepine pharmacology and central nervous system-mediated effects. Ochsner J. 2013;13(2):214–23.
37. Belliston S, Sundararajan J, Hammond N, Newell K, Lynch S. Reversible cerebral vasoconstriction syndrome in association with fingolimod use. Int J Neurosci. 2017;127(9):831–4. https://doi.org/10.1080/00207454.2016.1257991.
38. Schwarz A, Korporal M, Hosch W, Max R, Wildemann B. Critical vasospasm during fingolimod (FTY720) treatment in a patient with multiple sclerosis. Neurology. 2010;74(24):2022–4. https://doi.org/10.1212/WNL.0b013e3181e3972b.
39. Rot U, Ledinek AH. Interferons beta have vasoconstrictive and procoagulant effects: a woman who developed livedo reticularis and Raynaud phenomenon in association with interferon beta treatment for multiple sclerosis. Clin Neurol Neurosurg. 2013;115(Suppl 1):S79–81. https://doi.org/10.1016/j.clineuro.2013.09.027.
40. Strohm T, Chaudhry B, Willis MA, Shook S. Reversible cerebral vasoconstriction syndrome associated with interferon beta-1a use for multiple sclerosis. Mult Scler. 2016;22(12):1626–8. https://doi.org/10.1177/1352458516641774.
41. Wang X, Zhang Y, You H, Zhu T, Zhou D. A case of reversible cerebral vasoconstriction syndrome triggered by high-dose methotrexate in a boy with lymphoma. Headache. 2020;60(8):1767–72. https://doi.org/10.1111/head.13526.
42. Rozen TD, Bhatt AA. Reversible cerebral vasoconstriction syndrome developing after an erenumab injection for migraine prevention. Cephalalgia. 2022;42(3):250–6. https://doi.org/10.1177/03331024211037277.
43. Mi X, Ran L, Chen L, Qin G. Recurrent headache increases blood-brain barrier permeability and VEGF expression in rats. Pain Physician. 2018;21(6):E633–42.
44. Liu J, Guo M, Beegle RD, Miao R, Manoucheri MA. Case report of reversible cerebral vasoconstriction syndrome in a patient with systemic scleroderma. Cureus. 2022;14(4):e24364. https://doi.org/10.7759/cureus.24364.
45. Shima A, Maki T, Mimura N, et al. A case of reversible cerebral vasoconstriction syndrome associated with anti-phospholipid antibody syndrome and systemic lupus erythematosus. eNeurologicalSci. 2021;24:100351. https://doi.org/10.1016/j.ensci.2021.100351.
46. Atsumi T, Khamashta MA, Haworth RS, et al. Arterial disease and thrombosis in the antiphospholipid syndrome: a pathogenic role for endothelin 1. Arthritis Rheum. 1998;41(5):800–7. https://doi.org/10.1002/1529-0131(199805)41:5<800::AID-ART5>3.0.CO;2-J.
47. Kawanabe Y, Takahashi M, Jin X, et al. Cilostazol prevents endothelin-induced smooth muscle constriction and proliferation. PLoS One. 2012;7(9):e44476. https://doi.org/10.1371/journal.pone.0044476.
48. Maeda S, Saito S, Toda K, et al. A case of tacrolimus-induced reversible cerebral vasoconstriction syndrome after heart transplantation. Gen Thorac Cardiovasc Surg. 2020;68(12):1483–6. https://doi.org/10.1007/s11748-020-01309-2.
49. Khan WJ, Asif M, Aslam S, Nadeem I, Rossing W. Reversible cerebral vasoconstriction syndrome associated With oxybutynin use; a brief review of pathophysiology. J Community Hosp Intern Med Perspect. 2023;13(4):31–4. https://doi.org/10.55729/2000-9666.1192.
50. Yeboah K, Bittar J, Almajali M, Soudagar Turkey M, Ramiro J. Transfusion-related acute brain injury: a case report on reversible cerebral vasoconstriction syndrome. Cureus. 2020;12(7):e9077. https://doi.org/10.7759/cureus.9077.
51. Maddula M, Sprigg N, Bath PM, Munshi S. Cerebral misery perfusion due to carotid occlusive disease. Stroke Vasc Neurol. 2017;2(2):88–93. https://doi.org/10.1136/svn-2017-000067.
52. Liang H, Xu Z, Zheng Z, Lou H, Yue W. Reversible cerebral vasoconstriction syndrome following red blood cells transfusion: a case series of 7 patients. Orphanet J Rare Dis. 2015;10:47. https://doi.org/10.1186/s13023-015-0268-z.
53. Kothari N, Acharya S, Banode P. Reversible cerebral angiopathy after blood transfusion. Asian J Transfus Sci. 2012;6(1):56–8.
54. Short K, Emsley HCA. Illicit drugs and reversible cerebral vasoconstriction syndrome. Neurohospitalist. 2021;11(1):40–4. https://doi.org/10.1177/1941874420953051.
55. Calic Z, Choong H, Schlaphoff G, Cappelen-Smith C. Reversible cerebral vasoconstriction syndrome following indomethacin. Cephalalgia. 2014;34(14):1181–6. https://doi.org/10.1177/0333102414530526.
56. Summ O, Andreou AP, Akerman S, Goadsby PJ. A potential nitrergic mechanism of action for indo-

methacin, but not of other COX inhibitors: relevance to indomethacin-sensitive headaches. J Headache Pain. 2010;11(6):477–83. https://doi.org/10.1007/s10194-010-0263-7.
57. Schertz AR, Sarma AK, Datar S, Miller PJ. Reversible cerebral vasoconstriction syndrome (RCVS) caused by over-the-counter calcium supplement ingestion. BMJ Case Rep. 2021;14(1):e233877. https://doi.org/10.1136/bcr-2019-233877.
58. Feske SK. Posterior reversible encephalopathy syndrome: a review. Semin Neurol. 2011;31(2):202–15. https://doi.org/10.1055/s-0031-1277990.
59. Ospina JA, Duckles SP, Krause DN. 17beta-estradiol decreases vascular tone in cerebral arteries by shifting COX-dependent vasoconstriction to vasodilation. Am J Physiol Heart Circ Physiol. 2003;285(1):H241–50. https://doi.org/10.1152/ajpheart.00018.2003.
60. Soo Y, Singhal AB, Leung T, et al. Reversible cerebral vasoconstriction syndrome with posterior leucoencephalopathy after oral contraceptive pills. Cephalalgia. 2010;30(1):42–5. https://doi.org/10.1111/j.1468-2982.2009.01868.x.
61. Freilinger T, Schmidt C, Duering M, Linn J, Straube A, Peters N. Reversible cerebral vasoconstriction syndrome associated with hormone therapy for intrauterine insemination. Cephalalgia. 2010;30(9):1127–32. https://doi.org/10.1177/0333102409360675.
62. Choi S, Lee JY, Bae JS, Song HK, Lee JH, Kim Y. Reversible cerebral vasoconstriction syndrome associated with levonorgestrel-releasing intrauterine system. Brain Sci. 2021;11(5):601. https://doi.org/10.3390/brainsci11050601.
63. Moussavi M, Korya D, Panezai S, Peeraully T, Gizzi M, Kirmani JF. Reversible cerebral vasoconstriction syndrome in a 35-year-old woman following hysterectomy and bilateral salpingo-oophorectomy. J Neurointerv Surg. 2012;4(6):e35. https://doi.org/10.1136/neurintsurg-2011-010122.
64. Pop A, Carbonnel M, Wang A, Josserand J, Auliac SC, Ayoubi JM. Posterior reversible encephalopathy syndrome associated with reversible cerebral vasoconstriction syndrome in a patient presenting with postpartum eclampsia: a case report. J Gynecol Obstet Hum Reprod. 2019;48(6):431–4. https://doi.org/10.1016/j.jogoh.2019.03.019.
65. Chen SP, Fuh JL, Lirng JF, Wang SJ. Hyperintense vessels on flair imaging in reversible cerebral vasoconstriction syndrome. Cephalalgia. 2012;32(4):271–8. https://doi.org/10.1177/0333102412437387.
66. Lee MJ, Cha J, Choi HA, et al. Blood-brain barrier breakdown in reversible cerebral vasoconstriction syndrome: implications for pathophysiology and diagnosis. Ann Neurol. 2017;81(3):454–66. https://doi.org/10.1002/ana.24891.
67. Mandell DM, Matouk CC, Farb RI, et al. Vessel wall MRI to differentiate between reversible cerebral vasoconstriction syndrome and central nervous system vasculitis: preliminary results. Stroke. 2012;43(3):860–2. https://doi.org/10.1161/STROKEAHA.111.626184.
68. Singhal AB, Topcuoglu MA, Fok JW, et al. Reversible cerebral vasoconstriction syndromes and primary angiitis of the central nervous system: clinical, imaging, and angiographic comparison. Ann Neurol. 2016;79(6):882–94. https://doi.org/10.1002/ana.24652.
69. Chen SP, Fuh JL, Wang SJ, et al. Magnetic resonance angiography in reversible cerebral vasoconstriction syndromes. Ann Neurol. 2010;67(5):648–56. https://doi.org/10.1002/ana.21951.
70. Komatsu T, Kimura T, Yagishita A, Takahashi K, Koide R. A case of reversible cerebral vasoconstriction syndrome presenting with recurrent neurological deficits: evaluation using noninvasive arterial spin labeling MRI. Clin Neurol Neurosurg. 2014;126:96–8. https://doi.org/10.1016/j.clineuro.2014.08.023.
71. Rosenbloom MH, Singhal AB. CT angiography and diffusion-perfusion MR imaging in a patient with ipsilateral reversible cerebral vasoconstriction after carotid endarterectomy. AJNR Am J Neuroradiol. 2007;28(5):920–2.
72. Chen SP, Fuh JL, Chang FC, Lirng JF, Shia BC, Wang SJ. Transcranial color Doppler study for reversible cerebral vasoconstriction syndromes. Ann Neurol. 2008;63(6):751–7. https://doi.org/10.1002/ana.21384.
73. Caria F, Zedde M, Gamba M, et al. The clinical spectrum of reversible cerebral vasoconstriction syndrome: The Italian Project on Stroke at Young Age (IPSYS). Cephalalgia. 2019;39(10):1267–76. https://doi.org/10.1177/0333102419849013.
74. Wolff V, Armspach JP, Lauer V, et al. Ischaemic strokes with reversible vasoconstriction and without thunderclap headache: a variant of the reversible cerebral vasoconstriction syndrome? Cerebrovasc Dis. 2015;39(1):31–8. https://doi.org/10.1159/000369776.
75. Ducros A, Fiedler U, Porcher R, Boukobza M, Stapf C, Bousser M. Hemorrhagic manifestations of reversible cerebral vasoconstriction syndrome: frequency, features, and risk factors. Stroke. 2010;41(11):2050–511. https://doi.org/10.1161/STROKEAHA.109.572313.
76. Kumar S, Goddeau RP Jr, Selim MH, et al. Atraumatic convexal subarachnoid hemorrhage: clinical presentation, imaging patterns, and etiologies. Neurology. 2010;74(11):893–9. https://doi.org/10.1212/WNL.0b013e3181d55efa.
77. Muehlschlegel S, Kursun O, Topcuoglu MA, Fok J, Singhal AB. Differentiating reversible cerebral vasoconstriction syndrome with subarachnoid hemorrhage from other causes of subarachnoid hemorrhage. JAMA Neurol. 2013;70(10):1254–60. https://doi.org/10.1001/jamaneurol.2013.3484.
78. Edlow JA. Managing patients with nontraumatic, severe, rapid-onset headache. Ann Emerg Med. 2018;71(3):400–8. https://doi.org/10.1016/j.annemergmed.2017.04.044.
79. Manning T, Bartow C, Dunlap M, Kiehl R, Kneale H, Walker A. Reversible cerebral vasoconstriction syndrome associated with fluoxetine. J Acad Consult

Liaison Psychiatry. 2021;62(6):634–44. https://doi.org/10.1016/j.jaclp.2021.07.013.
80. Singhal AB, Topcuoglu MA. Glucocorticoid-associated worsening in reversible cerebral vasoconstriction syndrome. Neurology. 2017;88(3):228–36. https://doi.org/10.1212/WNL.0000000000003510.
81. Rocha EA, Topcuoglu MA, Silva GS, Singhal AB. RCVS2 score and diagnostic approach for reversible cerebral vasoconstriction syndrome. Neurology. 2019;92(7):e639–47. https://doi.org/10.1212/WNL.0000000000006917.
82. Robert T, Kawkabani Marchini A, Oumarou G, Uské A. Reversible cerebral vasoconstriction syndrome identification of prognostic factors. Clin Neurol Neurosurg. 2013;115(11):2351–7. https://doi.org/10.1016/j.clineuro.2013.08.014.
83. Chen SP, Fuh JL, Lirng JF, Wang YF, Wang SJ. Recurrence of reversible cerebral vasoconstriction syndrome: a long-term follow-up study. Neurology. 2015;84(15):1552–8. https://doi.org/10.1212/WNL.0000000000001473.
84. John S, Singhal AB, Calabrese L, et al. Long-term outcomes after reversible cerebral vasoconstriction syndrome. Cephalalgia. 2016;36(4):387–94. https://doi.org/10.1177/0333102415591507.
85. Singhal AB, Kimberly WT, Schaefer PW, Hedley-Whyte ET. Case records of the Massachusetts General Hospital. Case 8-2009. A 36-year-old woman with headache, hypertension, and seizure 2 weeks post partum. N Engl J Med. 2009;360(11):1126–37. https://doi.org/10.1056/NEJMcpc0809063.

10 Neuroradiological Findings in Neurological Adverse Events of CAR T therapy

Federica Pondrelli, Simone Rossi, Gian Maria Asioli, Luca Spinardi, and Maria Guarino

10.1 Introduction

In the last decade, the development of immune-based therapies has revolutionized the treatment of both solid and haematological malignancies.

Immunotherapy represents a novel anticancer strategy promoting the activation of immune effector cells with the aim of improving their natural ability to fight cancer cells.

Among the various treatments developed in recent years, chimeric antigen receptor (CAR) T-cell therapy and immune checkpoint inhibitors (ICIs) have consistently proven their efficacy. These innovations have been able to significantly improve the standard of care of both solid and haematological neoplasms.

However, they are hampered by adverse events, including neurotoxicity, increasing the complexity in the management of oncological patients [1, 2].

Authors Federica Pondrelli and Simone Rossi have equally contributed to this chapter.

F. Pondrelli · S. Rossi · G. M. Asioli · M. Guarino (✉)
IRCCS Istituto delle Scienze Neurologiche di Bologna, Bologna, Italy
e-mail: federica.pondrelli@aosp.bo.it; maria.guarino@aosp.bo.it

L. Spinardi
IRCCS Azienda Ospedaliero-Universitaria di Bologna, Bologna, Italy
e-mail: luca.spinardi@aosp.bo.it

10.2 CAR T-Cell Therapy

CAR T-cell therapy has revolutionized the treatment of refractory haematological malignancies in recent years conferring complete remission responses in 33–57% of patients, up to 92% in acute lymphoblastic leukaemia (B-ALL) [3]. CAR T cells are created starting from the apheresis of autologous lymphocytes. T lymphocytes are then genetically engineered via a viral vector to express the Chimeric Antigen Receptor (CAR) protein. At this point, after in vitro expansion of the CAR T cells and the administration of conditioning chemotherapy, they are reinfused in one single shot.

Several tumour antigens have been investigated as targets of CAR T cells. Among these, CD19-targeted CAR T cells are the most advanced in clinical development and are currently approved by the U.S. Food and Drug Administration (FDA) for various B-cell malignancies: B-cell acute lymphoblastic leukaemia, large B-cell lymphoma, follicular lymphoma, mantle cell lymphoma, and chronic lymphocytic leukaemia.

More recently, BCMA-targeting CAR T cells have also been approved for the treatment of multiple myeloma (MM). Moreover, attempts to expand the clinical use of CAR T cells in the treatment of solid cancers, autoimmune disorders, and chronic infections are currently a hot field of research [4].

M. Zedde, R. Pascarella (eds.), *Neuroimaging of Treatment-Related Conditions in the Brain*,
https://doi.org/10.1007/978-3-032-23618-0_10

Besides the promising efficacy of these therapies, the problem of toxicities has emerged. These are driven by the activation of infused CAR T cells leading to exaggerated cytokine-mediated inflammatory responses. Cytokine release syndrome (CRS) is the most frequent form of toxicity, characterized by systemic symptoms, usually occurring within 48 h of the infusion and possibly evolving to multi-organ failure.

Immune Effector Cell-Associated Neurotoxicity Syndrome (ICANS) is another frequent life-threatening complication almost consistently occurring after CRS. However, it presents in a minority of patients and usually a few days later in respect of CRS, supporting at least in part a different pathogenesis.

Strong evidence supports a cytokine-mediated neuroinflammatory process as the underlying mechanism, where the peripheral inflammation leads to blood-brain barrier disruption and endothelial dysfunction, resulting in astrocyte and microglia activation.

ICANS consists of a wide spectrum of acute neurological manifestations up to fulminant cerebral oedema.

In this clinical context, neuroimaging can aid in diagnosing and monitoring neurotoxicity in CAR T-cell recipients. In addition, nuclear medicine and advanced techniques of magnetic resonance are currently a hot field of research with the aim of better understanding ICANS pathophysiology and provide possible biomarkers.

10.2.1 Epidemiology and Risk Factors of ICANS

The incidence of ICANS widely varies between studies ranging from 37.5% to 77% [5]. A recent systematic review reports a pooled incidence of ICANS with CAR T-cell therapy of 26.9% for all-grade and 10.5% for high-grade (≥ grade 3) [6].

Risk factors for ICANS development in CAR T-cell therapy have been investigated by several studies without univocal results. However, they can be classified into three main categories: factors related to the type of malignancy and treatment, factors related to the host, and factors related to inflammatory state:

1. *Factors Related to the Type of Malignancy and Treatment:*
   - *Lymphoma Subtype*: aggressive lymphomas (i.e., diffuse large B-cell lymphoma (DLBCL) and primary mediastinal B-cell lymphoma (PMBCL)) are associated with a higher risk of ICANS.
   - *Tumour Burden*: a higher tumour burden at the time of infusion.
   - *CAR T-Cell Product*: constructs containing CD28 costimulatory domain (i.e., Axi-cel and Brexu-cel) confer a faster kinetics of T-cell activations.
   - *Dose of CAR T Cells*: higher doses are linked to increased neurotoxicity risk.
2. *Factors Related to the Host:*
   - *Age*: some studies found older patients at higher risk hypothetically due to blood-brain barrier (BBB) dysfunction.
   - *Pre-Existing Neurological Conditions*: patients with a history of CNS disorders may have a higher risk (but there was high variability between studies in definitions).
   - *Performance Status*: Poor baseline performance status correlates with a higher risk of ICANS.
3. *Factors Related to Inflammatory State:*
   - *Baseline Inflammatory Markers*: elevated inflammatory markers (e.g., ferritin, C-reactive protein) prior to treatment initiation indicate an inflammatory state at baseline, which seem consistently associated with a higher risk of ICANS.
   - *Cytokine Release Syndrome* (CRS): CRS almost invariably precedes ICANS onset suggesting a common pathophysiological pathway. However, their interconnection is complex and not clarified yet, as supported by different treatment strategies (at least in part).

Understanding these risk factors is crucial for identifying patients at higher risk of developing ICANS and consequently strictly monitoring them to implement therapeutic strategies if necessary.

10.2.2 Pathophysiology of ICANS

The pathophysiology of ICANS is intricately linked to the immune activation seen in CAR T-cell therapy and other immune effector cell therapies and is believed to be initiated by an exaggerated systemic production of pro-inflammatory mediators, typical of CRS. This is supported by the observation that CRS almost invariably precedes ICANS onset, which has been observed to occur in isolation only in rare cases showing mild manifestations.

The inflammatory cytokines and chemokines (interleukin (IL)-1β, IL-6, IL-10, CXCL8, CCL2, interferon-γ, granulocyte macrophage colony-stimulating factor (GMC-SF) and tumour necrosis factor (TNF)) are massively released in response to the activation of CAR T cells and macrophages in the tumour microenvironment [7]. Among them, IL 6 may have a central role in the complex interplay between CRS and ICANS by promoting cellular functions between CAR T cell and macrophage [8].

Besides cytokine-driven inflammation, blood-brain barrier disruption is a key feature of ICANS. In fact, the systemic production of pro-inflammatory factors leads to endothelial cell activation and disruption of the BBB. This allows for the entry of cytokines and immune effector cells into the brain parenchyma, inducing in severe cases neuronal swelling with risk of irreversible damage.

Another crucial element is represented by microglial activation, resulting in the production of more pro-inflammatory factors and reactive oxygen species (ROS). These can contribute to neuronal dysfunction and consequent impairment of neurotransmission with excitotoxicity.

Interestingly, an on-target off-tumour effect has also been postulated considering some evidence of CD19 expression in human brain mural cells (pericytes and vascular smooth muscle cells) [9].

In conclusion, while much remains to be learned about the exact mechanisms of ICANS, current evidence points to a complex interaction between immune system activation, cytokine release, BBB disruption, and microglial activation [8].

10.2.3 Clinical Presentation of ICANS

The core clinical feature of ICANS is represented by encephalopathy of various grades typically associated with signs of frontal lobe dysfunction (language disturbances, dysgraphia, apraxia) [10–12].

The course is extremely heterogeneous with some patients experiencing only mild neurological manifestations and spontaneous recovery, while a subgroup worse manifesting seizures, akinetic mutism, and coma, rarely until death due to fulminant cerebral oedema.

Neurotoxicity, which is almost constantly preceded by CRS, typically manifests in the first week after CAR-T-cell administration although in rare cases later onset has been reported [13, 14]. The hallmark symptoms of ICANS include the following:

- *Cognitive Impairment*: confusion, aphasia, attention deficits, and apraxia. These cognitive changes typically reflect a frontal lobe dysfunction ranging from subtle to more severe forms (i.e., akinetic mutism).
- *Dysgraphia*: writing difficulties characterized by grammatical errors or letter sizing are very frequent in patients affected by neurotoxicity. In addition, paligraphia has been observed to precede the clinical onset of severe ICANS, representing a possible specific predictor [15].
- *Seizures*: manifestation of severe ICANS (grade 3 per definition), possibly a marker of increased intracranial pressure. They can be focal or generalized and progress to status epilepticus.
- *Altered Mental Status*: this may range from mild ideo-motor slowing to coma, with some

patients exhibiting fluctuating levels of consciousness.

- *Other Symptoms*: Headache (not specific but alarming since it may indicate increased intracranial pressure and risk of diffuse cerebral oedema); tremor (not specific but very frequently observed as an early symptom of neurotoxicity).

ICANS is graded by the ASTCT consensus criteria using the immune effector cell-associated encephalopathy assessment tool (ICE score) (Table 10.1), which comprehends specific items on writing, orientation, attention, naming, and following commands. ICE score together with the level of consciousness and other clinical elements (i.e., seizures or signs of elevated intracranial pressure) determines the final ICANS grade of severity[1] (Table 10.2).

Since ICANS manifestations are not generally specific, other conditions, such as infections, metabolic disturbances, and stroke, must be considered. In this scenario, diagnostic tools such as neuroimaging can aid in the differential diagnosis.

10.2.4 Management of ICANS

Early recognition of ICANS is essential to allowing correct management and significantly impact patient outcomes. In this regard, close monitoring of CAR T-cell recipients is crucial to detect early signs of neurological deterioration and implement adequate supportive treatments.

Table 10.1 ICE score

Orientation: orientation to year, month, city, hospital: 4 points
Naming: ability to name 3 objects (eg. point to clock, pen, button): 3 points
Following commands: ability to follow simple commands (eg. "Show me 2 fingers" or "close your eyes and stick out your tonguw"): 1 point
Writing: ability to write a standard sentence (eg. "Our national bird is bald eagle"): 1 point
Attention: ability to count backwards from 100 by 10: 1 point

In mild ICANS (grade 1) the approach is supportive. Instead, corticosteroids are the cornerstone of the treatment for more severe cases (from ICANS grade 2). Importantly, reassuring data are emerging on the impact of corticosteroids on CAR T-cell therapy efficacy [16–18]. Thus, they are implemented from grade 2 and promptly tapered to intravenous high doses in case of deterioration or persistence of neurotoxicity. Concomitantly, an ICU admission is usually required.

At this point, if a satisfactory response is not obtained, it is possible to implement the use of monoclonal antibodies able to block the action of cytokines: higher doses of anakinra targeting IL-1 receptor and siltuximab targeting IL-6 [19]. Even if trials are lacking, these agents seem to be effective in the treatment of both CRS and ICANS [20, 21].

On the contrary, tocilizumab, an IL-6 receptor antagonist, does not have a clear therapeutic impact on ICANS patients. Moreover, it may actually have a detrimental effect since the IL-6 remaining in circulation can massively enter into the CNS.

10.2.5 Neuroimaging in ICANS

Neuroimaging can provide valuable information on the structural and functional changes occurring within the brain during ICANS helping clinicians in differential diagnosis [22]. In clinical practice, computed tomography (CT) and magnetic resonance imaging (MRI) are the most used techniques while, in the field of research, also positron emission tomography (PET) and advanced MRI are of great interest.

10.2.5.1 CT Imaging in ICANS

CT scans are often the first-line imaging modality due to their rapid acquisition time and widespread availability. However, CT scan has limited sensitivity compared to MRI in detecting subtle changes associated with neuroinflammation and generally results unremarkable. However, CT scan can reveal acute cerebral oedema in the rare

Table 10.2 ICANS grade

Neurotoxicity Domain	Grade 1	Grade 2	Grade 3	Grade 4
ICE score	7–9	3–6	0–2	0 (patient is unarousable and unable to perform ICE)
Depressed level of consciousness	Awakens spontaneously	Awakens to voice	Awakens only to tactile stimulus	Patient is unarousable or requires vigorous or repetitive tactile stimuli to arouse. Stupor or coma
Seizure	N/A	N/A	Any clinical seizure focal or generalized that resolves rapidly or nonconvulsive seizures on EEG that resolve with intervention	Life-threatening prolonged seizure (>5 min); or Repetitive clinical or electrical seizures without return to baseline in between
Motor findings	N/A	N/A	N/A	Deep focal motor weakness such as hemiparesis or paraparesis
Elevated ICP/ cerebral edema	N/A	N/A	Focal/local edema on neuroimaging	Diffuse cerebral edema on neuroimaging; decerebrate or decorticate posturing; or cranial nerve VI palsy; or papilledema; or Cushing's triad

cases presenting with fulminant intracranial hypertension [23] (Fig. 10.1). Moreover, it can play a role in the differential diagnosis with ischemic changes or haemorrhagic lesions [24].

10.2.5.2 Brain MRI in ICANS

Even if only small case series have been described, it emerged that brain MRI is usually not informative in ICANS patients. In fact, in a recent description of a CD19-targeted CAR T-cell recipient cohort by Pensato et al. 2021 [12], brain MRI during the acute phase was altered in 26% of ICANS patients. Similar results have been reported in the cohort described by Gust et al. 2017 [25], showing 30% of pathological MRI in ICANS patients. However, in severe ICANS (grade 3 or higher), the probability to observe pathological findings seems to increase (up to 53% in Gust et al. 2017 [25]).

Although not pathognomonic, recurrent patterns of structural changes have been found during ICANS:

- *Symmetric T2/FLAIR Hyperintensities in Deep White and Grey Matter*: bilateral thalami, the external capsules, the dorsal brainstem, and the hippocampi (Fig. 10.2). These are predominantly detected during the acute phase of severe ICANS (generally with grade $\geq$ 3) and seem to be reversible in patients with good outcomes, as we described in a previous report. [26] ICANS grades 1–2 seem less associated with these kinds of alterations [25].

  Interestingly, this pattern resembles those seen in the Central Variant of Posterior Reversible Encephalopathy Syndrome (PRES) and Wernicke encephalopathy [27]. Based on this observation, it has been hypothesized that these regions may be more susceptible to endothelial or metabolic injury due to their rich vascularization.
- *Supratentorial White Matter T2/FLAIR Hyperintensities*: they may occur in the periventricular or juxtacortical locations, isolated or multifocal, sometimes showing diffusion restriction. These are extremely non-specific findings whose significance, as well as whose clinical correlates, are not well defined. Some authors highlighted the similarity with small vessel disease or pre-infusion chemotherapeutic toxicity (methotrexate or fludarabine). However, pre-infusion MRI data, which could help in better clarifying the underlying pathogenesis of these alterations, is currently lacking (Fig. 10.3).
- *Leptomeningeal Enhancement*: diffuse or patchy leptomeningeal enhancement has been reported in high-grade neurotoxicity, probably expressing blood-brain barrier disruption (Fig. 10.4).

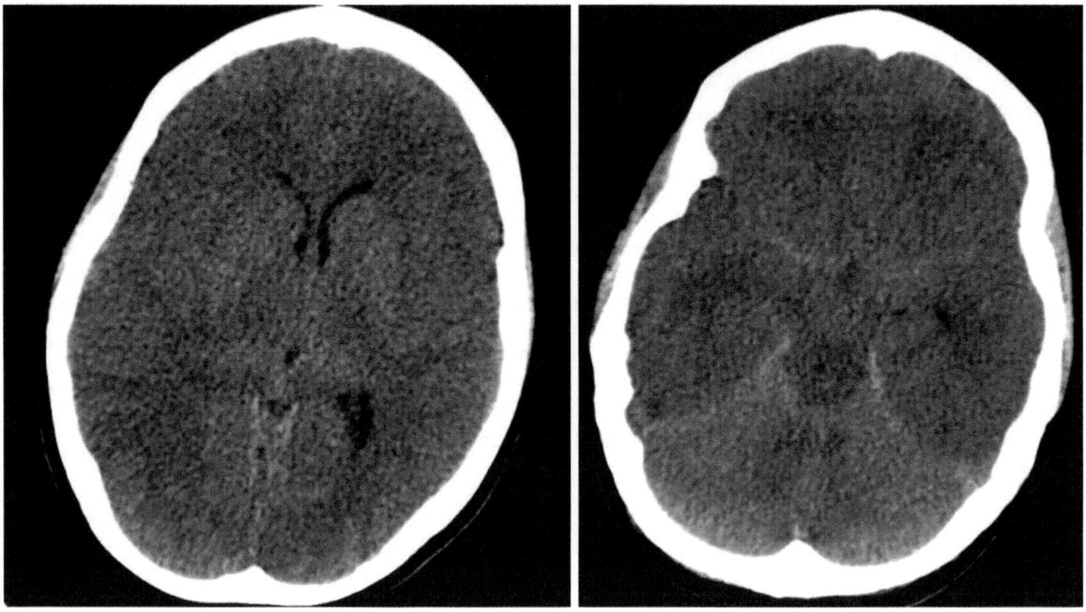

Fig. 10.1 CT scan in a patient with fulminant cerebral oedema

- *Cerebral Oedema*: this finding reflects a life-threatening condition, needing a prompt therapeutic intervention. In MRI study, it consists of widespread or focal T2/FLAIR hyperintensity with altered diffusion (increased for vasogenic oedema or restricted for cytotoxic oedema). This finding is documented generally in patients with ICANS grade $\geq$ 3 (Fig. 10.5).

10.2.5.3 Positron Emission Tomography (PET)

Data on brain FDG-PET in CAR T-cell therapy recipients are scant, but quite uniform. In fact, the observations made in case reports [28, 29] and two small cohorts [12, 30] point to a hypometabolism in the cortex of patients affected by ICANS. No specific patterns have been identified; however, it seems that there may be a prevalence of involvement of the frontal lobes, which is consistent with the clinical manifestation of encephalopathy with frontal dysfunction. An example is represented in Fig. 10.5.

10.2.5.4 Advanced MRI Techniques

To date, only one study [31] analysed the potential of the application of advanced MRI techniques in patients developing ICANS. They applied resting-state functional MRI (rsfMRI) on a small cohort of ICANS patients and they consistently found an increased dysconnectivity index (DCI), particularly pronounced in the language-dominant hemisphere (Figs. 10.6, 10.7, 10.8, and 10.9).

10.2.6 Late-Onset Toxicities Associated with BCMA-Targeted CAR T Cells

In recipients of CAR T-cell therapy targeting BCMA antigen, a rare acute-subacute neurotoxicity syndrome with delayed onset (2–6 months after infusion) has been reported. Since it is characterized by extrapyramidal movement disorders and cognitive impairment, it has been named "movement and neurocognitive treatment-emergent adverse events" (MNTs).

MNTs exhibit a rapidly progressive course and poor responsiveness to both symptomatic treatments (dopaminergic drugs, acetylcholinesterase inhibitors) and immunotherapy.

The underlying pathogenetic mechanism seems related to an "on-target, off-tumour" phe-

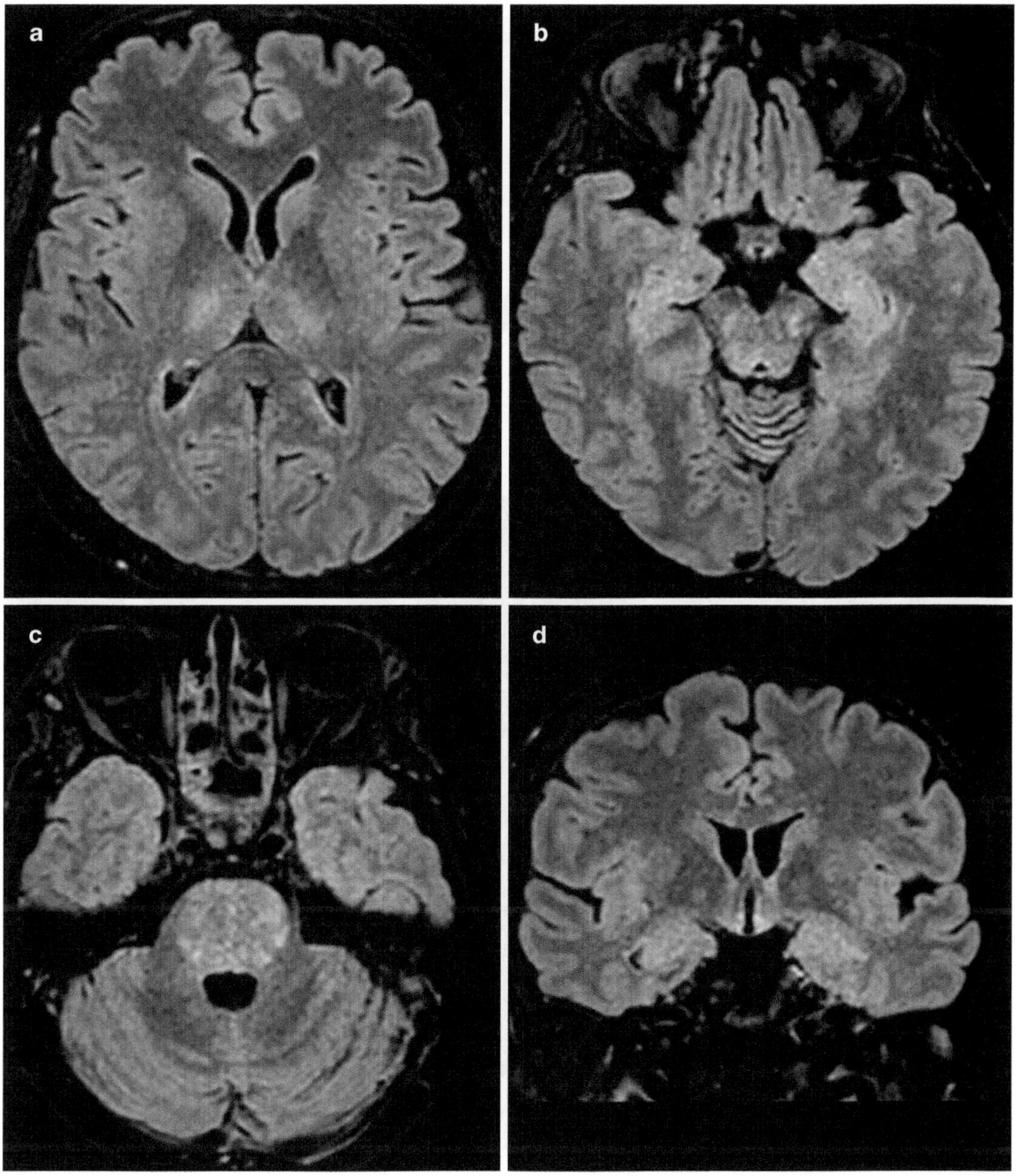

Fig. 10.2 Brain MRI findings in a patient with ICANS grade 3: bilateral and symmetrical T2/FLAIR hyperintensities in the thalami (**a**), hippocampi (**b–d**), pons (**c**)

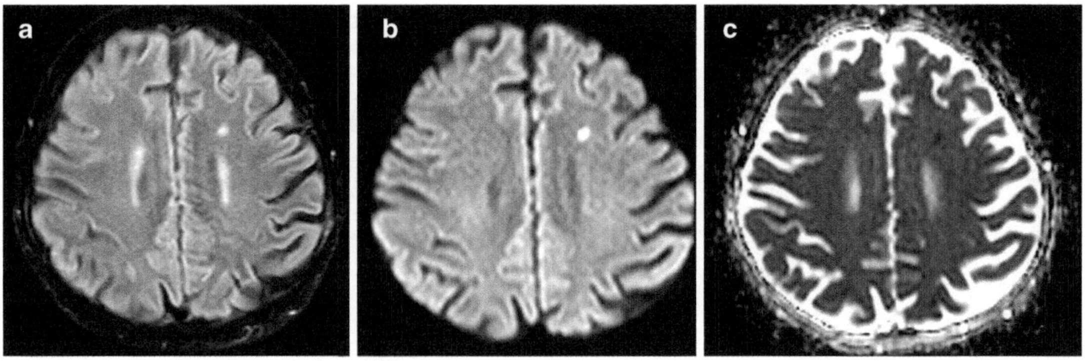

Fig. 10.3 Brain MRI findings at 40 days from infusion in a patient who previously developed ICANS grade 2: a small ovoidal area of T2/FLAIR hyperintensity (**a**) in the right subcortical frontal region, showing altered diffusion in DWI (**b**) with low value of ADC (**c**), thus consisting with cytotoxic oedema

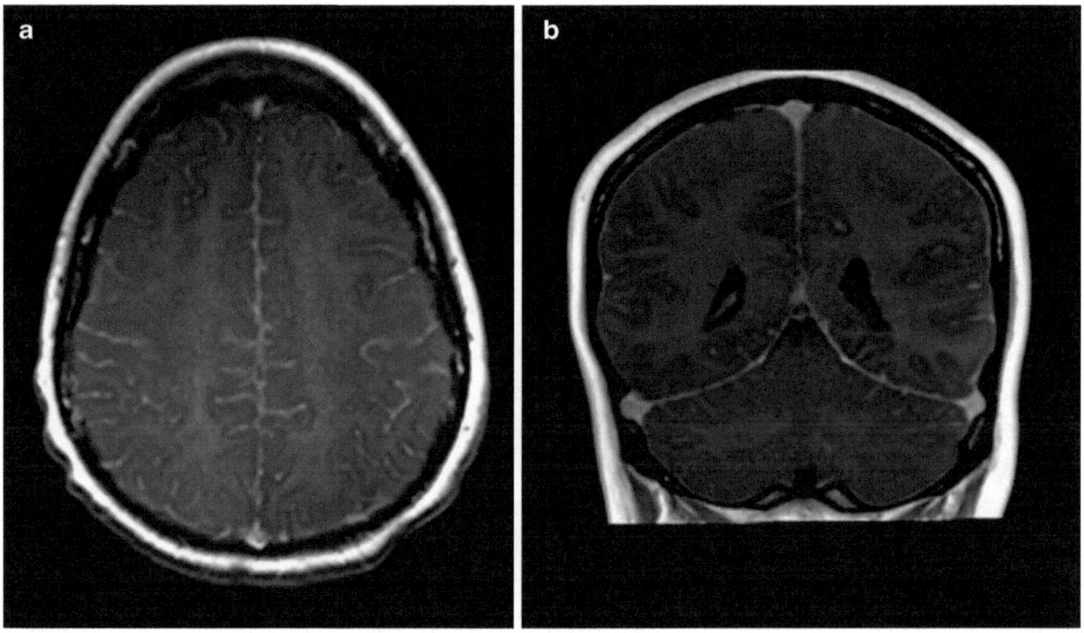

Fig. 10.4 Brain MRI findings in a comatose patient with fulminant cerebral oedema who subsequently succumbed: diffuse leptomeningeal enhancement on T1 with gadolinium sequences

nomenon, due to the expression of the target antigen on healthy cells and tissues. BCMA-targeted CAR T cells, after crossing the BBB, bind to BCMA-expressing basal ganglia cells, leading to their destruction, as demonstrated in anatomopathological studies on the brains of deceased patients [32].

In this context, brain MRI and cerebral DatScan are almost invariably unremarkable. Only anecdotal cases [33, 34] have been reported to show bilateral T2/FLAIR hyperintensities in the caudate head, the putamen, and the globus pallidus with a reversible course.

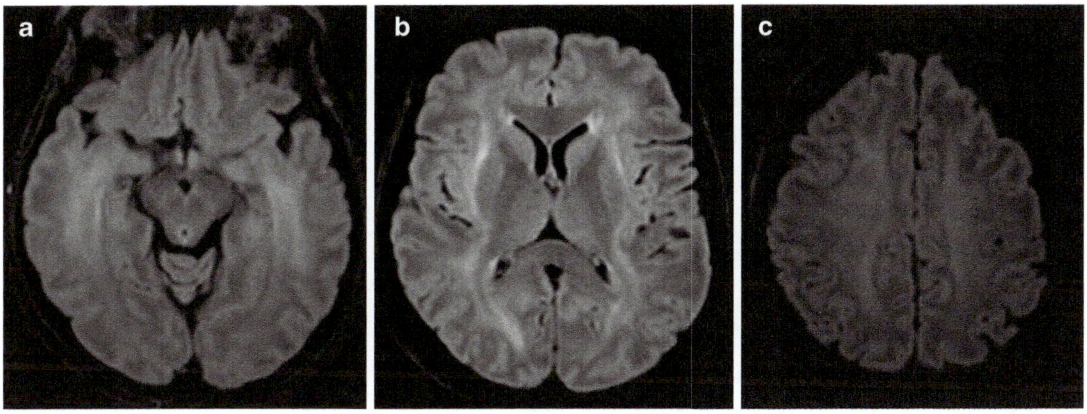

Fig. 10.5 Brain MRI findings during ICANS grade 4 manifesting with non-convulsive status epilepticus: diffuse bilateral T2/FLAIR hyperintensities in the white matter consisting of cerebral oedema

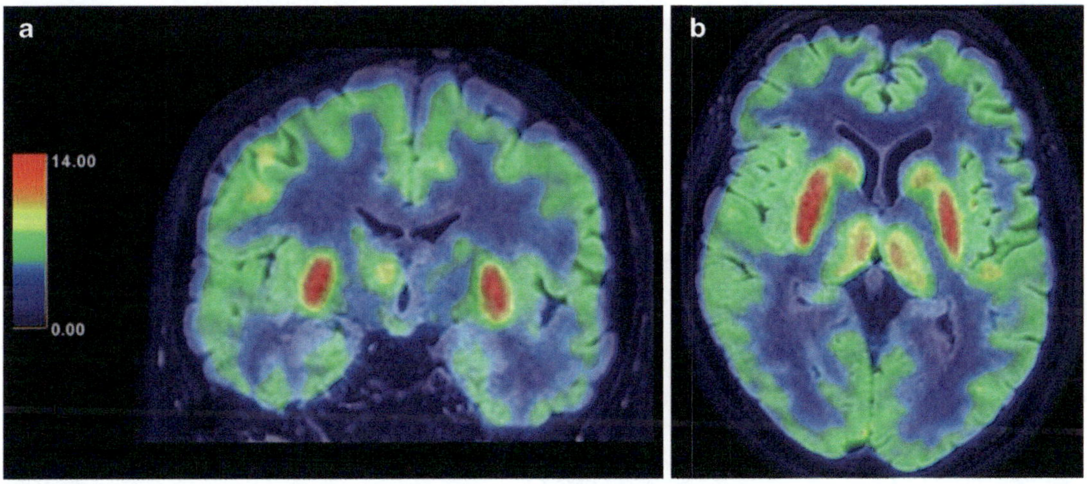

Fig. 10.6 Brain [18F]-fluorodeoxyglucose PET showing diffuse cortical hypofixation during ICANS 3

10.2.7 Differential Diagnosis and the Role of Neuroimaging in the Diagnostic Work-Up

Neuroimaging plays an adjuvant role in diagnosing and monitoring ICANS, offering insights into the underlying neurotoxic processes and aiding in clinical decision-making. It plays a role in excluding alternative causes of CNS dysfunction and to detect alterations being the expression of neuroinflammation, blood-brain barrier disruption, and microglial activation.

The principal differential diagnosis are as follows:

- CNS Infections: The underlying haematological disorder and lymphodepleting therapy can lead to significant immunosuppression with risk of both systemic and CNS-related infective complications. These are characterized by suggestive signs on MRI, such as diffuse meningeal enhancement, T2/FLAIR hyperintensities in viral encephalitis (HHV6, HSV1–2), or cerebritis and abscesses in fungal or bacterial infections.

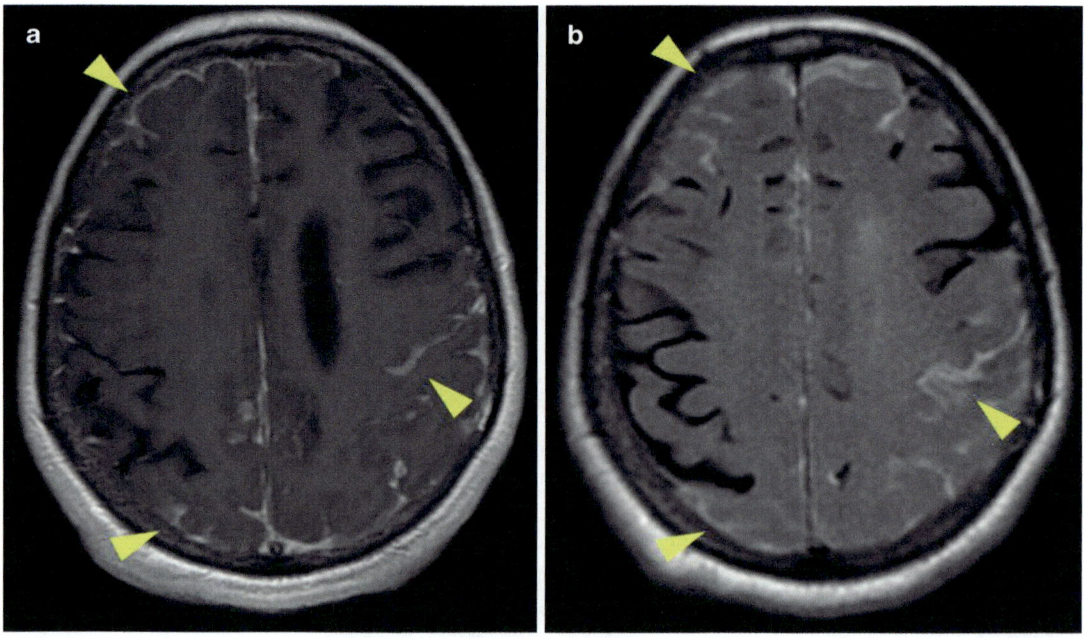

Fig. 10.7 Post-contrast T1 (**a**) and post-contrast FLAIR (**b**) axial sequences showing leptomeningeal enhancement in a 77-year-old male patient with immune-related meningoencephalitis following 6 cycles of pembrolizumab for non-small cell lung cancer. Note the diffuse and linear aspect of enhancement

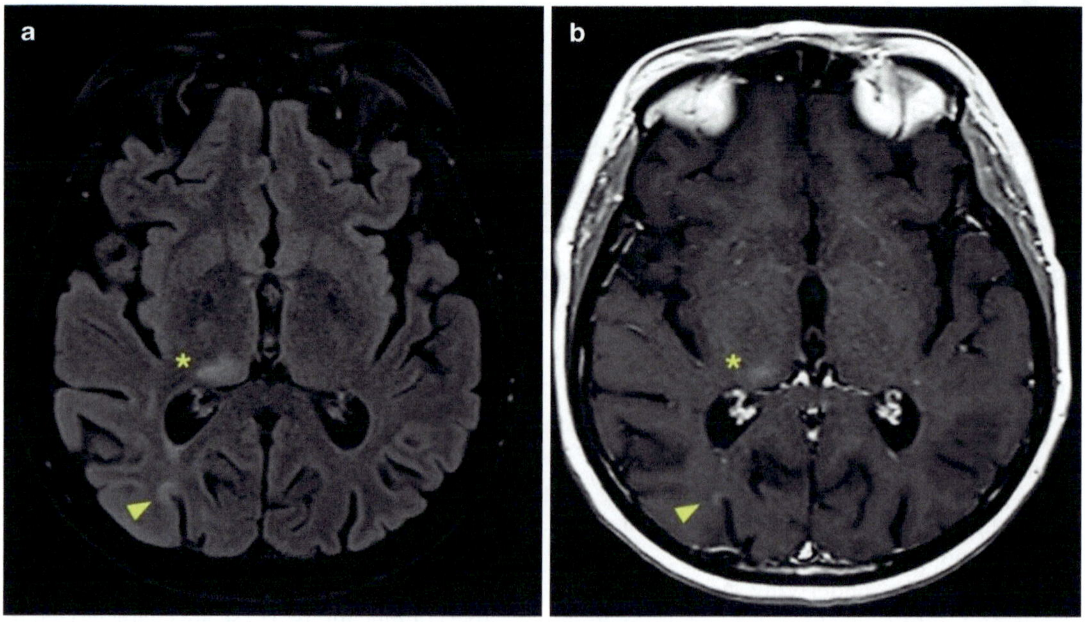

Fig. 10.8 Axial FLAIR sequence showing patchy and multifocal hyperintense lesions in cortical-subcortical parietal lobes and thalamic nuclei, in a 53-year-old female patient presenting with diffuse encephalopathy and focal parieto-occipital seizures following 12 cycles of pembrolizumab for non-small cell lung cancer. In post-contrast T1 images, the lesions present a blurry and faint gadolinium enhancement

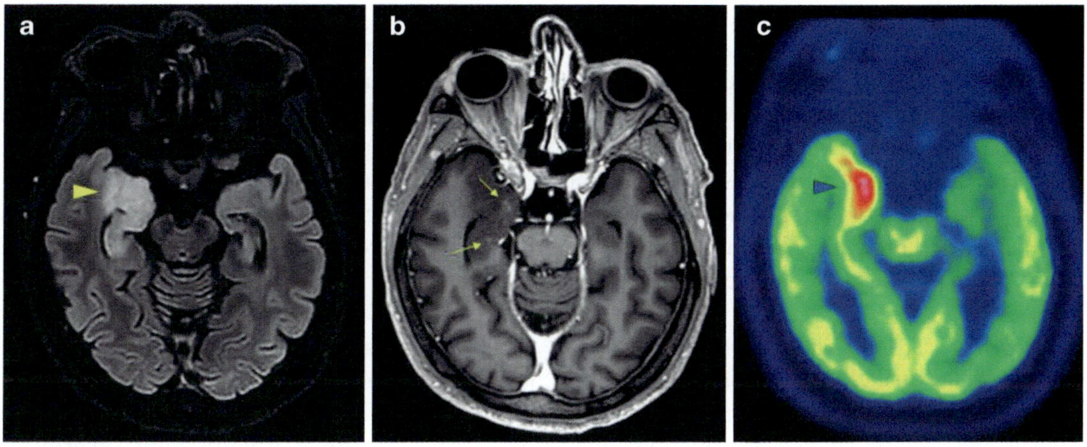

Fig. 10.9 Axial FLAIR showing a left temporal lobe hyperintense lesion with prominent swelling (**a**), with corresponding spotty foci of gadolinium enhancement (**b**), in a 59-year-old male patient who developed subacute behavioural changes and focal left temporal seizures following 10 cycles of atezolizumab for small cell lung cancer. Interestingly, 18-FDG-PET demonstrated a corresponding highly hypermetabolic area (**c**)

– Ischemic Stroke: The risk of ischemic stroke appears to be increased in patients who have received CAR-T-cell therapy, primarily due to the hypercoagulability induced by the treatment. Therefore, in the context of a new acute-onset focal neurological deficit, it is crucial to including vascular imaging (such as CT angiography or MRI angiography) as part of the diagnostic work-up.
– Cerebral Haemorrhage: Patients receiving CAR-T-cell therapy are often markedly thrombocytopenic following lymphodepleting chemotherapy. CT scan can easily rule out this complication.
– Other Causes of Encephalopathy: In case of normal neuroimaging study, it is crucial to consider in the differential diagnosis also side effects of analgesic drugs (e.g., opioids) commonly used for neoplastic pain, metabolic encephalopathy (renal or hepatic), and progression of the haematological disease at the leptomeningeal or parenchymal level.

10.3 Immune Checkpoint Inhibitors

Immune checkpoint inhibitors (ICIs) are monoclonal antibodies that target negative regulators of T-cell activation, including cytotoxic T-lymphocyte antigen-4 (CTLA-4), programmed death-1 (PD-1), programmed death ligand-1 (PD-L1), and lymphocyte activation gene 3 (LAG-3) [35]. By blocking these down-regulators of immunity, ICIs enhance anti-tumour T-cell response, thus producing a clinically notable effect on several types of cancers, including lung cancer, melanoma, and renal cell carcinoma. However, the immune system activation triggered by ICIs is non-specific and can lead to immune-mediated toxicities, which are collectively termed immune-related adverse events (ir-AEs) and may involve every organ or system tissue, including the nervous system [36]. Neurological ir-AEs (n-irAEs) manifest along a wide clinical spectrum and may involve both peripheral and central nervous system (CNS-irAEs) [37].

Neuromuscular ir-AEs, including myositis, polyradiculoneuropathy, and myasthenia gravis, are three times more common than CNS-irAEs [38]. The diagnosis of neuromuscular ir-AEs is mostly based on laboratory and neurophysiological findings and neuroimaging has a limited role, which will not be further deepened in the following sections.

CNS-irAEs are very rare, manifesting in about 1% of patients treated with ICIs, and their identification represents a diagnostic conundrum, due to their non-specific clinical presentation and to the extensive list of differential diagnosis [39]. Notwithstanding, the prompt recognition of CNS-irAEs is of paramount importance, given their high disability burden and fatality rate (10–20% in patients with ICI-related encephalitis).

Most CNS-irAEs manifest as acute or subacute new-onset neurological symptoms of CNS dysfunction and appear in close temporal relationship with the initiation of ICI treatment [40]: although late-onset toxicities have been reported, the vast majority of CNS-irAEs occur within 3–4 months from treatment initiation (i.e., 6–8 ICI cycles), and no later than 12 months from the last ICI infusion [41]. From a clinical standpoint, CNS-irAEs may be classified into *meningoencephalitis*, which manifest with meningeal involvement and/or diffuse encephalic dysfunction, and *focal encephalitis syndromes*, which present as isolated limbic, cerebellar, or brainstem involvement; *myelitis* accounts for a minority of CNS-irAEs. In the following paragraphs, we will describe the clinical features of CNS-irAEs, analyse their neuroradiological findings, and briefly discuss the diagnostic approach to these challenging presentations.

10.3.1 Meningoencephalitis

Meningoencephalitis refers to a diffuse CNS dysfunction as opposed to focal syndromes with limbic, brainstem, or cerebellar involvement and accounts for one-third of CNS-irAEs. ICI-induced meningoencephalitis manifests with altered mental status, seizures, language disturbances, and signs of meningeal irritation (e.g., headache, neck stiffness) [42]. When signs of brain parenchymal dysfunction are absent, the term *meningitis* is preferred; anyway, meningitis and meningoencephalitis probably represent a continuum of the same disease spectrum and the distinction between the two is artificial. The occurrence of meningoencephalitis has been associated with younger age, female sex, underlying melanoma, and treatments with CTLA-4 inhibitors [37, 40]. Despite a usually high severity at clinical nadir, meningoencephalitis present a favourable neurological outcome after ICI withdrawal and corticosteroid treatment in most of the patients (50–90%), without neurological sequelae.

Brain MRI is unremarkable in almost two-thirds of the cases (67% in a recent study [43]). When altered, it may show two patterns of alteration:

(a) Leptomeningeal enhancement [44–46] in post-contrast T1-weighted and FLAIR sequences (Fig. 10.1a, b). Notably, contrast-enhanced FLAIR images have been shown to be highly effective in the detection of leptomeningeal enhancement, as the suppression of CSF signal intensity on FLAIR sequences enables a better delineation of meningeal lesions that abut the border of the CSF. Moreover, the fact that slow-flowing blood is not usually hyperintense on post-contrast FLAIR images (contrary to post-contrast T1-weighted images), post-contrast FLAIR can account for a clearer distinction between enhancing meninges and enhancing cortical veins [47].

(b) Brain parenchymal hyperintense lesions in T2-weighted sequences, which usually present with patchy distribution, mostly involving the subcortical white matter in non-limbic areas. These lesions often present a "shaded" aspect and a variable, nuanced, gadolinium enhancement [42, 44, 48] (Fig. 10.2a, b).

Cerebrospinal fluid analysis (CSF) shows inflammatory findings in nearly all the patients, with marked pleocytosis (the median cell count was 30 cells/mm3 [range: 6–261] in one study [43]). Neuronal antibodies are usually absent (63% of patients), although a subset of patients may present anti-GFAP antibodies. Notably, patients with ICI-induced GFAP-encephalitis share similar clinical and radiological features with those with ICI-naïve GFAP-encephalitis, including markedly elevated CSF cell count and periventricular white-matter T2/FLAIR hyperintensities [43].

10.3.2 Focal Encephalitis Syndromes

Focal encephalitis syndromes are the most common clinical presentation of ICI-encephalitis, accounting for two-thirds of the cases, and can present as limbic encephalitis, rapidly progressive cerebellar ataxia (RPCA), and brainstem encephalitis, which could be either isolated or combined.

Limbic Encephalitis
Limbic encephalitis manifests with the classical clinical triad of subacute anterograde amnesia, temporal lobe seizures, and behavioural alterations. ICI-induced limbic encephalitis closely resembles spontaneous paraneoplastic neurological syndromes (PNS), and, as so, is associated with poor response to immune-active treatments, with high mortality rate [37] and long-term neurological sequelae [49]. Contrary to their spontaneous counterparts, ICI-induced PNSs can occur in patients with cancer types not typically associated with PNSs (e.g., clear renal cell carcinoma, mesothelioma) [50, 51] and usually present in patients with advanced and metastatic cancers [52].

Contrary to meningoencephalitis, brain MRI is altered in about 60–70% of the cases and shows T2/FLAIR hyperintensities and swelling of the mesial temporal lobe, which can present patchy gadolinium enhancement in a minority of the cases ($\approx$ 20%; Fig. 10.3a, b). In some cases, focal hippocampal atrophy or associated patchy leptomeningeal enhancement may be seen [43].

Notably, brain positron emission tomography (PET) with 18-fluorodexossiglucose (18-FDG) may show corresponding metabolic focal hypermetabolism (Fig. 10.3c) and may be a useful diagnostic tool, as in idiopathic autoimmune encephalitis [53].

CSF examination is less informative than in ICI-meningoencephalitis and shows a mild pleocytosis (median: 10 WBC/mm^3) in only half of the patients. On the contrary, patients with ICI-induced limbic encephalitis often present high-risk PNS antibodies (which are detected in >80% of the patients, in particular anti-Hu and anti-Ma2 antibodies [54, 55]).

Cerebellar Encephalitis
Cerebellar involvement is very rare in the post-ICI context and may be isolated or associated with limbic encephalitis, brainstem involvement, or cranial neuropathies (most often affecting the oculomotor nerves). From a clinical standpoint, ICI-cerebellitis manifests as a classic rapidly progressive cerebellar syndrome with limb and trunk ataxia, dysarthria, and oculomotor dysfunction (e.g., nystagmus, skew deviation, saccadic undershoot). Sometimes, immune-related cerebellitis may be associated with oculomotor nerve involvement [49]. ICI suspension and immune-active treatment led to neurological improvement or even remission in up to two-thirds of the patients.

Brain MRI is unrevealing in up to half of the cases. When altered, cerebellar hyperintensities are the most common findings, followed by cerebellar atrophy and cerebellar edema [56, 57].

Brainstem Encephalitis
ICI-induced brainstem encephalitis is anecdotical, with only a couple of cases being reported in the literature. Clinical presentation may be varied, including diplopia, vertigo, dysarthria, gait ataxia, facial numbness, and hiccups. Brain MRI may show T2-FLAIR brainstem hyperintensity in some patients but is more often unremarkable. The search for antineuronal antibodies might dis-

close unusual specificities, as antibodies targeting Kelch-like protein-11 (KLHL11) [58] and antibodies binding to the surface of rodent hippocampal neuron cultures [59].

Myelitis

Immune-related myelitis is an extremely rare complication of ICI, accounting for nearly 2% of all neurotoxicities [37]. Contrary to most of n-irAEs, myelitis is not invariably an early event, with some reported cases manifesting >6 months from ICI initiation [26]. Clinical presentation is typical of transverse myelitis and includes upper and/or lower limb weakness, sensory disturbances, sphincter dysfunction, and pyramidal signs. Interestingly, up to half of the patients received thoracic radiotherapy, suggesting that—by increasing local susceptibility to inflammation—radiotherapy might indeed represent a predisposing factor to ICI-induced myelitis [60].

In most patients, spine MRI reveals T2-FLAIR hyperintensity, which could present in the form of long-extensive transverse myelitis or with patchy distribution. The involved spine often shows a swelling appearance and present variable contrast enhancement. Occasionally, inflammatory changes may extend to the brain parenchyma (i.e., encephalomyelitis) or the caudal nerve roots (i.e., myeloradiculitis) [61]. CSF analysis often shows inflammatory findings, including raised proteins and pleocytosis. Conversely, neuronal antibodies are often negative, although in some patients anti-GFAP, anti-aquaporin-4, and anti-MOG have been reported.

10.3.3 Differential Diagnosis and the Role of Neuroimaging in the Diagnostic Work-Up

Several reasons make the diagnosis of CNS-irAEs a clinical challenge. First, patients treated with ICIs typically harbour an advanced-stage cancer and have received previous standard or targeted oncological therapies, which predispose them to a broad list of differential aetiologies of CNS disfunction (e.g., brain metastases or leptomeningeal carcinomatosis; neuro-infectious disorders due to chemotherapy-induced neutropenia; cerebrovascular disorders due to both cancer-induced hypercoagulability and chemotherapy-induced thrombocytopenia; metabolic encephalopathy related to liver or kidney failure, either due to neoplastic involvement or as chemotherapy-induced toxicities). Second, diagnostic procedures are often unrevealing (e.g., brain MRI and CSF analysis are often normal in ICI-induced focal encephalitis syndromes). Finally, even when altered, either laboratory or radiological findings are non-specific for an immune-mediated aetiology.

In this tangled context, neuroimaging has two key roles: the exclusion of alternative causes of CNS dysfunction and the demonstration of ongoing inflammation.

If the exclusion of alternative aetiologies is straightforward in the case of cerebrovascular disorders (e.g., ischemic stroke or intracerebral haemorrhage) or brain metastases, the same cannot be said for leptomeningeal carcinomatosis (LC), as the leptomeningeal enhancement seen in LC is often undistinguishable to those seen in ICI-meningoencephalitis. Of note, leptomeningeal enhancement in LC has more often a thick nodular—rather than linear and diffuse—appearance, with prominent involvement of occipital lobes and cerebellar convexities, and is more frequently associated with concomitant parenchymal metastases and cranial nerve enhancement [62]. Interestingly, internal acoustic canal enhancement was associated with carcinomatous rather than inflammatory leptomeningeal involvement in a recent study and could be a valuable tool in differentiating between LC and ICI-meningoencephalitis [63].

Finally, neuroimaging may be a useful tool to indirectly demonstrate an inflammatory pathophysiological mechanism. The stronger neuroradiological correlate of ongoing CNS inflammation is gadolinium enhancement. Unfortunately, contrast-enhancing lesions are found in only a minority of patients with CNS-irAEs, and the demonstration of an ongoing CNS inflammation often relies on CSF findings or remains hypothetical.

References

1. Lee DW, Santomasso BD, Locke FL, et al. ASTCT consensus grading for cytokine release syndrome and neurologic toxicity associated with immune effector cells. Biol Blood Marrow Transplant. 2019;25(4):625–38. https://doi.org/10.1016/j.bbmt.2018.12.758.
2. Burton LB, Eskian M, Guidon AC, et al. A review of neurotoxicities associated with immunotherapy and a framework for evaluation. Neurooncol Adv. 2021;3(Suppl 5):v108–20. https://doi.org/10.1093/noajnl/vdab107.
3. Elmarasi M, Elkonaissi I, Elsabagh AA, et al. CAR-T cell therapy: efficacy in management of cancers, adverse effects, dose-limiting toxicities and long-term follow up. Int Immunopharmacol. 2024., ISSN 1567-5769; https://doi.org/10.1016/j.intimp.2024.112312.
4. Yang Z, Ha B, Wu Q, et al. Expanding the horizon of CAR T cell therapy: from cancer treatment to autoimmune diseases and beyond. Front Immunol. 2025;16:1544532. https://doi.org/10.3389/fimmu.2025.1544532.
5. Grant SJ, Grimshaw AA, Silberstein J, et al. Clinical presentation, risk factors, and outcomes of immune effector cell-associated neurotoxicity syndrome following chimeric antigen receptor t cell therapy: a systematic review. Transplant Cell Ther. 2022;28(6):294–302. https://doi.org/10.1016/j.jtct.2022.03.006.
6. Han MW, Jeong SY, Suh CH, et al. Incidence of immune effector cell-associated neurotoxicity among patients treated with CAR T-cell therapy for hematologic malignancies: systematic review and meta-analysis. Front Neurol. 2024;15:1392831. https://doi.org/10.3389/fneur.2024.1392831.
7. Morris EC, Neelapu SS, Giavridis T, et al. Cytokine release syndrome and associated neurotoxicity in cancer immunotherapy. Nat Rev Immunol. 2022;22(2):85–96. https://doi.org/10.1038/s41577-021-00547-6.
8. Gu T, Hu K, Si X, et al. Mechanisms of immune effector cell-associated neurotoxicity syndrome after CAR-T treatment. WIREs Mech Dis. 2022;14(6):e1576. https://doi.org/10.1002/wsbm.1576.
9. Parker KR, Migliorini D, Perkey E, et al. Single-cell analyses identify brain mural cells expressing CD19 as potential off-tumor targets for CAR-T immunotherapies. Cell. 2020;183(1):126–142.e17. https://doi.org/10.1016/j.cell.2020.08.022.
10. Santomasso BD, Park JH, Salloum D, et al. Clinical and biological correlates of neurotoxicity associated with CAR T-cell therapy in patients with B-cell acute lymphoblastic leukemia. Cancer Discov. 2018;8:958–71. https://doi.org/10.1158/2159-8290.CD-17-1319.
11. Pensato U, Muccioli L, Cani I, et al. Brain dysfunction in COVID-19 and CAR-T therapy: cytokine storm-associated encephalopathy. Ann Clin Transl Neurol. 2021;8:968–79. https://doi.org/10.1002/acn3.51348.
12. Pensato U, Amore G, Muccioli L, et al. CAR t-cell therapy in BOlogNa-NEUrotoxicityTReatment and assessment in lymphoma (CARBON-NEUTRAL): proposed protocol and results from an Italian study. J Neurol. 2023;270(5):2659–73. https://doi.org/10.1007/s00415-023-11595-4.
13. Cordeiro A, Bezerra ED, Hirayama AV, et al. Late events after treatment with CD19-targeted chimeric antigen receptor modified T cells. Biol Blood Marrow Transplant. 2020;26(1):26–33. https://doi.org/10.1016/j.bbmt.2019.08.003.
14. Jung S, Greiner J, von Harsdorf S, et al. Fatal late-onset CAR T-cell-mediated encephalitis after axicabtagene-ciloleucel in a patient with large B-cell lymphoma. Blood Adv. 2021;5(19):3789–93. https://doi.org/10.1182/bloodadvances.2021004889.
15. Pensato U, Amore G, D'Angelo R, et al. Frontal predominant encephalopathy with early paligraphia as a distinctive signature of CAR T-cell therapy-related neurotoxicity. J Neurol. 2022;269(2):609–15. https://doi.org/10.1007/s00415-021-10766-5.
16. Lakomy T, Akhoundova D, Nilius H, et al. Early use of corticosteroids following CAR T-cell therapy correlates with reduced risk of high-grade CRS without negative impact on neurotoxicity or treatment outcome. Biomolecules. 2023;13(2):382. https://doi.org/10.3390/biom13020382.
17. Liu S, Deng B, Yin Z, et al. Corticosteroids do not influence the efficacy and kinetics of CAR-T cells for B-cell acute lymphoblastic leukemia. Blood Cancer J. 2020;10(2):15. https://doi.org/10.1038/s41408-020-0280-y.
18. Pensato U, Muccioli L, Taurino D, et al. Impact of neurotoxicity and steroid therapy on cancer progression-free survival in lymphoma patients treated with anti-CD19 CAR T cells. Neuro-Oncol Pract. 2024;npae128 https://doi.org/10.1093/nop/npae128.
19. Hayden PJ, Roddie C, Bader P, et al. Management of adults and children receiving CAR T-cell therapy: 2021 best practice recommendations of the European Society for Blood and Marrow Transplantation (EBMT) and the joint accreditation committee of ISCT and EBMT (JACIE) and the European haematology association (EHA). Ann Oncol. 2022;33(3):259–75. https://doi.org/10.1016/j.annonc.2021.12.003.
20. Strati P, Ahmed S, Kebriaei P, et al. Clinical efficacy of anakinra to mitigate CAR T-cell therapy-associated toxicity in large B-cell lymphoma. Blood Adv. 2020;4(13):3123–7. https://doi.org/10.1182/bloodadvances.2020002328.
21. Jain MD, Smith M, Shah NN. How I treat refractory CRS and ICANS after CAR T-cell therapy. Blood. 2023;141(20):2430–42. https://doi.org/10.1182/blood.2022017414.

22. Pinto SN, Liu CJ, Nelson MD Jr, et al. Neuroimaging of complications arising after CD19 chimeric antigen receptor T-cell therapy: a review. J Neuroimaging. 2023;33(5):703–15. https://doi.org/10.1111/jon.13138.
23. Pensato U, Muccioli L, Zinzani P, et al. Fulminant cerebral oedema following CAR T-cell therapy: case report and pathophysiological insights from literature review. J Neurol. 2022;269(8):4560–3. https://doi.org/10.1007/s00415-022-11117-8. Epub 2022 Apr 8. Erratum in: J Neurol. 2022 Aug;269(8):4564. doi:10.1007/s00415-022-11156-1
24. Lapidus AH, Anderson MA, Harrison SJ, et al. Neuroimaging findings in immune effector cell associated neurotoxicity syndrome after chimeric antigen receptor T-cell therapy. Leuk Lymphoma. 2022;63(10):2364–74. https://doi.org/10.1080/10428194.2022.2074990.
25. Gust J, Hay KA, Hanafi LA, et al. Endothelial activation and blood-brain barrier disruption in neurotoxicity after adoptive immunotherapy with CD19 CAR-T cells. Cancer Discov. 2017;7:1404–19.
26. Asioli GM, Castioni CA, Zinzani PL, et al. Intracranial pressure management in fulminant cerebral oedema after CAR T-cell therapy: not all is lost! Br J Haematol. 2024;204(3):1109–13. https://doi.org/10.1111/bjh.19270.
27. Santomasso BD, Gust J, Perna F. How I treat unique and difficult-to-manage cases of CAR T-cell therapy-associated neurotoxicity. Blood. 2023;141(20):2443–51. https://doi.org/10.1182/blood.2022017604.
28. Vernier V, Ursu R, Belin C, et al. Hypometabolism on brain FDG-PET as a marker for neurotoxicity after CAR T-cell therapy: a case report. Rev Neurol (Paris). 2022;178(3):282–4. https://doi.org/10.1016/j.neurol.2021.01.019.
29. Paccagnella A, Farolfi A, Casadei B, et al. 2-[18F] FDG-PET/CT for early response and brain metabolic pattern assessment after CAR-T cell therapy in a diffuse large B cell lymphoma patient with ICANS. Eur J Nucl Med Mol Imaging. 2022;49(3):1090–1. https://doi.org/10.1007/s00259-021-05562-2.
30. Morbelli S, Gambella M, Raiola AM, et al. Brain FDG-PET findings in chimeric antigen receptor T-cell therapy neurotoxicity for diffuse large B-cell lymphoma. J Neuroimaging. 2023;33(5):825–36. https://doi.org/10.1111/jon.13135.
31. Stoecklein S, Wunderlich S, Papazov B, et al. Functional connectivity MRI provides an imaging correlate for chimeric antigen receptor T-cell-associated neurotoxicity. Neurooncol Adv. 2023;5(1):vdad135. https://doi.org/10.1093/noajnl/vdad135. PMID: 38024243; PMCID: PMC10673700
32. Van Oekelen O, Aleman A, Upadhyaya B, et al. Neurocognitive and hypokinetic movement disorder with features of parkinsonism after BCMA-targeting CAR-T cell therapy. Nat Med. 2021;27(12):2099–103. https://doi.org/10.1038/s41591-021-01564-7.
33. Gudera JA, Baehring JM, Karschnia P. Parkinsonism following chimeric antigen receptor T cell therapy. JAMA Neurol. 2024; https://doi.org/10.1001/jamaneurol.2024.2506.
34. Couturier A, Escoffre M, Leh F, et al. Parkinson-like neurotoxicity in female patients treated with idecabtagene-vicleucel. Hema. 2024;8(7):e131. https://doi.org/10.1002/hem3.131.
35. Ribas A, Wolchok JD. Cancer immunotherapy using checkpoint blockade. Science. 2018;1979(359):1350–5.
36. Postow MA, Sidlow R, Hellmann MD. Immune-related adverse events associated with immune checkpoint blockade. N Engl J Med. 2018;378:158–68.
37. Marini A, et al. Neurologic adverse events of immune checkpoint inhibitors: a systematic review. Neurology. 2021;96:754–66. https://doi.org/10.1212/WNL.0000000000011795.
38. Rossi S, et al. Peripheral nervous system adverse events associated with immune checkpoint inhibitors. J Neurol. 2023;270:2975–86.
39. Vogrig A, Muñiz-Castrillo S, Farina A, Honnorat J, Joubert B. How to diagnose and manage neurological toxicities of immune checkpoint inhibitors: an update. J Neurol. 2022;269:1701–14.
40. Farina A, et al. Neurological outcomes in immune checkpoint inhibitor-related neurotoxicity. Brain Commun. 2023;5
41. Guidon AC, et al. Consensus disease definitions for neurologic immune-related adverse events of immune checkpoint inhibitors. J Immunother Cancer. 2021;9:e002890.
42. Farina A, Villagrán-García M, Vogrig A, Joubert B. Central nervous system adverse events of immune checkpoint inhibitors. Curr Opin Neurol. 2024;37:345–52. https://doi.org/10.1097/WCO.0000000000001259.
43. Farina A, et al. Diagnostic and prognostic biomarkers in immune checkpoint inhibitor-related encephalitis: a retrospective cohort study. Lancet Reg Health Eur. 2024;44
44. Vogrig A, et al. Central nervous system complications associated with immune checkpoint inhibitors. J Neurol Neurosurg Psychiatry. 2020;91:772–8.
45. Fonseca E, et al. Neurological adverse events related to immune-checkpoint inhibitors in Spain: a retrospective cohort study. Lancet Neurol. 2023;22:1150–9.
46. Valencia-Sanchez C, et al. Immune checkpoint inhibitor-associated central nervous system autoimmunity. Eur J Neurol. 2023;30:2418–29.
47. Parmar H, Sitoh Y-Y, Anand P, Chua V, Hui F. Contrast-enhanced flair imaging in the evaluation of infectious leptomeningeal diseases. Eur J Radiol. 2006;58:89–95.
48. Velasco R, et al. Encephalitis induced by immune checkpoint inhibitors. JAMA Neurol. 2021;78:864.
49. Rossi S, et al. Clinical course of neurologic adverse events associated with immune checkpoint inhibitors:

focus on chronic toxicities. Neurol Neuroimmunol Neuroinflamm. 2024;11:e200314.
50. Kopecký J, et al. Nivolumab induced encephalopathy in a man with metastatic renal cell cancer: a case report. J Med Case Rep. 2018;12:262.
51. Du Rusquec P, Peyre A, Toulgoat F, Honnorat J, Raimbourg J. Fatal anti-Ma2 encephalitis related to treatment of malignant pleural mesothelioma with a combination of anti-programmed death 1 and anti–cytotoxic T-lymphocyte associated protein 4 antibodies. J Thorac Oncol. 2019;14:e174–6.
52. Farina A, et al. Neurological adverse events of immune checkpoint inhibitors and the development of paraneoplastic neurological syndromes. Lancet Neurol. 2024;23. www.thelancet.com/neurology
53. Kassubek J, Juengling FD, Nitzsche EU, Lücking CH. Limbic encephalitis investigated by [18] FDG-PET and 3D MRI. J Neuroimaging. 2001;11:55–9.
54. Vogrig A, et al. Increased frequency of anti-Ma2 encephalitis associated with immune checkpoint inhibitors. Neurol Neuroimmunol Neuroinflamm. 2019;6
55. Farina A, et al. Anti-Hu antibodies in patients with neurologic side effects of immune checkpoint inhibitors. Neurol Neuroimmunol Neuroinflamm. 2023;10
56. Dinoto A, Mantovani E, Ferrari S, Mariotto S, Tamburin S. Cerebellar involvement associated with immune checkpoint inhibitors: a systematic review. Eur J Neurol. 2023;30:774–81.
57. Dentoni M, et al. Immune checkpoint inhibitor-related cerebellar toxicity: clinical features and comparison with paraneoplastic cerebellar ataxia. Cerebellum. 2024;23:2308–23.
58. Aboseif A, et al. Immune checkpoint inhibitor-associated Kelch-like protein-11 IgG brainstem encephalitis. Neurol Neuroimmunol Neuroinflamm. 2024;11
59. Damato V, et al. Association between a distinctive autoantibody-associated brainstem sensory syndrome and immune checkpoint inhibitors. JAMA Neurol. 2022;79:949.
60. Chatterton S, et al. Case series: immune checkpoint inhibitor-induced transverse myelitis. Front Neurol. 2023;14
61. Picca A, et al. Longitudinally extensive myelitis associated with immune checkpoint inhibitors. Neurol Neuroimmunol Neuroinflamm. 2021;8
62. Debnam JM, et al. Most common sites on MRI of intracranial neoplastic leptomeningeal disease. J Clin Neurosci. 2017;45:252–6.
63. Peker E, et al. Discrimination of leptomeningeal carcinomatosis and meningeal inflammation/infection with internal acoustic canal enhancement. Eur J Radiol. 2024;171:111299.

11 Drug-Induced Intracranial Hypertension

Marialuisa Zedde, Francesco Causin, and Rosario Pascarella

11.1 Introduction

Idiopathic intracranial hypertension (IIH), also known as pseudotumor cerebri, was first identified by Quinke in 1893. It is characterized by increased intracranial pressure (ICP) without evidence of space-occupying lesions or secondary causes. The diagnosis of IIH relies primarily on neuroimaging, particularly magnetic resonance imaging (MRI), to rule out other conditions. While certain imaging findings, such as increased ICP, may be incidentally present in asymptomatic individuals, their role in diagnosing IIH must be carefully evaluated on a case-by-case basis. The earliest diagnostic framework, the Modified Dandy Criteria, was based on head computed tomography (CT) imaging findings [1]. Over time, advancements in neuroimaging, including MRI and magnetic resonance venography (MRV), enhanced the ability to exclude secondary causes, and MRI findings were incorporated into the diagnostic criteria for IIH without papilledema in 2002 [2]. According to the latest international diagnostic criteria [3], MRI markers play a critical role in diagnosing IIH in the absence of papilledema or when unilateral or bilateral abducens nerve palsy is present. Key MRI findings include empty sella, posterior globe flattening, distention of the perioptic subarachnoid space (with or without optic nerve tortuosity), and transverse venous sinus stenosis.

Being the MRI signs of the disease similar in iatrogenic and idiopathic cases, it is strongly suggested to consider excluding iatrogenic subtypes of the disease, although their course and treatment have not been fully assessed, in order to remove the causative drug.

11.2 Iatrogenic Causes of Intracranial Hypertension

Iatrogenic causes of intracranial hypertension, fully mimicking the so-called idiopathic subtype, have been reported, mainly with medications such as retinol (vitamin A) and its derivatives, amiodarone, tetracyclines, and corticosteroids [4]. This last category includes secondary adrenal insufficiency following withdrawal of inhaled corticosteroids, reported in 2.5% of patients taking inhaled corticosteroids [5]. Several drugs have been reported in the literature as having a

M. Zedde (✉)
Neurology Unit, Stroke Unit, Azienda Unità Sanitaria Locale-IRCCS di Reggio Emilia, Reggio Emilia, Italy
e-mail: zedde.marialuisa@ausl.re.it

F. Causin
Neuroradiology Unit, Department of Women's and Children's Health, University Hospital of Padua, Padua, Italy

R. Pascarella
Neuroradiology Unit, Ospedale Santa Maria della Misericordia, AULSS 5 Polesana, Rovigo, Italy

M. Zedde, R. Pascarella (eds.), *Neuroimaging of Treatment-Related Conditions in the Brain*,
https://doi.org/10.1007/978-3-032-23618-0_11

causative association with raised intracranial pressure [6, 7]. A general list is provided in Table 11.1 [8, 9].

The natural history and therapeutic approach of iatrogenic cases, other than discontinuation, where possible, of the drug implicated as the causative agent, are unknown.

A recent systematic review [9] addressed this issue focusing on commonly used medications in dermatology, especially those for acne vulgaris, proposing specific risk categories for drugs as a guide for clinicians. The authors found 259 verifiable cases of drug-induced IH (DIIH). Vitamin A derivatives, tetracycline-class antibiotics, recombinant growth hormone, and lithium were found to be most strongly associated (Categories IV and V). Corticosteroids were moderately associated with DIIH (Category III). Drugs that were weakly associated with DIIH (Categories I and II) include cyclosporine, progestin-only contraceptives, combined oral contraceptives, second- and third-generation fluoroquinolones, sulfentrazone, gonadotropin-releasing hormones and luteinizing hormone-releasing hormone agonist, nalidixic acid, amiodarone, stanozolol, danazol, divalproic acid, sulfasalazine, ketoconazole, and ustekinumab. The most immediate consequence of this categorization is that patients who started taking high-risk medications might be educated on the signs and symptoms of intracranial hypertension [9]. The main findings of this review are summarized in Table 11.2.

Table 11.1 Drugs associated with raised intracranial pressure

Fluoroquinolones
Tetracycline-class antibiotics (tetracycline, minocycline, doxycycline)
Sulfa antibacterials
Corticosteroid and corticosteroid withdrawal
Danazol
Vitamin A derivatives (including isotretinoin and all-transretinoic acid)
Levothyroxine sodium (in children)
Nalidixic acid
Tamoxifen
Ciclosporin
Levonorgestrel implant
Leuprorelin (LHRH analog)
Lithium
Growth hormone
Indomethacin
Cimetidine
Amiodarone
Ketoconazole
Ustekinumab

Addressing some drugs in more details, the authors reported the following remarks:

– Vitamin A and Derivatives

Vitamin A derivatives are commonly used in dermatology and oncology. Drug-induced intracranial hypertension (DIIH) has been associated with vitamin A and its derivatives, with symptoms often occurring within days of starting treatment. Vitamin A alters the 11β-hydroxysteroid pathway, increasing CSF production and reducing reabsorption by the arachnoid body [10, 11]. Patients on vitamin A therapy should avoid further supplementation due to additive effects.

– Vitamin A Supplementation

Excessive vitamin A supplementation (>25,000 IU) can cause hypervitaminosis A, leading to symptoms such as xerosis, alopecia, and hepatosplenomegaly. DIIH occurred in 50% of hypervitaminosis A cases, particularly in children, possibly due to lower body fat and different metabolic processing [12]. One DIIH case involved concurrent isotretinoin use for acne [13].

– Isotretinoin

Isotretinoin, used for acne vulgaris, has been linked to 15 DIIH cases in patients aged 14–38, with onset between 4 and 8 weeks [14]. Two cases involved concurrent tetracycline-class antibiotics [15]. A further 173 cases were reported, with 153 resolving after discontinuation [16]. A 7-day washout period is recommended between isotretinoin and tetracyclines, though not clinically verified [17].

Table 11.2 Drugs and strength of association with IH [9]

Category (no. of verified cases)	Medication class	Patients	Associations/comments
V (≥20 cases)	Vitamin A and derivatives	84	Excessive vitamin A supplementation, treatment for acne
	Isotretinoin		
	Tretinoin		
	Tetracycline-class antibiotics	71	Treatment for acne, malaria prophylaxis
	Minocycline		
	Tetracycline		
	Doxycycline		
	Recombinant growth hormone	24	In children or among athletes (doping)
IV (15–19 cases)	Lithium	17	
III (10–14 cases)	Corticosteroids	14	In children, DIIH occurs after withdrawal from chronic use
II (5–9 cases)	Sulfentrazone	9	
	First-generation fluoroquinolone	7	
	Nalidixic acid		
	Cyclosporine	7	
	GnRH/LHRH agonists	6	
	Leuprorelin		
	Triptorelin		
	Amiodarone	5	
	Progestin-only contraceptives	4a	Subcutaneous implantable device
	Norplant®		
	Nexplanon®		
I (1–4 cases)	Second- and third-generation fluoroquinolones	4	Cases in this category may be coincidental
	Ciprofloxacin		
	Levofloxacin		
	Ofloxacin		
	Combined oral contraceptives	3	
	Stanozolol	1	
	Danazol	1	
	Divalproic acid	1	
	Sulfasalazine	1	
	Ketoconazole	1	
	Ustekinumab	1	

– Tretinoin (All-Trans Retinoic Acid)

Tretinoin, used in acne treatment and leukemia chemotherapy, was linked to 44 DIIH cases. Around 9% of leukemia patients treated with tretinoin developed increased ICP.

– Other Vitamin A Derivatives

Other derivatives like acitretin and etretinate have rarely been linked to DIIH. Acitretin is less lipophilic than etretinate, which has been withdrawn due to teratogenicity. No DIIH cases have been reported with alitretinoin or bexarotene, suggesting these may not affect choroid plexus and arachnoid granulation physiology.

– Tetracycline-Class Antibiotics

Tetracyclines are used for various infections and conditions. DIIH has been associated with minocycline, tetracycline, and doxycycline, with onset ranging from 2 weeks to several months [8, 18]. Combining tetracyclines with retinoids or lithium increases DIIH risk [19, 20]. A 7-day washout period is suggested between tetracyclines and isotretinoin, but lacks clinical evidence [21].

– Minocycline

Minocycline is most strongly linked to DIIH, especially during acne treatment. Women of childbearing age are most affected. Discontinuing minocycline and starting isotretinoin years later without recurrence has been reported [19, 22].

– Tetracycline

Tetracycline was associated with 24 DIIH cases, primarily in adolescents using it for acne treatment. One case involved delayed DIIH 1 month after discontinuing tetracycline [23].

– Doxycycline

Doxycycline has the fewest DIIH reports. Most cases involved long-term use for acne or malaria prophylaxis. Shorter courses, such as for Lyme borreliosis, were not associated with DIIH, except one case [24].

– Recombinant Growth Hormone

DIIH was reported in 24 pediatric patients receiving recombinant growth hormone, especially those with renal insufficiency or genetic growth impairments. No cases were reported in adults.

– Lithium

Seventeen cases of DIIH were linked to lithium use in both adults and children. Lithium, which competes with sodium for channels, could theoretically alter CSF production, though this mechanism has not been directly studied.

– Corticosteroids

DIIH has been associated with corticosteroid withdrawal, particularly in children. Twelve cases were reported after cessation of systemic corticosteroids for bronchitis or asthma, with two cases in infants after long-term use of topical betamethasone. Other reports suggest corticosteroid use in inflammatory bowel disease could be linked to increased ICP, but these cases had alternative explanations for elevated ICP. Corticosteroids are considered a rare cause of DIIH, particularly in pediatric patients.

– Sulfentrazone

Sulfentrazone, a sulfa antibiotic, was linked to nine cases of DIIH in Italian infants and adolescents, typically with transient symptoms. The sulfa group is unlikely to be directly responsible for DIIH since acetazolamide, a sulfa drug, is used to treat DIIH.

– Nalidixic Acid

Nalidixic acid, a first-generation fluoroquinolone, was associated with seven cases of DIIH, primarily in adults and children treated for non-CNS infections. Further reports are needed to clarify the relationship.

– Cyclosporine

Cyclosporine, used in organ transplants and psoriasis treatment, was linked to seven cases of DIIH. The exact mechanism remains unclear, though no cases were found in renal transplant patients receiving cyclosporine and systemic vitamin A derivatives for skin cancer prevention.

– GnRH/LHRH Agonists

GnRH/LHRH agonists like leuprorelin and triptorelin were linked to six cases of DIIH, with no sequelae after discontinuation. These medications are likely low-risk for DIIH.

– Amiodarone

Five cases of DIIH were associated with amiodarone use for ventricular arrhythmias. The pathophysiology is unclear, and cases may involve misclassification, particularly in the context of amiodarone-induced optic neuropathy.

– Progestin-Only Contraceptives

Forty-two cases of IIH were reported in association with progestin-only contraceptives, including Norplant® (discontinued in 2008). Studies suggest a potential increased risk, but more data are needed to confirm the association, especially with levonorgestrel intrauterine devices (Mirena®) [25–28].

– Second- and Third-Generation Fluoroquinolones

Only four cases of DIIH were linked to second- and third-generation fluoroquinolones (ciprofloxacin, levofloxacin, ofloxacin), suggesting a rare association with DIIH.

– Combined Oral Contraceptives (OCP)

Few verified cases of DIIH were linked to OCP use, mostly in obese women of childbearing age. Larger case-control studies show no significant increased risk of IIH with OCP use, making the association weak [29–32].

– Other Medications

Trimethoprim-sulfamethoxazole was linked to four cases of DIIH but lacks sufficient evidence for causality. Other medications such as anabolic steroids, divalproic acid, sulfasalazine, ketoconazole, and ustekinumab have single reports of DIIH, likely representing spurious associations. Notably, ketoconazole may contribute to DIIH through its effect on cortisol levels. Desmopressin injection, though associated with a single case of DIIH, was deemed more likely incidental due to the patient's multiple risk factors [33].

In addition, the authors proposed a set of diagnostic criteria for DIIH (Table 11.3).

Table 11.3 Proposed diagnostic criteria for drug-induced intracranial hypertension [9]

A diagnosis of DIIH can be made if the patient meets the diagnostic criteria for IIH *and* at least four of the following:	
A	Signs or symptoms of increased ICP are not due to any pre-existing clinical condition
B	Signs or symptoms of increased ICP developed within a reasonable time interval of drug administration
C	Upon discontinuation of suspected drug, signs or symptoms of increased ICP improved after five half-lives[a] with subsequent resolution
D	Signs or symptoms of increased ICP recurred on re-challenge of suspected drug
E	The suspected drug has been previously reported to be associated with increased ICP

[a]Five half-lives would correspond to an approximate drug clearance of 97%

11.3 Clinical Issues and Pathogenesis

The main information is available on IIH and less is known about iatrogenic IH. IIH predominantly affects women and is strongly associated with obesity, although its underlying pathogenesis remains incompletely understood. The diagnostic criteria for IIH include elevated intracranial pressure without hydrocephalus or mass lesions, normal CSF composition, and the absence of an identifiable underlying cause. These criteria are widely accepted for diagnosing IIH [1, 3]. Recent data indicate that the annual incidence of IIH is increasing, with an age- and gender-adjusted rate of 2.4 per 100,000 individuals reported between 2002 and 2014 [3].

The majority of IIH patients experience headaches that become progressively more severe and frequent. These headaches, as classified by the International Classification of Headache Disorders, 3rd Edition (ICHD-3), often present with highly variable phenotypes that can mimic other primary headache disorders [34]. Additional symptoms may include transient visual symptoms (brief unilateral or bilateral vision dimming lasting seconds), pulsatile tinnitus, back pain, neck pain, dizziness, visual blurring, cognitive disturbances, radicular pain, and typically horizontal diplopia [1, 3]. However, none of these symptoms are pathognomonic for IIH [35].

Clinical uncertainty persists in the diagnosis of IIH, and cases of misdiagnosis remain a concern [36]. A 2015 Cochrane review concluded that there is insufficient evidence to provide clear guidance on the pharmacological treatment of IIH [37]. The rarity of the condition, the incomplete understanding of its underlying pathological mechanisms, and the limited availability of disease-modifying therapies have contributed to the infrequency of randomized clinical trials in this field.

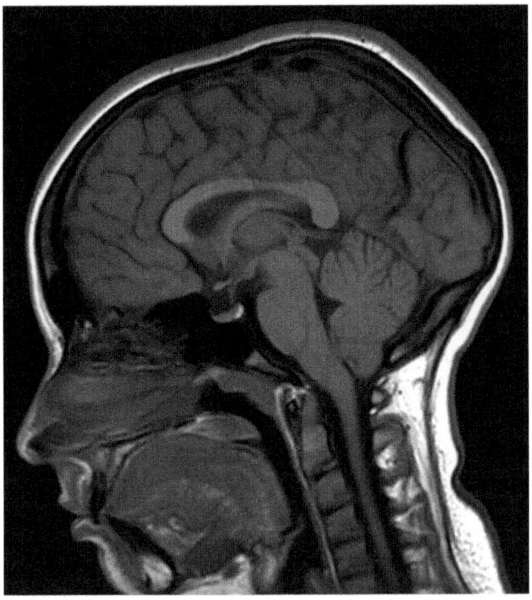

Fig. 11.1 T1W brain MRI in sagittal view showing a partially empty sella

11.4 Neuroimaging Diagnosis

Diagnostic criteria for IIH (for iatrogenic forms too) include negative findings on neuroimaging, mainly MRI. Conversely "positive" neuroimaging findings are associated with increased ICP, but they can also be incidentally found in asymptomatic subjects. Therefore, their role in diagnosis of IIH has to be defined in individual cases. The first proposed diagnostic criteria for IIH (the Modified Dandy Criteria) are based on head CT [1], but progressively brain MRI and MRV has been used as neuroimaging technique to exclude secondary causes and MRI findings were incorporated in diagnostic criteria for IIH without papilledema in 2002 [2]. According to the last available international diagnostic criteria [3], MRI markers of IIH are mandatory for the diagnosis if the patient does not have papilledema and/or have a unilateral or bilateral abducens nerve palsy, including empty sella (Fig. 11.1), flattening of the posterior aspect of the globe (Fig. 11.2), distention of the perioptic subarachnoid space with or without a tortuous optic nerve (Fig. 11.2), and transverse sinus stenosis (Fig. 11.3).

IIH without papilledema (IIHWOP) is a less well-recognized condition, but is specifically recognized as a category of headache by the International Headache Society classification in 2004 [38], and has published diagnostic criteria [3]. The majority of patients with IIHWOP are described as phenotypically similar to those with IIH, but it could be postulated that chronic daily headache (CDH), which occurs in approximately 4% of the population and 6.8% of individuals with morbid obesity, could be undiagnosed IIHWOP [39]. The prevalence of transverse sinus stenosis (TSS) in refractory chronic headache patients [40] is a further issue to support this hypothesis. Particularly in IIHWOP patients, neuroimaging findings often include CSF leaks and fistulas at the skull base, which are often missed if no definite suspicion is posed in the neuroimaging evaluation [41].

Diagnostic criteria of IIH are summarized in Table 11.4.

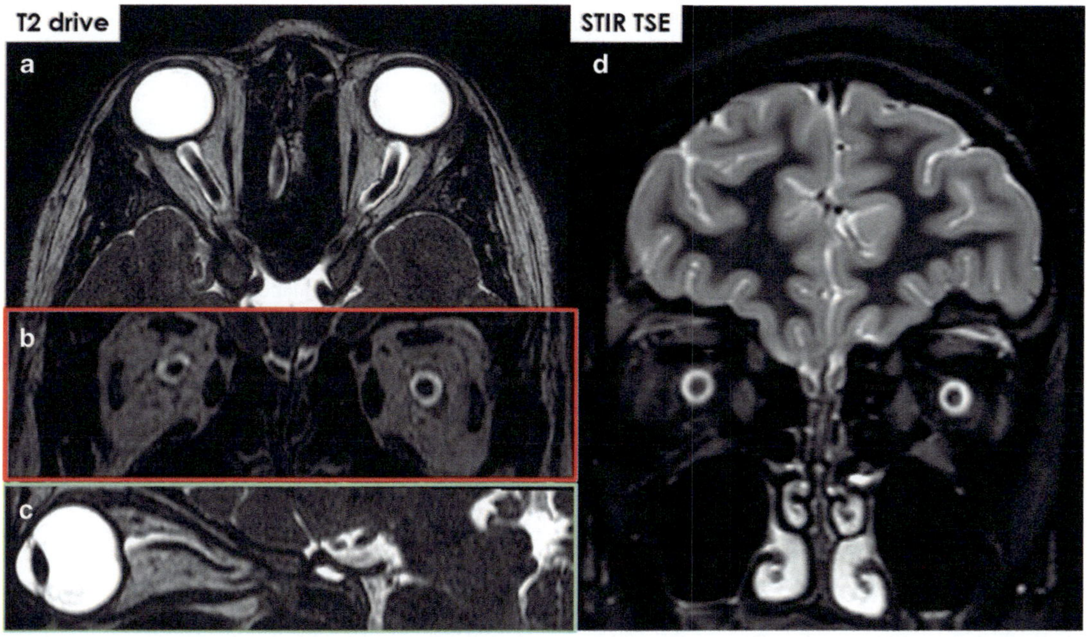

Fig. 11.2 MRI at the orbital level with distension and widening of the perioptic sheaths both in T2 Drive sequence (panels **a**–**c**) and in STIR TSE sequence in coronal plane (panel **d**)

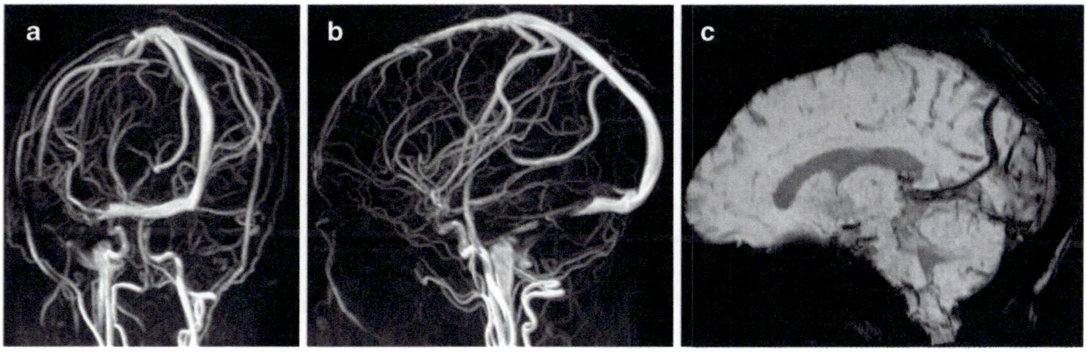

Fig. 11.3 3D Phase Contrast MRV reconstructed in oblique and lateral views (panels **a** and **b**, respectively) and SWI reconstructed in sagittal view (panel **c**). The left transverse sinus is hypoplasic and the right one shows a flow gap in the transverse-sigmoid transition, but this appearance should not be assumed as stenosis without a contrastographic confirmation. In addition, in all panels, a persistent falcine sinus is evident, associated with aplasia of the straight sinus and of the inferior sagittal sinus

Table 11.4 Original and modified Dandy criteria and the criteria used in the Idiopathic Intracranial Hypertension Treatment Trial

A: Modified Dandy criteria for idiopathic intracranial hypertension [2]
1. Signs and symptoms of increased ICP (headaches, nausea, vomiting, transient visual obscurations, or papilledema)
2. Absence of localized findings in neurological examination (except for false localizing signs such as abducens nerve palsy)
3. Normal CT/MRI findings without evidence of hydrocephalus or mass lesion
4. CSF opening pressure >25 cm H_2O with normal CSF cytological and chemical findings
5. No other causes of elevated intracranial pressure identified
B: Idiopathic intracranial hypertension treatment trial—modified Dandy criteria [42]
1. Signs and symptoms of increased ICP
2. Absence of localizing findings on neurologic examination
3. Absence of deformity, displacement, or obstruction of the ventricular system and otherwise normal neurodiagnostic studies, except for evidence of increased CSF pressure (>200 mm H_2O); abnormal neuroimaging except for empty sella turcica, optic nerve sheath with filled-out CSF spaces, and smooth-walled non-flow-related venous sinus stenosis or collapse should lead to another diagnosis
4. Awake and alert
5. No other cause of increased ICP
If the CSF opening pressure was 200–250 mm H_2O, at least one of the following was also required: Pulse synchronous tinnitus CN VI palsy Frisen grade II papilledema Echography for drusen-negative and no other disc anomalies mimicking disc edema present MRV with lateral sinus collapse/stenosis preferable using auto-triggered elliptic centric-ordered technique Partially empty sella on coronal or sagittal views and optic nerve sheaths with filled-out CSF spaces next to globe on T2-weighted axial scans

11.5 Neuroimaging Features of IIH

MRI is a non-invasive tool to assess the globe, optic nerve, optic tract, and the brain for associated signs leading to raised ICP.

Neuroimaging signs of IH are summarized in Table 11.5 (the main neuroradiological signs are labeled in light green).

Table 11.5 Neuroimaging signs of IH

Empty sella (defined as a pituitary grade of ≥3) [43]
Protrusion of the optic nerve head
Flattening of the posterior sclera
Increased CSF in the perioptic sheaths
Vertical tortuosity of the intraorbital optic nerve
Optic nerve head hyperintensity in DWI MRI
Enlarged Meckel caves
Cephaloceles
Cerebellar tonsillar herniation (>5 mm under McRae line)
Sigmoid sinus wall abnormalities (SSWAs)
Bilateral transverse sinus stenosis on contrast-enhanced imaging with at least 50% narrowing [44]
Optic nerve head enhancement in post-contrast imaging
Size of the optic canal
Enlargement of the foramen ovale
Enlargement of Dorello's canal
Jugular bulb dehiscence
Prominent posterior fossa emissary veins
CSF leaks and fistulas at the skull base
Cerebellar tonsillar ectopia more than 5 mm below the foramen magnum (opisthion-basion line)

Empty sella is a neuroimaging finding in which the sella turcica is partially or fully filled with CSF. Primary empty sella is associated with IIH. Initially it was thought it was caused by herniation of the subarachnoid space into the sella turcica from intracranial hypertension resulting in compression of the pituitary gland. Actually the main hypothesis is that it may partially be related to the bony enlargement of the sella turcica, caused by chronic increased ICP, the floor of the bony sella turcica being extremely thin (less than 1 mm in thickness). On MRI, an empty sella contains a flattened pituitary gland surrounded by a CSF-intensity signal (Fig. 11.4) [45]. The finding of partial empty sella in IIH has been reported to be reversible, depending on the chronicity of the increased intracranial pressure and on the structural integrity of the sella turcica at baseline.

Orbital findings associated with IIH include protrusion of the optic nerve head, flattening of the posterior sclera, increased perioptic CSF (ON sheath distension) (Fig. 11.4), and vertical/horizontal tortuosity of the intraorbital optic nerve. Optic nerve protrusion, i.e., the swelling of the optic nerve head because of increased CSF pressure in the optic nerve sheath, correlates with papilledema in fundoscopic examination and with optic nerve edema on OCT [46]. MRI without contrast medium do not show changes in signal intensity of optic nerve head, but with contrast a focal hyperintensity at the optic nerve head can be seen [47]. Quantitative analysis of MRI using 2D mapping showed that optic nerve protrusion is a clinically relevant marker of papilledema risk in IIH, linearly related to the papilledema grade [48].

Optic nerve appears tortuous or kinked because of the fixation of the nerve at proximal and distal points and increased CSF pressure in the optic nerve sheath. Its detection depends on the MRI slice thickness and orientation and a horizontal and vertical tortuosity can be distinguished; horizontal tortuosity is less common but more specific for increased ICP than vertical tortuosity. Vertical tortuosity is often associated with a "smear sign," being the middle portion of the optic nerve covered by the orbital fat [47]. Distension of the ONS presumably occurs because of the high CSF pressure in the ONS and appears on imaging as a widened ring of CSF surrounding an optic nerve [49] with a threshold >2 mm [50]. The balance between the intracranial and intraocular pressure maintains the normal convexity of the posterior globe. Posterior globe flattening is the straightening out of the curvature of the posterior sclera where it attaches to the optic nerve. It may be due to the transmission of increased CSF pressure from the subarachnoid space through the ONS to the posterior globe [50]. Enhancement of the optic disc on post-contrast axial T1 orbital MRI is one of the less sensitive findings in IIH, likely because of the small size of the region of interest [51].

More recently diffusion-weighted imaging (DWI) MRI was applied to orbital scan and few studies showed that optic nerve head (ONH) hyperintensity seen on DWI can be a potential sign of papilledema on imaging with a specificity of 100% but a low sensitivity and a significant correlation between the clinical grade of papilledema and hyperintensity of ONH on DWI in patients with IIH [52, 53]. Due to technical limitations these studies have several pitfalls. In a more recent application of a newer technique of DWI based on read out-segmented, multi-shot EPI sequences (rs-EPI) [54], a correlation between the clinical grade of papilledema and qualitative grading of ONH hyperintensity as well as with mean ADC value of ONH was investigated in patients with papilledema. The authors found a significant correlation between ONH hyperintensity and mean ADC value of ONH with clinical grades of papilledema and that

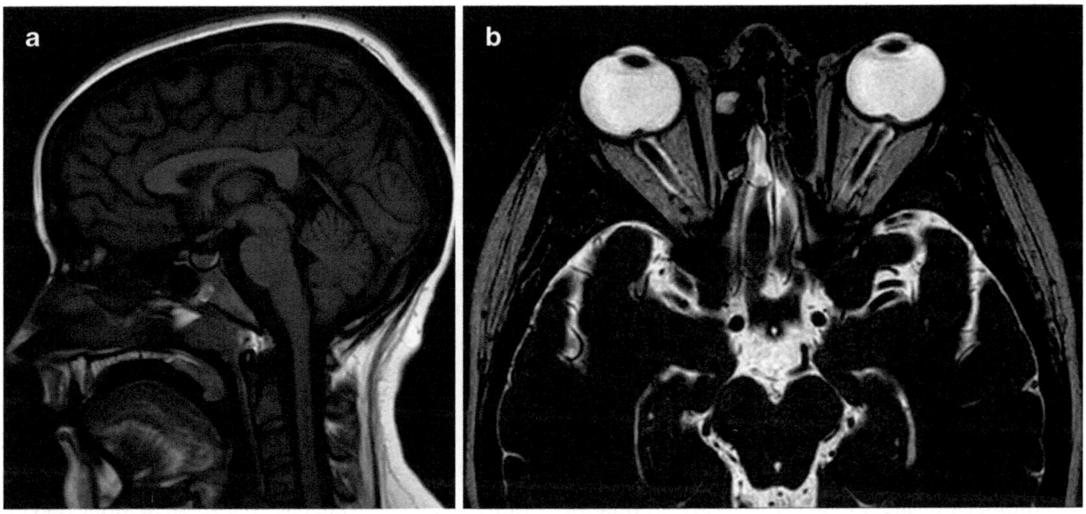

Fig. 11.4 Another patient with empty sella (panel **a**, sagittal T1W MRI) and widening of the perioptic sheaths (T2 Drive MRI in panel **b**)

between cases and control groups. ONH hyperintensity was found to be a highly sensitive (87.5% for both) and specific (specificity 97.1% and 98.6% for two observers) sign of papilledema. A mean cut-off ONH ADC value was found to have high sensitivity (96.83%) and specificity (95.31%) to distinguish between the cases and controls.

The measure of the size of the optic canal is rarely performed with MRI and more easily done on orbital CT. It has been suggested that optic canal may be larger on the side of the worse papilledema in selected patients with very asymmetric papilledema from IIH [55]. It is unclear, however, whether a larger canal is congenital (and therefore may contribute to asymmetric papilledema by facilitating the transmission of CSF pressure to the lamina cribrosa, leading to worse papilledema) or may develop over time in patients with chronic untreated IIH because of bony erosion.

One of the potential clinical manifestations of IIH is pulsatile tinnitus (PT). Several venous abnormalities can be observed in both conditions, including sigmoid sinus wall abnormalities (SSWA), transverse and sigmoid sinus stenosis, jugular bulb abnormalities, and prominent posterior fossa emissary veins [56]. In particular, there seems to be an overlap of clinical features among patients with IIH and patients with SSWA [57]. A similar morphological change can be found on the jugular bulb that is normally separated from the posterior hypotympanum by the bony jugular plate. It receives venous blood from the sigmoid sinus and transmits most of the flow inferiorly to the internal jugular vein [58]. A high-riding jugular bulb is a normal anatomic variant, more commonly seen on the right, which can be identified on axial CT images when the roof of the bulb is seen at or above the same level of the basal turn of the cochlea [58]. A focal outpouching from the jugular bulb is occasionally identified and is termed a jugular bulb diverticulum; this structure usually protrudes superiorly and medially into the petrous temporal bone.

Another nonspecific neuroimaging sign is the prominence of the posterior fossa emissary veins, mainly the posterior condylar emissary vein and the mastoid emissary vein. Mastoid emissary veins course from the midportion of the sigmoid sinus to join extracranial venous structures such as the deep cervical vein or a posterior auricular vein to join the vertebral venous plexus [59]. The posterior condylar emissary vein courses from the medial lower end of the sigmoid or marginal sinus to the vertebral venous plexus traveling through the osseous condylar canal in the occipital condyle. Variant venous anatomy, such as a hypoplastic jugular vein, can result in primary dural sinus drainage through an enlarged emissary vein to the vertebral plexus [60]. Several case reports have shown an association between a dilated posterior fossa emissary vein and PT [61]. In IIH and PT cohorts, Sundarajan et al. [62] assessed the presence of prominent emissary veins on MRV and corroborated subsequent conventional venography. The three subtypes classified were condylar arising from the internal jugular bulb, mastoid arising from the sigmoid sinus, and occipital arising from the torcula.

The presence of internal jugular vein diverticula or prominent emissary veins was uniformly distributed across IIH and PT cohorts, presumably related to pressure-induced vessel dilation and collateral redistribution in the setting of stenosis [62]. The prominence of emissary veins may not be uniquely specific to the diagnosis of IIH, given their similar prominence in patients with both IIH and isolated venous PT, as previously reported with regard to the occipital emissary vein [63].

The primary role of intracranial vascular imaging in patients suspected of IIH is to exclude cerebral venous thrombosis [64] and, more rarely, dural fistulas. More recently, bilateral transverse sinus stenosis on MRV emerged as the cause of IIH and consequence of increased ICP. A 3D gadolinium-enhanced MRV is considered more sensitive than conventional MRV for detecting areas of subtle cerebral venous stenosis (Figs. 11.5, 11.6, and 11.7) [65]. The transverse sinuses can be particularly susceptible to stenosis as ICP increases, because of absent or diminished bony grooves adjacent to the structures and in some patients, congenital or acquired narrowing of the venous sinuses contributes to IIH by

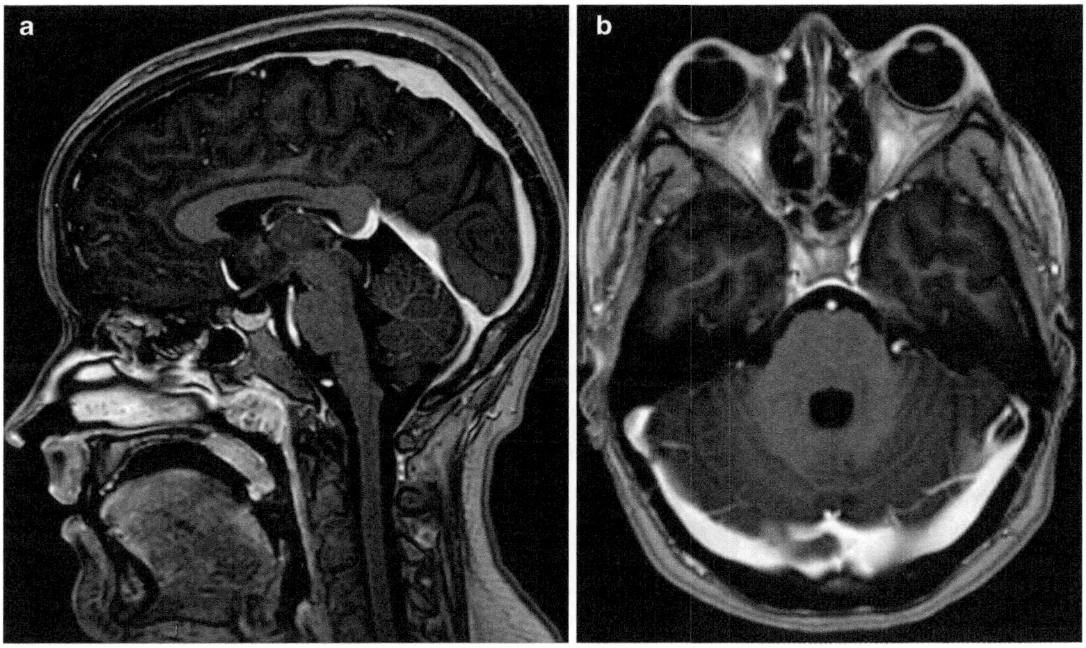

Fig. 11.5 Post-contrast T1W MRI with partially empty sella (panel **a**, sagittal view) and lateral sinus stenosis on the right side (panel **b**)

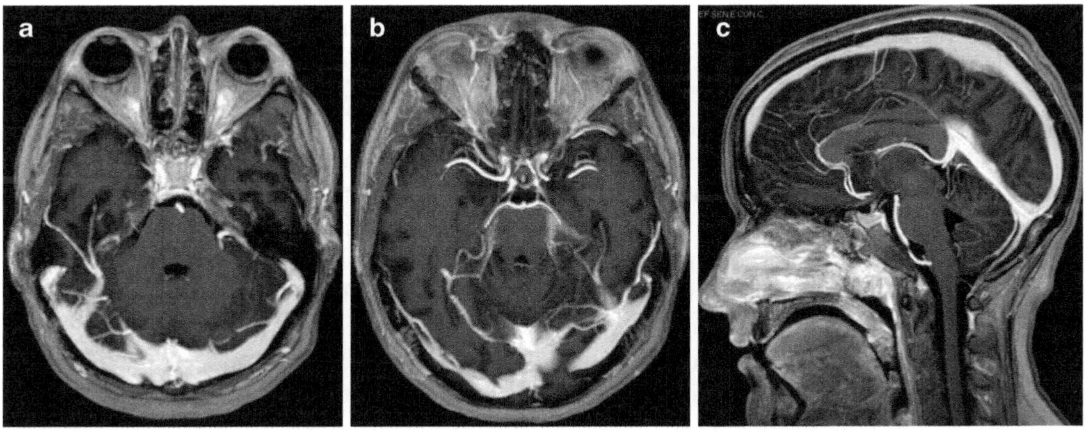

Fig. 11.6 Post-contrast 3D T1W TFE, reconstructed with MIP/MPR protocol in axial plane (panels **a** and **b**, at sequential levels) and sagittal plane (panel **c**). A long longitudinal sepimentum can be seen in the right transverse sinus, responsible for an intrinsic stenosis

increasing cerebral venous pressure. The reversibility of stenosis with treatment of the increased ICP supports the hypothesis that it is a secondary finding in some patients [66].

Bilateral transverse TSS greater than 50% is an extremely sensitive imaging marker of IIH [66]. Kelly et al. [67] addressed the prevalence of TSS among individuals with normal ICP [68], finding it incidentally in 7/240 adult subjects. Checking MRI and clinical records, all patients were obese women (mean age: 41; mean BMI: 37.1) with CSF opening pressures at the upper limit of normal (22–25 cmH_2O). All had bilateral TSS; six had short TSS and an empty sella; one

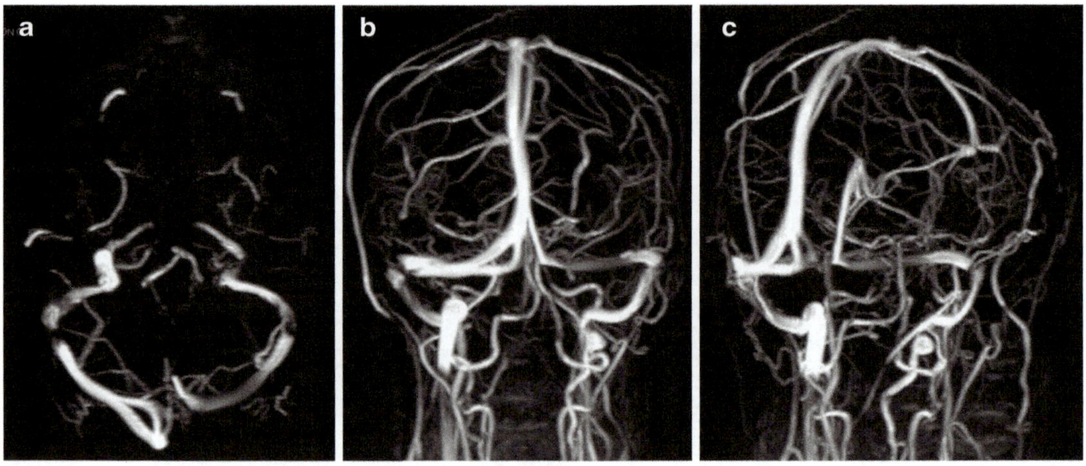

Fig. 11.7 Contrast-enhanced Phase Contrast MRV, reconstructed in axial plane (panel **a**) from 2D source images, and in volume rendering in panels **b** and **c**. A stenosis of the distal transverse sinus is visible on both sides

had long TSS and no empty sella; one had flattening of the posterior sclera; two had prominence of peri-optic nerve CSF.

In 2003 Farb et al. [65] proposed a grading scheme for the assessment of the degree of transverse-sigmoid sinus stenosis, the combined conduit score (CCS); the score was developed in the setting of IIH with auto-triggered elliptic-centric-ordered 3D gadolinium-enhanced MR venography (ATECO MRV). It was a prospective study on 29 patients with established IIH and 59 controls, and the assessment of transverse sinus stenosis was performed in a blinded manner on maximum intensity projection (MIP) reconstructions from gadolinium-enhanced MRV images (projections: RAO, LAO, and rotational cine loop MIPs), as time-of-flight artifacts overestimate stenosis. The patency of transverse-sigmoid sinus was graded for each side in Table 11.6.

Table 11.6 Combined conduit score [65]

Score	Description
0	Discontinuity (gap) or aplastic segment
1	Hypoplasia or severe stenosis within a segment of the conduit estimated as <25% of the cross-sectional diameter of the lumen of the distal superior sagittal sinus
2	Moderately stenosed segment of the conduit (25–50%)
3	Mildly narrowed segment (50–75%)
4	No significant narrowing (75–100%)

The highest degree from the torcula through to the distal sigmoid sinus determines the score on each side. Usually the CCS value is the sum of the right and left scores (range 0–8), and the cut-off of 4 is suggested to define significant stenosis. The first proposal of Farb et al. assessed a sensitivity and specificity of 93% for CCS score. It was suggested [69] that all patients with TSS on MRV should undergo fundoscopy to assess for papilledema.

This finding supported a role of venous hypertension in patients with IIH, as suggested by previous manometric studies which found pressure gradients across transverse sinus stenoses in patients with IIH [70, 71]. It has been proposed that bilateral TSS, or stenosis of a dominant transverse sinus, might lead to the following series of events: decreased venous outflow drainage > cerebral venous hypertension > CSF passive resorption impairment > further raising CSF pressure resulting in external compression of the distal portion of the transverse sinuses > leading to worsening of the venous stenosis and perpetuation of this vicious cycle [72, 73]. Bilateral TSS also is often found in patients with intracranial hypertension not due to IIH [74].

More recently a unifying theory has been proposed, taking into account the manometric measurements performed during sinus catheterization and stenting [75]. The proposed theory is centered around four core principles: (1) elevations in ICP have a diffuse impact on venous sinuses and their calibers; (2) there is variability in susceptibility to ICP-mediated stenosis in different regions of the sinuses, with the lateral transverse sinus being most susceptible and the torcula being resistant; (3) venous sinus stenosis is mediated through a positive feedback loop resulting in upstream venous congestion and elevated intramural venous pressures; and (4) recurrent stenosis occurs after stenting due to the effect of ongoing ICP elevations on susceptible regions of the sinuses in the setting of lower intramural venous pressures, resulting in a new positive feedback loop. The final stenosis is an extramural stenosis. Other sinuses can be involved, e.g., the distal segment of the superior sagittal sinus stenosis.

The dynamic nature of this process is suggested by the demonstration of the increase in cerebral sinuses diameter after lumbar puncture [76].

West JL et al. [77] stated that an increase in trans-stenotic pressure (TPG) of 3.5 mmHg was seen for every 10% increase in TSS in IIH patients and this linear correlation between TSS and TPG was confirmed in PT patients [78], while the degree of TSS had a much smaller effect on TPG (this discrepancy may be related to the differences in the subjects included and measurement methods) and the greater the length of TSS, the larger the TPG. Dinkin M et al. [79] proposed that compared with the degree of TSS, the shape of TSS may have a more important impact on the clinical course of IIH patients and Lasley JA et al. [80] speculated that the association may exist between the shape of TSS and PT. However, ipsilesional TPG was significantly larger in patients with contralateral transverse sinus dysplasia, suggesting that TPG may be related to the dominant blood flow and alternative pathways [78].

Another difference between IIH and PT patients on TSS is suggested by Sundarajan et al. [62]. In this study MRVs of 115 patients with IIH and 43 patients with PT before venous sinus stent placement were reviewed, recording intrinsic or extrinsic stenosis, prominent emissary veins, optic nerve tortuosity, cephalocele, sella appearance, poststenotic fusiform enlargement versus saccular venous aneurysm, and internal jugular bulb diverticula. Most patients with IIH (75 of 115 sinuses, 65%) had extrinsic stenosis, and most patients with PT (37 of 45 sinuses, 82%) had intrinsic stenosis. Intrinsic stenosis refers to internal filling defects such as prominent arachnoid granulations that narrow the sinus. Extrinsic stenosis involves external compression of the sinus by adjacent brain parenchyma. Marked optic nerve tortuosity was more common in IIH. Cephaloceles were rare in both cohorts, with an increased trend toward the presence in IIH. Empty sellas were more common in IIH. Cerebellar tonsils were similarly located at the foramen magnum level in both cohorts. Saccular venous aneurysms were more common in PT patients. Internal jugular bulb diverticula were similarly common in both cohorts.

Assessing the sensitivity of bilateral TSS is challenging because of inconsistent definitions across studies and the use of various venous imaging techniques (flow-sensitive MRV, contrast-enhanced MRV, CTV). Moreover, the degree of stenosis predictive of a clinically significant pressure gradient (30–35%) in the venous sinuses is considerably lower than the arterial stenosis at which pathologic hemodynamic alterations occur. While highly predictive of a venous pressure gradient when a stenosis is identified, non-invasive imaging does not appear to be a suitable diagnostic evaluation for the purpose of ruling out clinically significant cerebral VSS [81].

However, TSS can be found incidentally in normal subjects [67]. It has been pointed out that, depending on the definition of TSS, 100% of patients with IIH have bilateral stenosis on MRV [82]. More recently, a grading scale of TSS was proposed: 0, normal; 1, stenosis <33%; 2, stenosis 33–66%; 3, stenosis >66%; and 4, hypoplasia or agenesis [56]. The index proposed in this study was termed the index of transverse sinus stenosis (ITSS). This index consisted of the product of the number of the stenosis scale for each transverse sinus, according to the following formula: ITSS = degree of stenosis of the right transverse

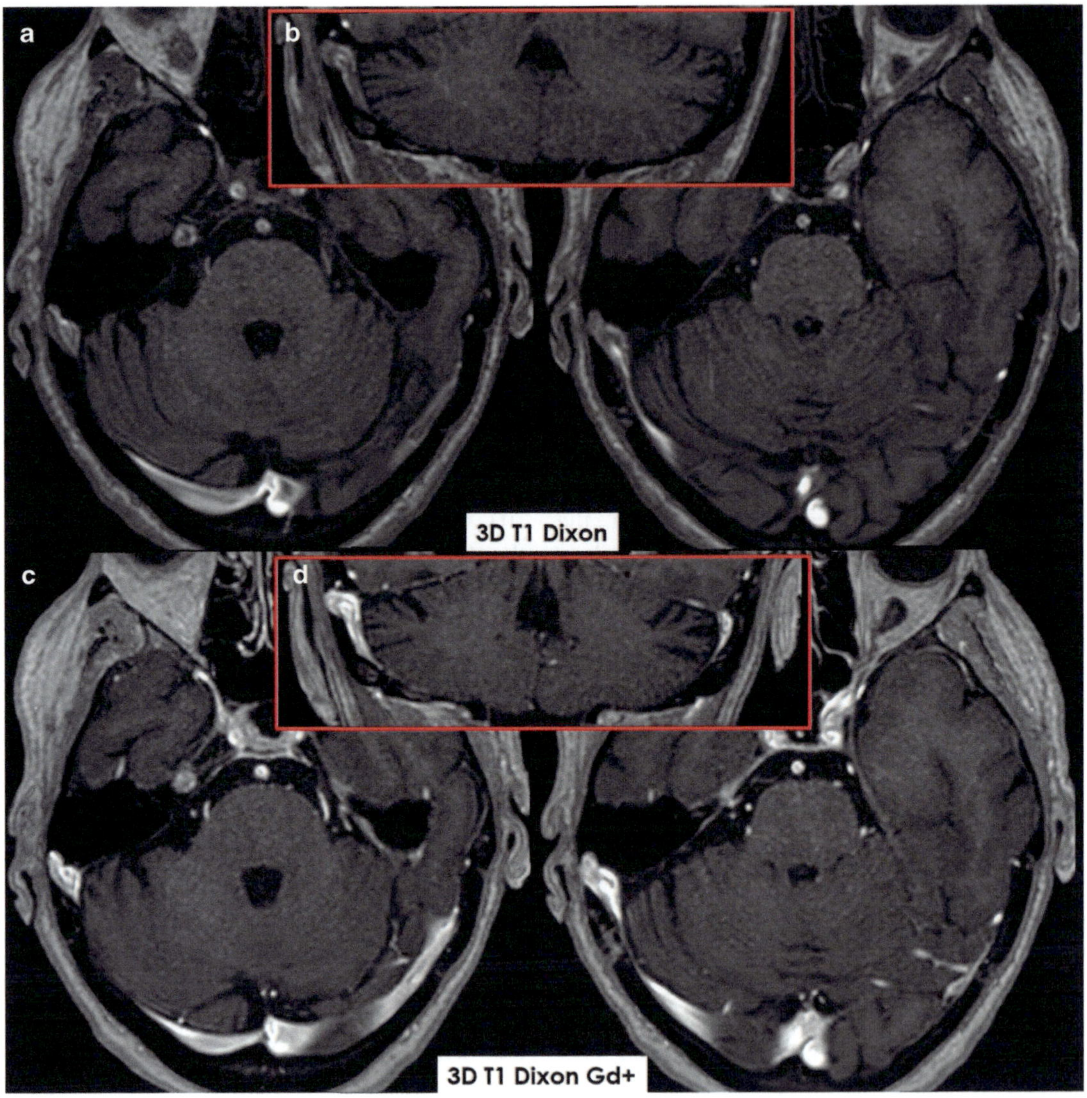

Fig. 11.8 SSWAs with right sigmoid diverticulum in 3D T1 Dixon sequence before (panels **a** and **b**) and after (panels **c** and **d**) contrast administration. Panels b and d show the corresponding coronal view

sinus × degree of stenosis of the left transverse sinus. It was applied in 63 individuals (32 diagnosed with IIH and 31 controls). Index values ≥4 for a diagnosis of IIH had a sensitivity and specificity of 94.7% and 93.5%, respectively.

SSWAs are an increasingly recognized diagnosis in the work-up of PT but they can also be associated with IIH (Figs. 11.8, 11.9, 11.10, 11.11, and 11.12). SSWAs range from a thin but intact sigmoid sinus plate to focal dehiscence of the sigmoid sinus plate, diverticulum formation with a focal protrusion of the vascular elements into the mastoid air cells, and ectasia with smooth bulging of the sigmoid sinus into the mastoid air cells without a focal diverticulum. Diverticula can be sessile outpouchings or narrow-necked, pedunculated structures, and more than one anomaly can be present. The most common abnormality is a diverticulum of the lateral surface of the sigmoid sinus (11 of 54 total patients with PT) [83]. The prevalence of SSWA in patients with PT was 23% versus 1.2% in asymp-

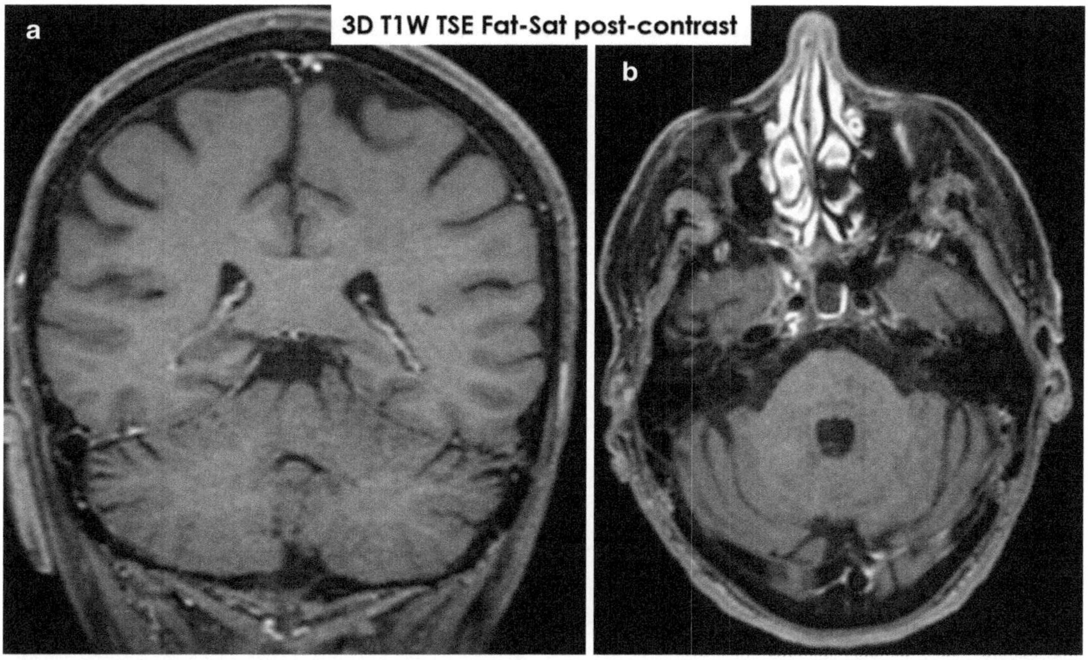

Fig. 11.9 Same patients as in the previous figure. T1W TSE fat sat shows similar findings with the confirmed sigmoid diverticulum, on the right side

tomatic patients [57]. The demographic features of these patients showed a significant overlap with the IIH patient population, suggesting a potential association between IIH and SSWA, and a possible explanation for PT in patients with IIH [84]. In a retrospective imaging study [85] aiming to evaluate the association between sigmoid sinus dehiscence/diverticulum (SSDD) and IIH, the PT patients with SSDD showed a significantly higher prevalence of empty sella ($p < 0.001$), flattened posterior sclera ($p = 0.001$), vertical tortuosity of the optic nerve ($p = 0.001$), protrusion of the optic nerve ($p = 0.006$), transverse sinus stenosis ($p = 0.011$), and distension of the optic nerve sheath ($p = 0.000$). In another recent retrospective neuroradiological study [86] investigating the correlation between transverse sinus stenosis and trans-stenotic pressure gradient (TPG) in unilateral PT patients with SSWA on 57 patients with unilateral venous PT using CT venography and catheter manometry, the mean value of ipsilesional TPG was 7.61 ± 0.52 mmHg. The degree and length of ipsilesional TSS were positively correlated with TPG ($p < 0.001$, $p' < 0.001$), respectively. TPG was significantly larger in patients with contralateral transverse sinus dysplasia than those without ($p = 0.023$) and significantly smaller in patients with ipsilesional sigmoid sinus diverticulum than those with isolated dehiscence ($p = 0.001$). Stepwise linear regression indicated that the degree ($\beta = 9.207$, 95% CI = 3.558–14.856), length ($\beta = 0.122$, 95% CI = 0.025–0.220) of ipsilesional TSS, and contralateral transverse sinus hypoplasia ($\beta = 1.875$, 95% CI = 0.220–3.530) were significantly correlated with TPG ($R^2 = 0.471$).

CT is the study of choice for the evaluation of potential SSWA. CT angiography timed to visualize both arterial and venous structures with temporal bone reconstructions is sensitive in identifying potential abnormalities [86]. CT images should be reconstructed for a high-resolution algorithm with a 0.67-mm section thickness, small field of view, and both axial and coronal reformats provided for analysis. Bone windows must be carefully scrutinized to evaluate the integrity of the sigmoid sinus plate. Subtle findings can be difficult to identify, especially in

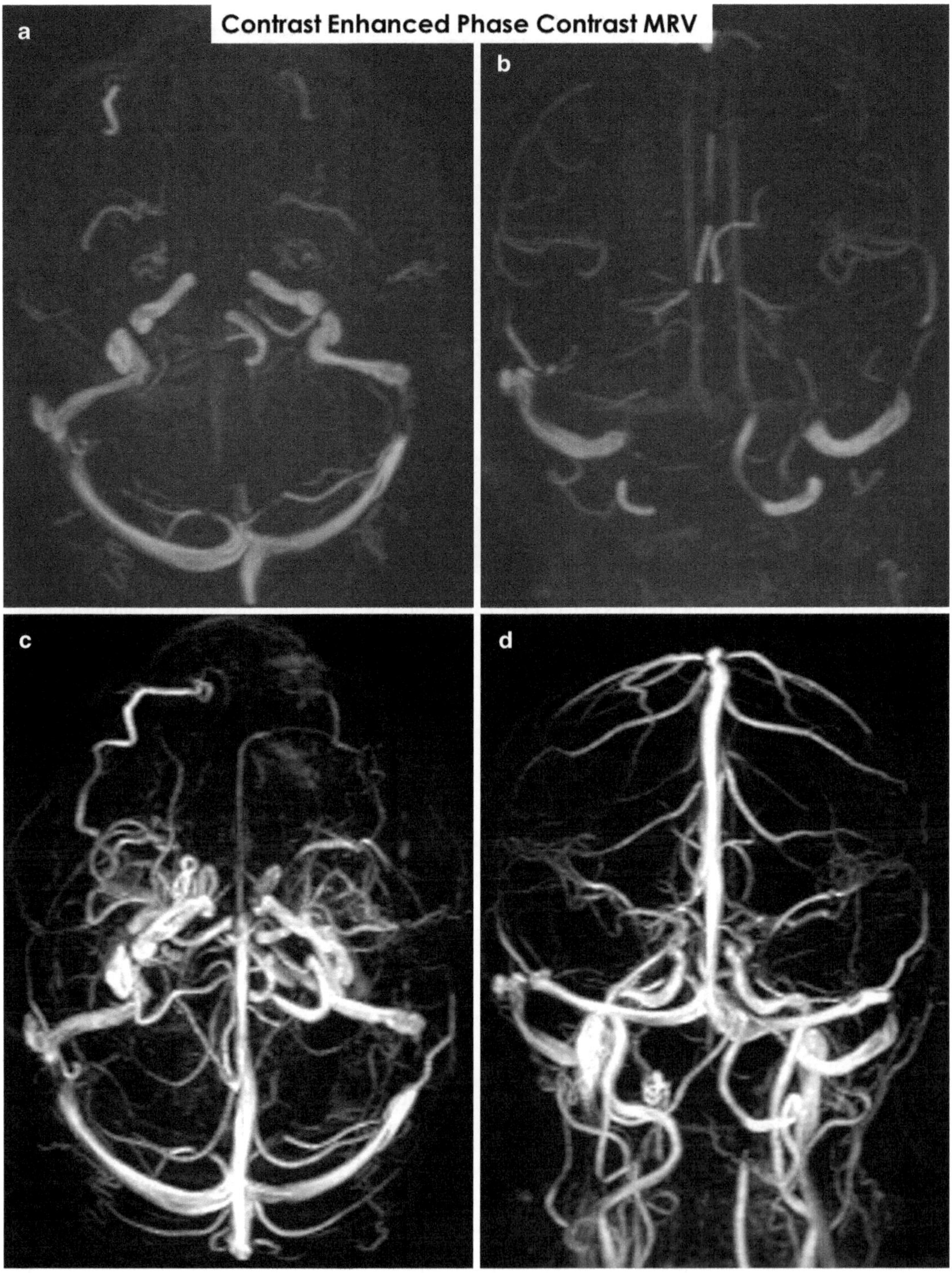

Fig. 11.10 In the same patient as in Figs. 11.8 and 11.9, the contrast-enhanced Phase Contrast MRV shows a bilateral transverse sinus stenosis (panels **a** and **b**: MIP/MPR reconstruction from the source images; panels **c** and **d**: volume rendering reconstruction)

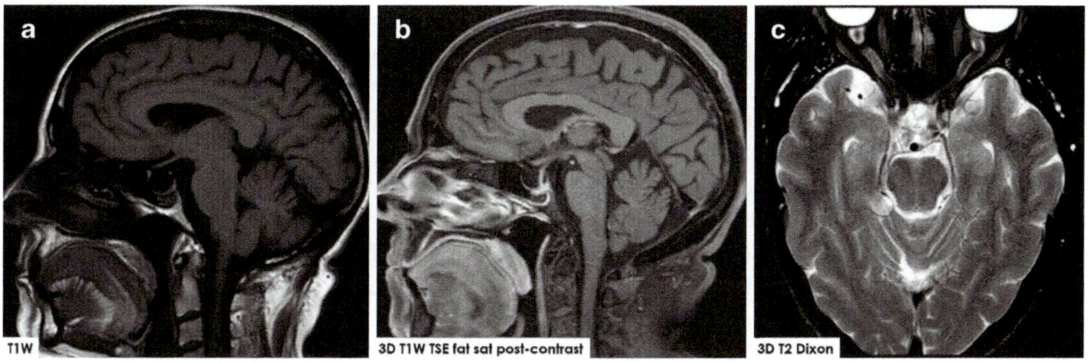

Fig. 11.11 In the same patient an empty sella is well visible (panels **a** and **b** in coronal view) and a tortuous course of the optic nerves imaged in panel **c**

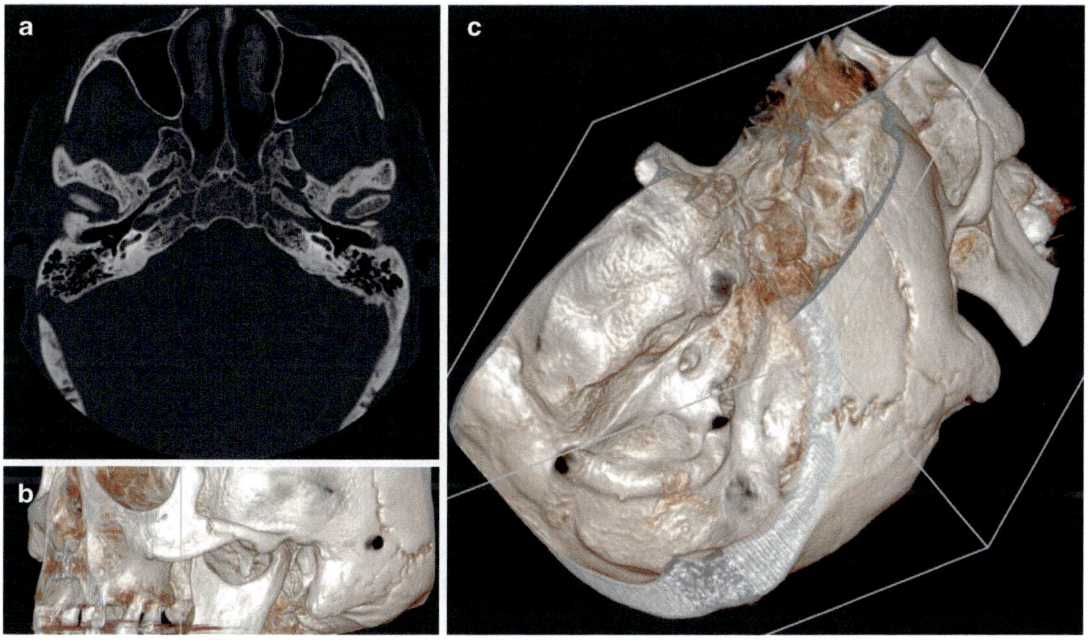

Fig. 11.12 High-resolution CT of the ear, showing a discontinuation of the temporal bone at the transverse-sigmoid transition on the right side as predisposing condition for diverticulum in IIH (panel **a**). In panels **b** and **c** there is a tridimensional reconstruction of the skull bone, highlighting the bone discontinuation

the case of bony dehiscence without diverticulum formation.

Useful imaging signs in the identification of SSWA [87] are

1. Irregularity of the semicircular contour of the bony sigmoid sinus wall.
2. Focal thinning of the calvarial cortex adjacent to the sigmoid sinus wall.
3. Absence of the thin layer of cortical bone overlying the sinus.
4. Air-on-sinus sign: direct contact of the mastoid air cells with the adjacent sinus.

Elevated ICP also pushes the structures into the skull base foramina and results in encephalocele/meningocele [88]. Protrusion of some structures such as the Meckel cave or cerebellar tonsils may also be seen through the skull base foramina. This may result in an indented or bilobed appearance of the Meckel cave. In a recent case-control study [89] on 75 IIH patients and 75 controls, the main aim was to investigate if the shape (bilobed or indented appearance of the Meckel cave) or the size/volume of the Meckel cave on T2-weighted MRI sequences could serve as a non-invasive diagnostic imaging marker for the diagnosis of IIH. The transverse diameter of Meckel cave was measured in the axial and coronal planes of T2-weighted MRI sequences (respectively 5.21 + 1.22 mm on the right side and 5.16 + 0.90 mm on the left side in cases and 3.89 + 0.62 mm vs. 4.09 + 0.68 mm in controls) (p value, 0.001). Fifty-seven (76%) of IIH patients showed an indented Meckel cave as opposed to 21 (28%) in the control group. The study revealed that enlargement of the Meckel cave has about 75% sensitivity and about 86% specificity for diagnosis of IIH, which has the third highest sensitivity and specificity among the preceding imaging findings after bilateral TSS and empty sella.

These patients are at risk for development of spontaneous CSF leaks via either the anterior or lateral skull base. The hypothesis is that IIH causes osseous erosions leading to CSF leak as a consequence of osseous dehiscences and arachnoid herniation. Osseous dehiscences in the skull base occur mainly in the cribriform plate, the sphenoid sinus, and the tegmen tympani, among other locations [41]. More controversial reports include expansion of the foramen ovale [90] and enlargement of Dorello's canal [91].

IIH is an increasingly recognized etiology of spontaneous skull base CSF leaks in the otolaryngology and neurosurgery literature [92–95]. Spontaneous skull base CSF leaks might represent a variant of IIH in patients who do not develop typical symptoms and signs of IIH because the leak acts as a "natural" CSF diversion. However, determining if a patient with spontaneous CSF leak may have IIH may be difficult, as signs and symptoms of raised ICP may be obviated by the leak [41].

Noncontrast high-resolution CT scan with thin sections allowing multiplanar reconstruction is the first-line imaging technique to localize bone defects at the skull base; in difficult cases, such as those with multiple defects or a negative CT scan despite an active CSF leak, CT or MR cisternography may help identify the site of the CSF leak [96, 97]. CSF leaks are associated with meningoceles and meningoencephaloceles in 50%–100% of cases [98]. When a CSF leak is diagnosed, brain MRI helps to differentiate herniated intracranial contents from sequestered secretions within the paranasal sinuses and allows screening for findings consistent with long-standing IIH, such as a partial or complete empty sella, reported in 66–100% of cases with spontaneous CSF leaks [99]. Pachymeningeal enhancement and sagging of the brain are uncommon in patients with CSF leaks presumed to be secondary to IIH [100].

An interesting association exists between IIH and the presence of spontaneous CSF fistulas. The underlying hypothesis is that the increased ICP leads to the development of prominent arachnoid granulations within the skull base and, when they develop over pneumatized bone, bony thinning and disruption of the dura can occur [101]. Typical locations are the tegmen tympani, floor of the middle cranial fossa, lateral wall of the sphenoid sinus, and cribriform plates [100, 101].

Widening of the foramen ovale, visualized best on axial high-resolution CT scan, likely is related to herniation of the contents of Meckel cave through the foramen ovale leading to bony remodeling. The utility of this finding on routine imaging for patients with presumed IIH remains unclear. One study evaluated the tendency of the foramen ovale (FO) to appear widened in patients with IIH.

Dorello's canal (DC) transmits the abducens nerve (CNVI) to the cavernous sinus and may undergo changes in the presence of increased ICP. The enlargement of DC is due to CSF evagination into it and was studied using Axial MRI FIESTA sequence, 3D-CISS MR cisternography. Additionally, some patients were observed to have visible DCs on only one side.

These findings could be relevant in individual cases because subjects with spontaneous CSF leaks had postclamping average ICP identical to controls with IIH and papilledema, and such evidence suggests that a CSF leak in this patient population provides sufficient pressure diversion to avoid the development of papilledema [101].

Tonsillar herniation is the caudal displacement of the cerebellar tonsils >5 mm into the upper cervical spinal canal through the foramen magnum and is best visualized on mid-sagittal T1 MRI [80]. Although tonsillar herniation is the hallmark of Chiari malformation Type I (CM1) [102], these two conditions are not synonymous. Up to 15% of the normal population have a small degree herniation of the tonsils (>2 mm and > 5 mm) below the foramen magnum (tonsillar ectopia) [103]. Cerebellar tonsillar herniation also has been reported after lumbar puncture and placement of a lumbar-peritoneal shunt. More recently, confusion has arisen with studies reporting patients with typical CM1 displaying radiologic findings of chronically increased ICP [104] and typical IIH patients with herniation of the cerebellar tonsils (some of whom met the criteria for CM1) [74]. It is unclear whether these patients have primary CM1 complicated by increased ICP, or IIH complicated by CM1-like tonsillar herniation, or both conditions.

The progressive enlargement of the foramen magnum with secondary caudal descent of the tonsils was hypothesized [105] but in a single center study, the foramen magnum size was not different between IIH patients and controls [106].

Referring to a lower than usual position of the cerebellar tonsils in IIH as "tonsillar descent" involves a dynamic process pushing the tonsils down, either because of low pressure below (such as in spontaneous intracranial hypotension) or high pressure above (such as in IIH). This association between tonsillar herniation and IIH is emerging, and the prevalence of IIH in tonsillar herniation and the direction of the causation, if any, between these two entities are still controversial. Bony remodeling associated with IIH may lead to herniation of meninges (meningocele) or brain tissue (meningoencephalocele) through skull base foramina or areas of thin bone of the skull base. Meningoceles and meningoencephaloceles are best demonstrated on MRI with contrast [107] and have been strongly associated with CSF leaks.

In the early descriptions of patients with IIH, before the era of modern neuroimaging, the radiologic finding of "slit-like" ventricles was emphasized as opposed to the dilated ventricles of patients with obstructive hydrocephalus. Although slit-like ventricles were reported in studies using older generation CT scan imaging [95], this finding has not been corroborated on more recent MRI studies [89, 108].

11.6 Diagnostic Accuracy of MRI Sign

The diagnostic yield of the above-described MRI sign of IIH is summarized in the following table (Table 11.7).

While suggestive, these findings are not diagnostic of active intracranial hypertension due to their occurrence in normal individuals [65] as well as only partial normalization following treatment.

The findings of MRI signs (empty sella, increased perioptic cerebrospinal fluid, optic nerve tortuosity, TSS) typically associated with IIH are also not rare in other conditions, ranging from patients with primary headache syndromes and asymptomatic individuals [41, 65, 119, 120]. For example, empty sella has a prevalence of 8–35% in general population and it is more common in women and obese individuals [121, 122].

The incidental findings of MRI signs typically associated with IIH may lead to over-referral of patients, sometimes to invasive testing and overdiagnosis, mainly in obese women [36]. In a recent prospective study aimed to address the prevalence of incidentally detected signs of IHH on MRI (empty sella, optic nerve head protrusion, posterior scleral flattening, increased perioptic cerebrospinal fluid, optic nerve tortuosity, enlarged Meckel caves, cephaloceles, cerebellar tonsillar descent, and bilateral transverse venous sinus stenosis) and their association with papilledema [123], among 296 subjects [median age 49.5 years (interquartile range, 37.8–62.0 years), 63.5% female] at least 1 radiographic sign of IH

Table 11.7 Diagnostic accuracy of MRI signs for IIH

Finding	Definition	Prevalence	Sensitivity	Specificity
Empty sella	The term "empty sella" refers to complete or partial CSF filling of the sella turcica associated with lack of visible pituitary gland on mid-sagittal T1 MRI	26.7% of people with IIH and 5.4% of controls [110]	26.7–80% (partially ES 53.3–65.1%) [109]	83–95% (partially ES 75–95.3%) [109]
Protrusion of the optic nerve head	Swelling of the optic nerve head because of increased CSF pressure in the optic nerve sheath	3.3% of people with IIH and 0% of controls [110]	3.3–37.2% [109]	95–100% [109]
Increased perioptic CSF	It appears as $a > 2$ mm widened ring of CSF surrounding an optic nerve	66.7% of people with IIH and 17.9% of controls	45–66.7% [109]	82.1–95% [109]
Tortuosity of the intraorbital optic nerve	Vertical tortuosity is more common but horizontal tortuosity, although less common, is more specific for increased ICP than vertical tortuosity	40% of people with IIH and 8.9% of controls [110] horizontal tortuosity (controls: 10%; pretreatment: IIH 80%; posttreatment: 20%) [112]	Horizontal 40.5% [111] Vertical 34.9–43% [109]	Horizontal 83.3% [111] Vertical 86–95% [109]
Optic nerve head enhancement	The association between papilledema grade and optic nerve hyperintensity is not well established [113]	NA	17% [55]	99% [55]
Flattening of the posterior sclera	Straightening out of the curvature of the posterior sclera where it attaches to the optic nerve	43.3% of people with IIH and 0% of controls [110]	43.3–80% [109]	95–100% [109]
DWI hyperintensity of the optic nerve head	ONH hyperintensity mean cut-off ONH ADC value	52.6–78.9% in at least one eye in IIH patients; 5–10% in controls [113, 114]	ONH hyperintensity 87.5% Mean ADC value 96.83%	ONH hyperintensity 97.1–98.6% Mean ADC value 95.31%
Transverse sinus stenosis	Transverse sinus stenosis multiplicative index ≥2 Transverse sinus stenosis index ≥4 Bilateral >50% transverse sinus stenosis Minimal cross-sectional area of left transverse sinus and mean cross-sectional area of right transverse sinus cut-off value 55% Combined transverse stenosis score <4 Bilateral transverse sinus flow gaps Combined venous conduit score ≤4.7	The prevalence of unilateral transverse sinus stenosis or hypoplasia in a sample of patients representing the general population was 33%, the prevalence of bilateral transverse sinus stenosis was 5%, and the prevalence of unilateral stenosis with contralateral hypoplasia was 1% [115, 116] Almost 100% of people with IIH, depending on the definition of transverse sinus stenosis [55]	Cumulative value 84.4 (65.9–93.9) 94.9 (91.7–96.9) [113] CCS score > 4: 93% [43]	Cumulative value 84.4 (65.9–93.9) 94.9 (91.7–96.9) [113] CCS score > 4: 93% [43]
Enlarged Meckel cave	Indented or bilobed appearance of the Meckel cave[b]	75% in IIH pts. vs. 14% in controls[b] [88]	75% [88]	86% [88]

Cerebellar tonsillar herniation	The caudal displacement of the cerebellar tonsils >5 mm into the upper cervical spinal canal through the foramen magnum		16% [55]	95% [55]
Meningoceles/ encephaloceles	Herniation of meninges (meningocele) or brain tissue (meningoencephalocele) through skull base foramina or areas of thin bone of the skull base	IIH cohort 5/115 [62]	11% [55]	NA [55]
Spontaneous cerebrospinal fluid leaks	Egress of CSF from the intracranial cavity through an osteodural disruption between the subarachnoid space and a pneumatized structure within the skull base	NA	CT 92% MR NA [55]	CT 100% MR NA [55]
Sigmoid sinus wall anomalies (SSWA)	This spectrum of anomalies includes a thin but intact sigmoid sinus plate, focal dehiscence of the sigmoid sinus plate, diverticulum formation with a focal protrusion of the vascular elements into the mastoid air cells, and ectasia with smooth bulging of the sigmoid sinus into the mastoid air cells without a focal diverticulum	The prevalence of SSWA in patients with PST was 23% versus 1.2% in asymptomatic patients [84] Among patients with IIH the incidence of SSWAs was significantly higher in subjects with PT than without (70% vs. 0%, $p = 0.02$) [117]	NA	NA
Internal jugular bulb diverticula	A focal outpouching from the jugular bulb. Internal jugular bulb diverticula were evaluated on coronal plane MRV imaging, with sizes graded according to height projecting above a line drawn perpendicular to the distal sigmoid sinus insertion into the internal jugular vein. Diverticula were categorized as either being small (≥5 mm in height) or prominent (<5 mm in height)	47/115 < 5 mm (40.87%) 68/115 ≥ 5 mm (59.13%) In IIH cohort [55]	NA	NA
Prominence of the posterior fossa emissary veins	Measurement of vein caliper on MRV	The prevalence of emissary veins in MRI was found in the right mastoid emissary vein (MEV) 82.7% and left MEV 81.4%. Occipital emissary vein (OEV) was present in 63 patients (28.6%) [118] IIH cohort Condylar 52/115 Occipital and condylar 28/115 Mastoid 6/115 Mastoid and condylar 5/115 Occipital, condylar, and mastoid 1/115 None 23/115 [55]	NA	NA
Optic canal size	Usually measured in CT		NA	NA

(continued)

Table 11.7 (continued)

Finding	Definition	Prevalence	Sensitivity	Specificity
Slit-like lateral ventricles	Narrowing or collapse of the walls of the lateral ventricles	3.3% of people with IIH and 0% of controls [108]	3.3–39.5%	79.1–100%
Tight subarachnoid spaces	Very small sulci and cisterns		6.1% [109]	97.1% [109]
Enlargement of Dorello's Canal	Radiographic patency of DC on MRI [109]	NA	NA	NA
Widening of the foramen ovale	Diameter of the foramen ovale ≥30 mm [102]	NA	50%	81%

[a] *ONH* optic nerve head

[b] The authors performed quantitative measurement for the transverse diameter of the Meckel cave in coronal T2 plane but they did not propose a threshold for it, finding a significantly larger transverse diameter in IIH patients versus controls. They also adopted a similar approach for the volume of the Meckel cave. In addition, they used a qualitative evaluation of the shape of the Meckel cave, finding an indented appearance in most IIH patients [88]

was present in 145 patients (49.0%): 98 patients (33.1%) had empty sella, 47 patients (15.9%) had enlarged Meckel caves, 32 patients (10.8%) had increased perioptic cerebrospinal fluid, 23 patients (7.8%) had optic nerve tortuosity, 2 patients (0.7%) had scleral flattening, 4 patients (1.4%) had cephaloceles, and 6 of 198 patients (3.0%) had bilateral transverse sinus stenosis. It is noteworthy that only five patients (1.7%) had papilledema, with a significantly higher body mass index and history of IIH, in addition to an increased prevalence of empty sella, optic nerve tortuosity, and TSS detected on MRI in comparison with the ones without papilledema. The prevalence of papilledema increased from 2.8% among patients with at least one MRI sign of IIH to 40.0% among patients with four or more MRI signs of IIH. The presence of papilledema therefore seems to characterize a cohort of patients with MRI signs of IIH deserving of a further diagnostic path.

In a recent systematic review and meta-analysis [113] addressing sensitivity and specificity of MRI signs of IIH, comprising a total of 724 patients with IIH, "empty" sella, posterior displacement of pituitary stalk, meningoceles, posterior globe flattening, optic nerve head protrusion, optic nerve enhancement, optic nerve sheath distension, optic nerve tortuosity, slit-like ventricles, tight subarachnoid spaces, and inferior position of cerebellar tonsils had pooled sensitivity ranging from 6.1% to 68.6%, and pooled specificity ranging from 84.0% to 99.2%. TSS had pooled sensitivity of 84.4% (95% CI: 65.9–93.9%) and pooled specificity of 94.9% (95% CI: 91.7–96.9%). Then, the first group of signs has overall high specificity but low sensitivity; TSS appears to be the most useful sign, because it has high specificity and high sensitivity. The presence of multiple imaging markers increases the likelihood of IIH diagnosis, although absence of these findings does not rule it out. Furthermore, several attempts have been performed in order to overcome the differential diagnosis between "true" TSS and anomalies (hypo-aplasia), avoiding over-diagnosis. One of them was recently published and proposed the quantitative measurement of transverse-sigmoid sinus and internal jugular bulb diameter on 3D post-contrast T1W sequence [124]. This consideration and the mention of the added value of post-contrast 3D T1W imaging is of paramount relevance in order to distinguish "true" transverse sinus stenosis from thrombotic and non-thrombotic filling defects, including anomalies and arachnoid granulations and septa [125].

11.7 Management

Iatrogenic intracranial hypertension was not systematically addressed in the literature, being a rare secondary cause of a rare condition. Basically, whenever possible, stopping the causative drug is an option and sometimes the clinical and neuroimaging signs fully or partially resolved [126–129]. In refractory cases, the same management of IIH is usually applied, the drug being a potential trigger on an underlying previously unknown condition.

11.8 Conclusions

Drug-induced intracranial hypertension is a rare condition, but it may have the same consequences of the IIH and deserves the same diagnostic pathway and treatment. The MRI signs of intracranial hypertension are not rare in the general population and they are not specific for the diagnosis if a related clinical context lacks. The diagnostic accuracy of a dedicated MRI investigation has been partially assessed and the knowledge of these issues might be of help in diagnosing the disease.

References

1. Smith J. Whence pseudotumor cerebri? J Clin Neuroophthalmol. 1985;5:55–6.
2. Friedman D, Jacobson D. Diagnostic criteria for idiopathic intracranial hypertension. Neurology. 2002;59:1492–5.
3. Friedman DI, Liu GT, Digre KB. Revised diagnostic criteria for the pseudotumor cerebri syndrome in adults and children. Neurology. 2013;81:1159–65.

4. Markey KA, Mollan SP, Jensen RH, et al. Understanding idiopathic intracranial hypertension: mechanisms, management, and future directions. Lancet Neurol. 2016;15:78–91.
5. Woods CP, Argese N, Chapman M, et al. Adrenal suppression in patients taking inhaled glucocorticoids is highly prevalent and management can be guided by morning cortisol. Eur J Endocrinol. 2015;173(5):633–42.
6. Friedman DI. Novel.utah.edu Walsh and Hoyt text, Chapter 5. In: Miller N, Newman NJ, editors. Walsh and Hoyt's clinical neuro-ophthalmology. 5th ed. Baltimore: Williams & Wilkins Ed; 1998. p. 237–91. https://collections.lib.utah.edu/details?id=190037#contents.
7. Mollan SP, Davies B, Silver NC, Shaw S, Mallucci CL, Wakerley BR, Krishnan A, Chavda SV, Ramalingam S, Edwards J, Hemmings K, Williamson M, Burdon MA, Hassan-Smith G, Digre K, Liu GT, Jensen RH, Sinclair AJ. Idiopathic intracranial hypertension: consensus guidelines on management. J Neurol Neurosurg Psychiatry. 2018;89(10):1088–100. https://doi.org/10.1136/jnnp-2017-317440.
8. Friedman DI. Medication-induced intracranial hypertension in dermatology. Am J Clin Dermatol. 2005;6(1):29–37. https://doi.org/10.2165/00128071-200506010-00004.
9. Tan MG, Worley B, Kim WB, Ten Hove M, Beecker J. Drug-induced intracranial hypertension: a systematic review and critical assessment of drug-induced causes. Am J Clin Dermatol. 2020;21(2):163–72. https://doi.org/10.1007/s40257-019-00485-z.
10. Kushida A, Tamura H. Retinoic acids induce neurosteroid biosynthesis in human glial GI-1 cells via the induction of steroidogenic genes. J Biochem. 2009;146:917–23.
11. Warner JE, Bernstein PS, Yemelyanov A, Alder SC, Farnsworth ST, Digre KB. Vitamin A in the cerebrospinal fluid of patients with and without idiopathic intracranial hypertension. Ann Neurol. 2002;52:647–50.
12. Lombaert A, Carton H. Benign intracranial hypertension due to A-hypervitaminosis in adults and adolescents. Eur Neurol. 1976;14:340–50.
13. Spector RH, Carlisle J. Pseudotumor cerebri caused by a synthetic vitamin A preparation. Neurology. 1984;34:1509–11.
14. Fraunfelder FW, Fraunfelder FT, Corbett JJ. Isotretinoin-associated intracranial hypertension. Ophthalmology. 2004;111:1248–50.
15. Lee AG. Pseudotumor cerebri after treatment with tetracycline and isotretinoin for acne. Cutis. 1995;55:165–73.
16. Fraunfelder FT, LaBraico JM, Meyer SM. Adverse ocular reactions possibly associated with isotretinoin. Am J Ophthalmol. 1985;100:534–7.
17. Caruana DM, Wylie G. 'Washout' period for oral tetracycline antibiotics prior to systemic isotretinoin. Br J Dermatol. 2016;174:929–30.
18. Chiu AM, Chuenkongkaew WL, Cornblath WT, Trobe JD, Digre KB, Dotan SA, et al. Minocycline treatment and pseudotumor cerebri syndrome. Am J Ophthalmol. 1998;126:116–21.
19. Tintle SJ, Harper JC, Webster GF, Kim GK, Thiboutot DM. Safe use of therapeutic-dose oral isotretinoin in patients with a history of pseudotumor cerebri. JAMA Dermatol. 2016;152:582–4.
20. Jonnalagadda J, Saito E, Kafantaris V. Lithium, minocycline, and pseudotumor cerebri. J Am Acad Child Adolesc Psychiatry. 2005;44:209.
21. Caruana D, Wylie G. "Wash-out" period for oral tetracycline antibiotics prior to systemic isotretinoin. Br J Dermatol. 2015;173:34–5.
22. Bettoli V, Borghi A, Mantovani L, Scorrano R, Minghetti S, Toni G, et al. Safe use of oral isotretinoin after pseudotumor cerebri due to minocycline. Eur J Dermatol. 2011;21:1024–5.
23. Law C, Yau GL, ten Hove M. Delayed development of intracranial hypertension after discontinuation of tetracycline treatment for acne vulgaris. J Neuroophthalmol. 2016;36:67–9.
24. Friedman DI, Gordon LK, Egan RA, Jacobson DM, Pomeranz H, Harrison AR, et al. Doxycycline and intracranial hypertension. Neurology. 2004;62:2297–9.
25. Bohm R, Hocker J, Cascorbi I, Herdegen T. OpenVigil-free eyeballs on AERS pharmacovigilance data. Nat Biotechnol. 2012;30:137–8.
26. Etminan M. Risk of intracranial hypertension with intrauterine levonorgestrel: reply. Ther Adv Drug Saf. 2016;7:25–6.
27. Rai R, Kirk B, Sanders J, Valenzuela R, Sundar S, Warner J, et al. The relationship between the levonorgestrel-releasing intrauterine system and idiopathic intracranial hypertension. Invest Ophthalmol Vis Sci. 2015;56:2228.
28. Koerner JC, Friedman DI. Inpatient and emergency service utilization in patients with idiopathic intracranial hypertension. J Neuroophthalmol. 2014;34:229–32.
29. Ireland B, Corbett JJ, Wallace RB. The search for causes of idiopathic intracranial hypertension. A preliminary case-control study. Arch Neurol. 1990;47:315–20.
30. Giuseffi V, Wall M, Siegel PZ, Rojas PB. Symptoms and disease associations in idiopathic intracranial hypertension (pseudotumor cerebri): a case-control study. Neurology. 1991;41:239–44.
31. Wall M. Idiopathic intracranial hypertension. Neurol Clin. 2010;28:593–617.
32. Reddy AR, Backhouse OC. Contraceptive, cerebral vein thrombosis and choked discs. Eur J Ophthalmol. 2007;17:669–70.
33. Neely DE, Plager DA, Kumar N. Desmopressin (DDAVP)-induced pseudotumor cerebri. J Pediatr. 2003;143:808.
34. Headache Classification Committee of the International Headache Society (IHS). The interna-

tional classification of headache disorders, 3rd edition. Cephalalgia. 2018;38(1):1–211.
35. Wall M, George D. Idiopathic intracranial hypertension. A prospective study of 50 patients. Brain. 1991;114(Pt 1):155–80.
36. Fisayo A, Bruce BB, Newman NJ, et al. Overdiagnosis of idiopathic intracranial hypertension. Neurology. 2016;86:341–50. https://doi.org/10.1212/WNL.0000000000002318.
37. Piper RJ, Kalyvas AV, Young AM, et al. Interventions for idiopathic intracranial hypertension. Cochrane Database Syst Rev. 2015:CD003434. https://doi.org/10.1002/14651858.CD003434.pub3.
38. International Headache Society Classification Subcommittee. International classification of headache disorders: 2nd edition. Cephalalgia. 2004;24:1–160.
39. Mollan SP, Chong YJ, Grech O, Sinclair AJ, Wakerley BR. Current perspectives on idiopathic intracranial hypertension without papilloedema. Life. 2021;11:472; Neurol Sci (2019) 40 (Suppl 1): S59–70.
40. Favoni V, Pierangeli G, Cirillo L, Toni F, Abu-Rumeileh S, La Morgia C, Messia M, Agati R, Cortelli P, Cevoli S. Transverse sinus stenosis in refractory chronic headache patients: an observational study. Front Neurol. 2019;10:1287.
41. Bidot S, Levy JM, Saindane AM, Oyesiku NM, Newman NJ, Biousse V. Do most patients with a spontaneous cerebrospinal fluid leak have Idiopathic intracranial hypertension? J Neuroophthalmol. 2019;39(4):487–95. https://doi.org/10.1097/WNO.0000000000000761.
42. Wall M, Corbett JJ. Revised diagnostic criteria for the pseudotumor cerebri syndrome in adults and children. Neurology. 2014;83(2):198–200.
43. Yuh WT, Zhu M, Taoka T, et al. MR imaging of pituitary morphology in idiopathic intracranial hypertension. J Magn Reson Imaging. 2000;12(6):808–13.
44. Riggeal BD, Bruce BB, Saindane AM, et al. Clinical course of idiopathic intracranial hypertension with transverse sinus stenosis. Neurology. 2013;80(3):289–95.
45. Guitelman M, Basavilbaso NG, Vitale M, et al. Primary empty sella (PES): a review of 175 cases. Pituitary. 2012;16:270–4.
46. Chang Y, Alperin N, Bagci A, et al. Relationship between optic nerve protrusion measured by OCT and MRI and papilledema severity. Investig Ophthalmol Vis Sci. 2015;56:2297.
47. Passi N, Degnan A, Levy L. MR imaging of papilledema and visual pathways: effects of increased intracranial pressure and pathophysiologic mechanisms. Am J Neuroradiol. 2012;34:919–24.
48. Alperin N, Bagci A, Lam B, Sklar E. Automated quantitation of the posterior scleral flattening and optic nerve protrusion by MRI in idiopathic intracranial hypertension. Am J Neuroradiol. 2013;34:2354–9.
49. Degnan A, Levy L. Pseudotumor cerebri: brief review of clinical syndrome and imaging findings. Am J Neuroradiol. 2011;32:1986–93.
50. Bidot S, Saindane A, Peragallo J, et al. Brain imaging in idiopathic intracranial hypertension. J Neuroophthalmol. 2015;35:400–11.
51. Brodsky MC, Glasier CM. Magnetic resonance visualization of the swollen optic disc in papilledema. J Neuroophthalmol. 1995;15:122–4; AJNR Am J Neuroradiol 40:334–39.
52. Viets R, Parsons M, Van Stavern G, et al. Hyperintense optic nerve heads on diffusion-weighted imaging: a potential imaging sign of papilledema. AJNR Am J Neuroradiol. 2013;34(7):1438–42.
53. Salvay DM, Padhye LV, Huecker JB, et al. Correlation between papilledema grade and diffusion-weighted magnetic resonance imaging in idiopathic intracranial hypertension. J Neuroophthalmol. 2014;34(4):331e5.
54. Ray N, Vyas S, Khandelwal N, Bansal R, Lal V. Papilloedema: diffusion-weighted imaging of optic nerve head. Clin Radiol. 2019;74(8):652.e11–9. https://doi.org/10.1016/j.crad.2019.05.005.
55. Bidot S, Bruce BB, Saindane AM, Newman NJ, Biousse V. Asymmetric papilledema in idiopathic intracranial hypertension. J Neuroophthalmol. 2015;35:31–6.
56. Mattox DE, Hudgins P. Algorithm for evaluation of pulsatile tinnitus. Acta Otolaryngol. 2008;128(4):427–31.
57. Harvey RS, Hertzano R, Kelman SE, et al. Pulse-synchronous tinnitus and sigmoid sinus wall anomalies: descriptive epidemiology and the idiopathic intracranial hypertension patient population. Otol Neurotol. 2014;35(1):7–15; Neuroradiology. 2015;57:747–53.
58. Ong CK, Fook-Hin CV. Imaging of jugular foramen. Neuroimaging Clin North Am. 2009;19(3):469–82.
59. Mortazavi MM, Tubbs RS, Riech S, et al. Anatomy and pathology of the cranial emissary veins: a review with surgical implications. Neurosurgery. 2012;70(5):1312–8.
60. Hoffmann O, Klingebiel R, Braun JS, et al. Diagnostic pitfall: atypical cerebral venous drainage via the vertebral venous system. AJNR Am J Neuroradiol. 2002;23(3):408–11.
61. Chauhan NS, Sharma YP, Bhagra T, et al. Persistence of multiple emissary veins of posterior fossa with unusual origin of left petrosquamosal sinus from mastoid emissary. Surg Radiol Anat. 2011;33(9):827–31.
62. Sundararajan SH, Ramos AD, Kishore V, Michael M, Doustaly R, DeRusso F, Patsalides A. Dural venous sinus stenosis: why distinguishing intrinsic-versus-extrinsic stenosis matters. AJNR Am J Neuroradiol. 2021;42(2):288–96. https://doi.org/10.3174/ajnr.A6890.
63. Dinkin MJ, Patsalides A. Venous sinus stenting for idiopathic intracranial hypertension: where are we now? Neurol Clin. 2017;35:59–81.

64. Biousse V, Ameri A, Bousser MG. Isolated intracranial hypertension as the only sign of cerebral venous thrombosis. Neurology. 1999;53:1537–42.
65. Farb R, Vanek I, Scott J, et al. Idiopathic intracranial hypertension: the prevalence and morphology of sinovenous stenosis. Neurology. 2003;60:1418–24.
66. Morris P, Black D, Port J, Campeau N. Transverse sinus stenosis is the most sensitive MR imaging correlate of idiopathic intracranial hypertension. Am J Neuroradiol. 2017;38:471–7.
67. Kelly LP, Saindane AM, Bruce BB, Ridha MA, Riggeal BD, Newman NJ, Biousse V. Does bilateral transverse cerebral venous sinus stenosis exist in patients without increased intracranial pressure? Clin Neurol Neurosurg. 2013;115(8):1215–9. https://doi.org/10.1016/j.clineuro.2012.11.004.
68. Wilson MH. Monro-Kellie 2.0: the dynamic vascular and venous pathophysiological components of intracranial pressure. J Cereb Blood Flow Metab. 2016;36(8):1338–50. https://doi.org/10.1177/0271678X16648711.
69. Kelly LP, Saindane AM, Bruce BB, Ridha MA, Riggeal BD, Newman NJ, et al. Does bilateral transverse cerebral venous sinus stenosis exist in patients without increased intracranial pressure? Clin Neurol Neurosurg. 2013;115:1215–9.
70. King JO, Mitchell PJ, Thomson KR, Tress BM. Cerebral venography and manometry in idiopathic intracranial hypertension. Neurology. 1995;45:2224–8.
71. King JO, Mitchell PJ, Thomson KR, Tress BM. Manometry combined with cervical puncture in idiopathic intracranial hypertension. Neurology. 2002;58:26–30.
72. Biousse V, Bruce BB, Newman NJ. Update on the pathophysiology and management of idiopathic intracranial hypertension. J Neurol Neurosurg Psychiatry. 2012;83:488–94.
73. McGeeney BE, Friedman DI. Pseudotumor cerebri pathophysiology. Headache. 2014;54:445–58.
74. Saindane AM, Bruce BB, Desai NK, Roller LA, Newman NJ, Biousse V. Transverse sinus stenosis in adult patients with Chiari malformation type I. AJR Am J Roentgenol. 2014;203:890–6.
75. Fargen KM. A unifying theory explaining venous sinus stenosis and recurrent stenosis following venous sinus stenting in patients with idiopathic intracranial hypertension. J Neurointerv Surg. 2021;13(7):587–92. https://doi.org/10.1136/neurintsurg-2020-017208.
76. Horev A, Hallevy H, Plakht Y, Shorer Z, Wirguin I, Shelef I. Changes in cerebral venous sinuses diameter after lumbar puncture in idiopathic intracranial hypertension: a prospective MRI study. J Neuroimaging. 2013;23(3):375–8. https://doi.org/10.1111/j.1552-6569.2012.00732.x.
77. West JL, Greeneway GP, Garner RM, et al. Correlation between angiographic stenosis and physiologic venous sinus outflow obstruction in idiopathic intracranial hypertension. J Neurointerv Surg. 2019;11(1):90–4.
78. Zhao P, Ding H, Lv H, Li X, Qiu X, Zeng R, Wang G, Wei J, Jin L, Yang Z, Gong S, Wang Z. CT venography correlate of transverse sinus stenosis and venous transstenotic pressure gradient in unilateral pulsatile tinnitus patients with sigmoid sinus wall anomalies. Eur Radiol. 2021;31(5):2896–902. https://doi.org/10.1007/s00330-020-07415-2.
79. Dinkin M, Oliveira C. Men are from Mars, idiopathic intracranial hypertension is from venous: the role of venous sinus stenosis and stenting in idiopathic intracranial hypertension. Semin Neurol. 2019;39(06):692–703.
80. Lansley JA, Tucker W, Eriksen MR, Riordan-Eva P, Connor SEJ. Sigmoid sinus diverticulum, dehiscence, and venous sinus stenosis: potential causes of pulsatile tinnitus in patients with idiopathic intracranial hypertension? Am J Neuroradiol. 2017;38(9):1783–8.
81. Riggeal BD, Bruce BB, Saindane AM, Ridha MA, Kelly LP, Newman NJ, Biousse V. Clinical course of idiopathic intracranial hypertension with transverse sinus stenosis. Neurology. 2013;80:289–95.
82. Carvalho GB, Matas SL, Idagawa MH, Tibana LA, de Carvalho RS, Silva ML, Cogo-Moreira H, Jackowski AP, Abdala N. A new index for the assessment of transverse sinus stenosis for diagnosing idiopathic intracranial hypertension. J Neurointerv Surg. 2017;9(2):173–7. https://doi.org/10.1136/neurintsurg-2016-012605.
83. Schoeff S, Nicholas B, Mukherjee S, et al. Imaging prevalence of sigmoid sinus dehiscence among patients with and without pulsatile tinnitus. Otolaryngol Head Neck Surg. 2014;150(5):841–6.
84. Liu Z, Dong C, Wang X, Han X, Zhao P, Lv H, Li Q, Wang Z. Association between idiopathic intracranial hypertension and sigmoid sinus dehiscence/diverticulum with pulsatile tinnitus: a retrospective imaging study. Neuroradiology. 2015;57(7):747–53. https://doi.org/10.1007/s00234-015-1517-5.
85. Krishnan A, Mattox DE, Fountain AJ, et al. CT arteriography and venography in pulsatile tinnitus: preliminary results. AJNR Am J Neuroradiol. 2006;27(8):1635–8.
86. Eisenman DJ. Sinus wall reconstruction for sigmoid sinus diverticulum and dehiscence: a standardized surgical procedure for a range of radiographic findings. Otol Neurotol. 2011;32(7):1116–9.
87. Bialer OY, Rueda MP, Bruce BB, et al. Meningoceles in idiopathic intracranial hypertension. AJR Am J Roentgenol. 2014;202:608–13.
88. Kamali A, Sullivan KC, Rahmani F, Gandhi A, Aein A, Arevalo O, Rabiei P, Choi SJ, Zhang X, Gabr RE, Riascos RF. Indentation and transverse diameter of the Meckel cave: imaging markers to diagnose idiopathic intracranial hypertension. AJNR Am J Neuroradiol. 2020;41(8):1487–94. https://doi.org/10.3174/ajnr.A6682.

89. Butros SR, Goncalves LF, Thompson D, Agarwal A, Lee HK. Imaging features of idiopathic intracranial hypertension, including a new finding: widening of the foramen ovale. Acta Radiol. 2012;53(06):682–8.
90. Eggerstedt M, Dua SG, Varelas AN, Bhabad SH, Batra PS, Tajudeen BA. Enlargement of Dorello's canal as a novel radiographic marker of Idiopathic intracranial hypertension. J Neurol Surg B Skull Base. 2020;81(3):232–6. https://doi.org/10.1055/s-0039-1688783.
91. Seth R, Rajasekaran K III, Luong A, Benninger MS, Batra PS. Spontaneous CSF leaks: factors predictive of additional interventions. Laryngoscope. 2010;120:2141–6.
92. Brainard L, Chen DA, Aziz KM, Hillman TA. Association of benign intracranial hypertension and spontaneous encephalocele with cerebrospinal fluid leak. Otol Neurotol. 2012;33:1621–4.
93. Aaron G, Doyle J, Vaphiades MS, Riley KO, Woodworth BA. Increased intracranial pressure in spontaneous CSF leak patients is not associated with papilledema. Otolaryngol Head Neck Surg. 2014;151:1061–6.
94. Rosenfeld E, Dotan G, Kimchi TJ, Kesler A. Spontaneous cerebrospinal fluid otorrhea and rhinorrhea in idiopathic intracranial hypertension patients. J Neuroophthalmol. 2013;33:113–6.
95. Lloyd KM, DelGaudio JM, Hudgins PA. Imaging of skull base cerebrospinal fluid leaks in adults. Radiology. 2008;248:725–36; 2013;33:113–16.
96. Selcuk H, Albayram S, Ozer H, Ulus S, Sanus GZ, Kaynar MY, Kocer N, Islak C. Intrathecal gadolinium-enhanced MR cisternography in the evaluation of CSF leakage. AJNR Am J Neuroradiol. 2010;31:71–5. Radiographics. 2013;33:553–70.
97. Prichard CN, Isaacson B, Oghalai JS, Coker NJ, Vrabec JT. Adult spontaneous CSF otorrhea: correlation with radiographic empty Sella. Otolaryngol Head Neck Surg. 2006;134:767–71.
98. Schievink WI. Spontaneous spinal cerebrospinal fluid leaks. Cephalalgia. 2008;28:1345–56.
99. Schlosser RJ, Woodworth BA, Wilensky EM, et al. Spontaneous cerebrospinal fluid leaks: a variant of benign intracranial hypertension. Ann Otol Rhinol Laryngol. 2006;115(7):495–500.
100. Alonso RC, de la Peña MJ, Caicoya AG, et al. Spontaneous skull base meningoencephaloceles and cerebrospinal fluid fistulas. Radiographics. 2013;33(2):553–70.
101. Aaron G, Doyle J, Vaphiades MS, Riley KO, Woodworth BA. Increased intracranial pressure in spontaneous CSF leak patients is not associated with papilledema. Otolaryngol Head Neck Surg. 2014;151(6):1061–6. https://doi.org/10.1177/0194599814551122.
102. Hadley DM. The Chiari malformations. J Neurol Neurosurg Psychiatry. 2002;72(suppl 2):ii38–40.
103. McVige JW, Leonardo J. Imaging of Chiari type I malformation and syringohydromyelia. Neurol Clin. 2014;32:95–126.
104. Barkovich AJ, Wippold FJ, Sherman JL, Citrin CM. Significance of cerebellar tonsillar position on MR. AJNR Am J Neuroradiol. 1986;7:795–9.
105. Aiken AH, Hoots JA, Saindane AM, Hudgins PA. Incidence of cerebellar tonsillar ectopia in idiopathic intracranial hypertension: a mimic of the Chiari I malformation. AJNR Am J Neuroradiol. 2012;33:1901–6.
106. Pérez MA, Bialer OY, Bruce BB, Newman NJ, Biousse V. Primary spontaneous cerebrospinal fluid leaks and idiopathic intracranial hypertension. J Neuroophthalmol. 2013;33:330–7.
107. Roller LA, Bruce BB, Saindane AM. Demographic confounders in volumetric MRI analysis: is the posterior fossa really small in the adult Chiari 1 malformation? AJR Am J Roentgenol. 2015;204:835–41.
108. Weisberg LA. Computed tomography in benign intracranial hypertension. Neurology. 1985;35:1075–8.
109. Hoffmann J, Huppertz HJ, Schmidt C, Kunte H, Harms L, Klingebiel R, Wiener E. Morphometric and volumetric MRI changes in idiopathic intracranial hypertension. Cephalalgia. 2013;33:1075–84.
110. Barkatullah AF, Leishangthem L, Moss HE. MRI findings as markers of idiopathic intracranial hypertension. Curr Opin Neurol. 2021;34(1):75–83. https://doi.org/10.1097/WCO.0000000000000885.
111. Agid R, Farb R, Willinsky R, et al. Idiopathic intracranial hypertension: the validity of cross-sectional neuroimaging signs. Neuroradiology. 2006;48:521–7.
112. Batur Caglayan H, Ucar M, Hasanreisoglu M, et al. Magnetic resonance imaging of idiopathic intracranial hypertension. J Neuroophthalmol. 2019;39:324–9.
113. Kwee RM, Kwee TC. Systematic review and meta-analysis of MRI signs for diagnosis of idiopathic intracranial hypertension. Eur J Radiol. 2019;116:106–15. https://doi.org/10.1016/j.ejrad.2019.04.023.
114. Salvay D, Padhye L, Huecker J, et al. Correlation between papilledema grade and diffusion-weighted magnetic resonance imaging in idiopathic intracranial hypertension. J Neuroophthalmol. 2014;34:331–5.
115. Viets R, Parsons M, Van Stavern G, Hildebolt C, Sharma A. Hyperintense optic nerve heads on diffusion-weighted imaging: a potential imaging sign of papilledema. AJNR Am J Neuroradiol. 2013;34(7):1438–42. https://doi.org/10.3174/ajnr.A3388.
116. Durst CR, Ornan DA, Reardon MA, Mehndiratta P, Mukherjee S, Starke RM, Wintermark M, Evans A, Jensen ME, Crowley RW, Gaughen J, Liu KC. Prevalence of dural venous sinus stenosis and hypoplasia in a generalized population. J Neurointerv Surg. 2016;8(11):1173–7. https://doi.org/10.1136/neurintsurg-2015-012147.
117. Kline NL, Angster K, Archer E, Raghavan P, Morales RE, Mathews MK, Eisenman DJ. Association of pulse synchronous tinnitus

and sigmoid sinus wall abnormalities in patients with idiopathic intracranial hypertension. Am J Otolaryngol. 2020;41(6):102675. https://doi.org/10.1016/j.amjoto.2020.102675.

118. Gulmez Cakmak P, Ufuk F, Yagci AB, Sagtas E, Arslan M. Emissary veins prevalence and evaluation of the relationship between dural venous sinus anatomic variations with posterior fossa emissary veins: MR study. Radiol Med. 2019;124(7):620–7. https://doi.org/10.1007/s11547-019-01010-2.
119. Mallery RM, Rehmani OF, Woo JH, et al. Utility of magnetic resonance imaging features for improving the diagnosis of idiopathic intracranial hypertension without papilledema. J Neuroophthalmol. 2019;39(3):299–307.
120. Saindane AM, Lim PP, Aiken A, Chen Z, Hudgins PA. Factors determining the clinical significance of an "empty" sella turcica. AJR AmJ Roentgenol. 2013;200(5):1125–31.
121. Chiloiro S, Giampietro A, Bianchi A, et al. Diagnosis of endocrine disease: primary empty sella: a comprehensive review. Eur J Endocrinol. 2017;177(6):R275–85. https://doi.org/10.1530/EJE-17-0505.
122. Guitelman M, Garcia Basavilbaso N, Vitale M, et al. Primary empty sella (PES): a review of 175 cases. Pituitary. 2013;16(2):270–4.
123. Chen BS, Meyer BI, Saindane AM, Bruce BB, Newman NJ, Biousse V. Prevalence of incidentally detected signs of intracranial hypertension on magnetic resonance imaging and their association with papilledema. JAMA Neurol. 2021;78(6):718–25. https://doi.org/10.1001/jamaneurol.2021.0710.
124. Korkmazer B, Karaman AK, Kızılkılıç EK, Unkun R, Arslan S, Uygunoğlu U, Kızılkılıç O, Koçer N, Islak C. Efficacy of dural sinus quantitative measurements in idiopathic intracranial hypertension: a practical diagnostic feature. Clin Neuroradiol. 2023;33(2):545–54. https://doi.org/10.1007/s00062-022-01244-0.
125. Zedde M, Pascarella R. Non-thrombotic filling defects in cerebral veins and sinuses: when normal structures mimic a disease. Neurol Int. 2025;17:9. https://doi.org/10.3390/neurolint17010009.
126. Visani G, Bontempo G, Manfroi S, Pazzaglia A, D'Alessandro R, Tura S. All-trans-retinoic acid and pseudotumor cerebri in a young adult with acute promyelocytic leukemia: a possible disease association. Haematologica. 1996;81(2):152–4.
127. Smith MB, Griffiths EA, Thompson JE, Wang ES, Wetzler M, Freyer CW. High pseudotumor cerebri incidence in tretinoin and arsenic treated acute promyelocytic leukemia and the role of topiramate after acetazolamide failure. Leuk Res Rep. 2014;3(2):62–6. https://doi.org/10.1016/j.lrr.2014.07.001.
128. Hokazono K, Cunha LP, Preti RC, Cabral Zacharias L, Ribeiro Monteiro ML. Optic nerve sheath fenestration as adjuvant treatment for severe pseudotumor cerebri syndrome induced by all-trans retinoic acid. Case Rep Ophthalmol. 2023;14(1):326–30. https://doi.org/10.1159/000531001.
129. Gallipoli P, Drummond MW. Pseudotumour cerebri as a manageable side effect of prolonged all-trans retinoic acid therapy in an adult patient with acute promyelocytic leukaemia. Eur J Haematol. 2009;82(3):242–3. https://doi.org/10.1111/j.1600-0609.2008.01185.x.

12 Contrast-Induced Encephalopathy

Alexander Stebner, Salome Bosshart, Nicolin Hainc, Nathalie Nierobisch, and Johanna Ospel

12.1 Introduction

Contrast-induced encephalopathy (CIE) is a rare adverse event associated with intravascular administration of iodine-containing contrast media used for diagnostic imaging to enhance visibility of anatomical structures and diagnostic or therapeutic endovascular procedures (see Fig. 12.1). CIE is acute neurotoxicity induced by iodine contrast media and manifests with a range of neurological symptoms. It can mimic acute ischemic stroke or acute encephalopathy with symptoms like hemiparesis, cortical blindness, and seizures [1, 2]. The most common procedures leading to this condition are neuroendovascular interventions and cardiac catheterization. Among neuroendovascular procedures, most cases are reported to be related to diagnostic angiography and aneurysm embolization, and less commonly to endovascular thrombectomy (EVT) [3]. It is important to differentiate CIE,

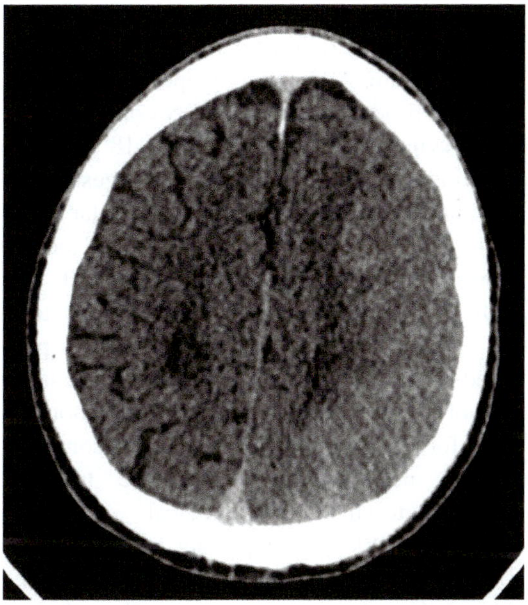

Fig. 12.1 CT-imaging of a patient who developed CIE with severe cortical swelling of the left hemisphere and contrast extravasation after an endovascular procedure

A. Stebner
Department of Clinical Neurosciences, Foothills Medical Centre, University of Calgary, Calgary, Canada

Institute of Radiology, Cantonal Hospital Münsterlingen, Münsterlingen, Switzerland

S. Bosshart
Department of Clinical Neurosciences, Foothills Medical Centre, University of Calgary, Calgary, Canada

N. Hainc · N. Nierobisch
Institute of Neuroradiology, University Hospital of Zurich, Zurich, Switzerland
e-mail: Nathalie.Nierobisch@usz.ch

J. Ospel (✉)
Department of Clinical Neurosciences, Foothills Medical Centre, University of Calgary, Calgary, Canada

Department of Radiology, University of Calgary, Calgary, Canada
e-mail: johanna.ospel@ucalgary.ca

M. Zedde, R. Pascarella (eds.), *Neuroimaging of Treatment-Related Conditions in the Brain*,
https://doi.org/10.1007/978-3-032-23618-0_12

which usually is a self-limiting disease, from other acute, treatable conditions, which require prompt specific therapies to avoid permanent morbidity. Although the outcome of CIE is generally favorable with most patients recovering fully, there are rare, documented cases where this condition has resulted in death [4, 5].

CIE is not a new phenomenon and has probably existed for several decades since angiography has been introduced [6]. Fischer-Williams et al. [7] described in 1970 a case that retrospectively might be considered a typical case of CIE. They reported on a 52-year-old woman who developed transient cortical blindness, a frequently observed symptom of CIE, following a cardiac catheterization procedure. Additional symptoms were nausea, mild headache, and difficulty concentrating. These symptoms lasted for about 18 h before resolving completely. The authors suggested that an embolus at the bifurcation of the basilar artery might have caused her symptoms. With today's knowledge, it was more likely a case of CIE.

To date, several more case reports and systematic reviews with meta-analyses have been published on this very rare disease, but there is still a lack of prospective studies. Various synonyms exist for this condition including "contrast-induced neurotoxicity" or "acute transient contrast-induced neurological deficits (ATCIND)" [8]. It is important to differentiate contrast-induced neurotoxicity, when using abbreviations from contrast-induced nephropathy (CIN) which is a more frequent and completely different complication of iodine-containing contrast agents [9].

The prevalence of CIE is rising due to the increasing frequency of endovascular procedures, particularly those performed for acute coronary disease and strokes [10]. However, CIE can also occur following any endovascular procedure and even routinely performed CT scans with iodine contrast [11]. A systematic review estimates the incidence of CIE to be 0.5% [8]. The incidence and risk vary depending on the type of the procedure. Higher incidence rates are observed when contrast media is administered directly into the aortic arch during endovascular interventions as opposed to small, peripheral arteries or veins, or when higher dosage and high-osmolar contrast agents are used [12]. These conditions increase the risk of developing CIE, emphasizing the need for careful selection of contrast-agent type and dosage during procedures. Still, case reports exist of CIE even after use of a minimal dosage of low-osmolar, non-ionic contrast media [13].

The average age of patients reported with CIE is around 60 years [3, 8, 14, 15], but there have also been rare cases of CIE reported in children [16]. Frequently reported comorbidities include hypertension and end-stage renal failure [1, 17], but a causal relationship to CIE cannot be inferred with certainty, since both these conditions are more often prevalent among patients with cardiovascular and cerebrovascular diseases, which therefore more often require procedures involving contrast media [2].

Our understanding of CIE remains incomplete. The pathophysiological mechanism is most likely due to a transient breakdown of the blood-brain barrier (BBB). This breakdown leads to the leakage of contrast media and plasma into the brain parenchyma and CSF spaces, resulting in neuronal dysfunction. This mechanism not only leads to the typical symptoms, such as altered mental status, seizures, and neurological deficits, due to neurotoxicity of the contrast media, but also results in the imaging findings observed in patients with CIE, such as contrast staining in the brain parenchyma and sulci, as well as the presence of vasogenic edema [18].

Many clinicians are unfamiliar with CIE, therefore hesitant to diagnose it and initiate the appropriate treatment [19]. Accurate diagnosis and timely treatment are important for patient safety and outcome. This highlights the importance of knowledge about this rare condition and the ability to recognizing its imaging patterns without mistaking it for other severe diseases.

This chapter summarizes the pathophysiological mechanisms, clinical and radiological presentations, and therapeutic possibilities for CIE, thereby enhancing clinicians' knowledge and confidence in diagnosing and treating this condition.

12.2 Contrast Media as a Causative Agent

This section focuses primarily on iodine--containing contrast agents, as these are the only types of contrast agents that appear to play a significant role in the pathogenesis of CIE. There are no reports in the literature of CIE cases associated with other types of contrast agents after intravascular administration to our knowledge. Iodine-containing contrast agents are used to enhance the visibility of structures in various imaging modalities that utilize X-rays such as computed tomography (CT), angiography for both diagnostic or interventional procedures, and fluoroscopy. In these procedures, the contrast agent may be administered into different compartments, including the intraarterial or intravenous compartments, oropharyngeal tract, rectal area, and intraarticular or intraosseous spaces to enhance visibility of different structures.

The first use of contrast media was reported for urography in the 1920s [20]. Since then, there has been significant progress in the development of contrast agents for various imaging modalities. These advancements have led to the creation of safer and more effective contrast agents, tailored to enhance the visualization of different structures. These developments have not only improved diagnostic accuracy but also helped to expand the spectrum of conditions that can be treated with interventional procedures, contributing to better patient outcomes. Even though the adverse event rate for iodine contrast agents is relatively low due to development of less toxic chemical formulations, the increasing utilization of contrast media in medical imaging and interventional procedures has led to a rise in the absolute number of adverse reactions [20].

Iodine contrast agents can be classified based on their chemical structure, ionic properties, and osmolality. Structurally, they are categorized as either monomeric or dimeric. Monomeric agents consist of single molecules, while dimeric are composed of two linked molecules, which results in a lower osmolality compared to monomeric agents, because the osmotic load is distributed across a larger molecule. Based on their ability to separate into ions in solution, iodine contrast agents are classified as ionic or non-ionic. Ionic agents dissociate into ions, whereas non-ionic agents do not, making them less likely to cause adverse reactions by causing alteration of the plasma tonicity. According to their osmolality, iodine contrast media are classified into high-osmolar (HOCM), which has a higher osmolality than serum, low-osmolar (LOCM) that is slightly higher than serum, and iso-osmolar (IOCM) which has a similar osmolality compared to serum [18, 20, 21].

Iodine contrast agents enhance medical imaging, by increasing the radiodensity of the tissues into which they are introduced, such as blood vessels during angiography or organs after the contrast diffuses into them over a short period of time. This enhancement occurs because iodine atoms have a high atomic number, leading to a greater absorption of X-rays compared to other body tissues with lower densities. Consequently, the area containing iodine contrast appears brighter on the scan [21].

Under normal circumstances, iodine contrast agents cannot pass the BBB, a structure with high, selective permeability that separates the circulating blood from the brain and extracellular fluid in the central nervous system. However, damage to the BBB caused by conditions like inflammation, tumors, or ischemia can lead to leakage of the contrast agent into brain tissue. Thus, contrast agents can enhance pathological conditions like tumors but can also lead to CIE (further explained in the pathophysiology section) due to neurotoxicity of the contrast agent [18, 22].

Non-ionic, low-osmolar iodine contrast agents are associated with a lower incidence of CIE compared to high-osmolar contrast agents. HOCM tend to increase the permeability of the BBB by disrupting the tight junctions between cells [22]. In contrast, low-osmolar agents have an osmolality closer to that of blood, which reduces the risk of BBB disruptions and thus adverse reactions. Additionally, non-ionic contrast agents do not dissociate into ions, which further decreases their neurotoxicity compared to ionic agents [22]. This characteristic makes non-ionic, low-osmolar contrast agents less likely to cause CIE. However, there are still reports of CIE symptoms occurring even with low amounts of these agents, indicating that while the risk is reduced, it is not completely eliminated [13]. It is recommended to use non-ionic, iso-osmolar or low-osmolar contrast agents with the lowest possible dosage to minimize the risk of CIE and other severe adverse events [15, 23].

12.3 Pathophysiology

The actual mechanism of CIE is still not fully understood. It is known that this rare disease occurs in the context of the use of iodine-containing contrast media and that a compromised BBB, which allows leakage of contrast media into the brain parenchyma, plays a significant role in the development of symptoms [18].

The BBB is a complex structure composed of endothelial cells, astrocytes, pericytes, neurons, and the extracellular matrix. Its integrity is maintained by intact tight junctions between the endothelial cells. However, various pathophysiological changes can alter these tight junctions and increase the permeability of the BBB [18, 22, 24]. Under normal conditions, the permeability for contrast agents is low, especially for non-HOCMs. However, when HOCM are used, their increased osmolality can cause swelling of the astrocyte foot processes, leading to an insufficiency of the BBB and making contrast-agent leakage more likely [18, 22, 24]. Conditions such as hypoxia during an ischemic stroke, inflammatory processes, or previous strokes that have already damaged the brain parenchyma and BBB make individual patients more susceptible to develop CIE [25].

Two main theories could explain the symptoms that occur after contrast agent passes the BBB. First, the glucose metabolism of the neurons is altered because the contrast-agent functions as a competitive inhibitor to hexokinase, an important enzyme in glucose metabolism [26]. As the cerebral energy metabolism relies predominantly on glucose, its inhibition results in neuronal malfunction. Second, iodine contrast agents have been shown to modify the electrical activity of neurons [27]. This modification can lead to suppression of neuronal activity, due to inhibitory effects, but it can also have epileptogenic effects, which might explain the seizures frequently observed in patients with contrast-induced encephalopathy [18].

The breakdown of the BBB also results in radiologically observed cerebral vasogenic edema. This edema occurs due to oncotic pressure created by the contrast media itself and the diffusion of molecules and fluids as a result of increased BBB permeability. The resulting mass effect from the edema leads to increased intracranial pressure. Edematous brain parenchyma with increased intracranial pressure can compress and displace adjacent brain structures, potentially leading to entrapment of critical structures (see Fig. 12.2). This entrapment could cause additional symptoms like severe headache, nausea and vomiting, altered consciousness, and neurological deficits. In extreme cases, the increased pressure can cause brain herniation, which is a life-threatening condition that can ultimately result in death [18].

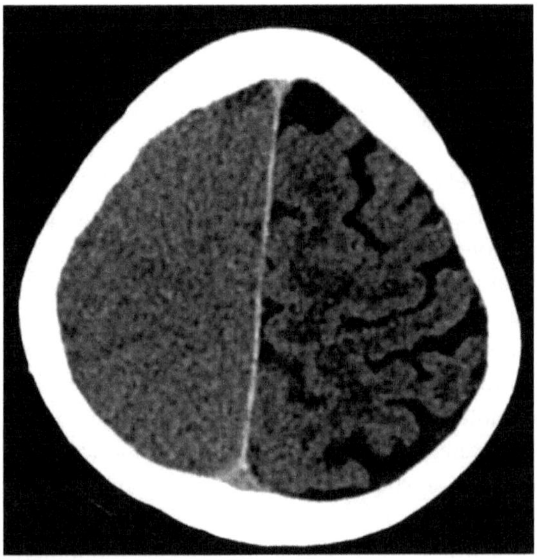

Fig. 12.2 Significant cerebral vasogenic edema in a patient with CIE

12.4 Risk Factors

Since the BBB plays an important role in maintaining brain function, any disturbance to its structure is a potential risk factor for CIE. Previous ischemic stroke, which directly damages the integrity of the BBB, is a potential risk factor for developing CIE [3, 8]. Other frequently observed comorbidities include hypertension and renal dysfunction [1].

> **Risk factors:**
>
> Hypertension
> Renaldys function
> Prior stroke
> Brain parenchymal damage
> Leukoencephalopathy

Hypertension is the most common comorbidity and risk factor in individuals who develop CIE [1]. Particularly, significant intraprocedural blood pressure variations seem to play a crucial role in its development [15, 28]. However, there is a potential bias, as hypertension is also frequently present in patients undergoing interventions such as cardiac catheterization for acute coronary syndrome or EVT for stroke [29]. This makes it challenging to determine whether hypertension is a direct risk factor for CIE or if it is merely a common comorbidity seen in the affected patient population without being causally related to CIE.

Severe renal failure is also a common comorbidity in patients with CIE, likely due to the slow clearance of contrast agents and therefore prolonged exposure to the contrast agent, which increases the risk of BBB alterations and neurotoxicity. Interestingly, acute kidney injury is also commonly associated with CIE [3]. Further research is needed to investigate the causal relationship between CIE and acute/chronic kidney damage (Fig. 12.3).

The posterior circulation is particularly vulnerable to contrast-induced damage due to its vascular anatomy and regulation of blood flow [30]. This increased vulnerability is also frequently observed in the related disease of posterior reversible encephalopathy syndrome (PRES), a condition in which patients develop vasogenic edema predominantly in the posterior regions of the brain. Both CIE and PRES share common triggers, such as hypertension and renal dysfunction and might have similar symptoms [31, 32].

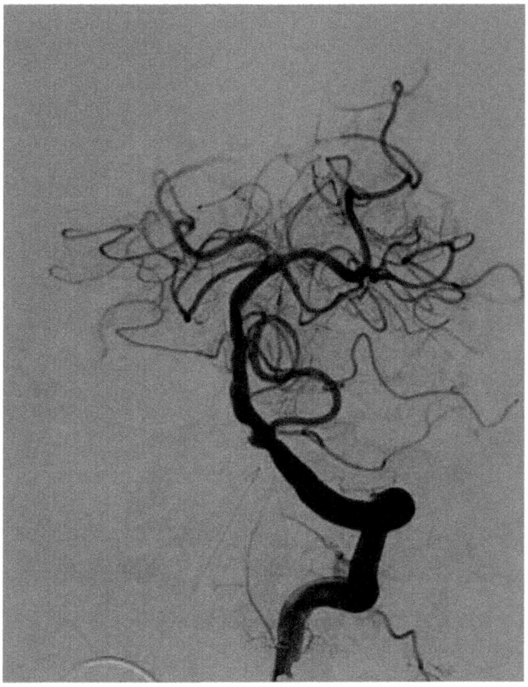

Fig. 12.3 Imaging of an endovascular procedure for the posterior circulation

12.5 Clinical Presentation

Symptoms commonly associated with CIE are cortical blindness, impaired consciousness, and seizures. While they are the most common findings, de facto any neurologic deficit can be a symptom of CIE. Similar to a transient ischemic attack, CIE is related hypofunction of the brain that is transient in most cases, and the symptoms are dictated by the affected brain area, i.e., the brain area with the highest exposure to contrast media. Predilection sites could be brain areas with a weakened BBB, e.g., due to ischemia, and it commonly affects perfusion territory of a vessel

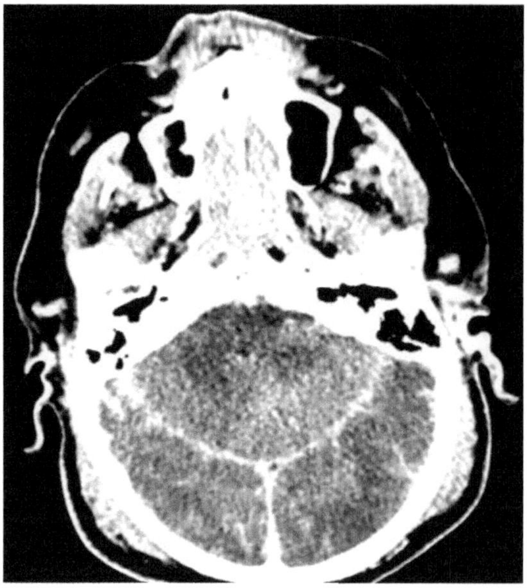

Fig. 12.4 CT showing contrast staining and swelling bilateral in the occipital region

that has undergone an intervention and therefore received higher doses of contrast media than the rest of the brain. Accordingly, cortical blindness (located in the occipital cortex) occurs significantly more often when contrast agent is injected in the posterior circulation (see Fig. 12.4) [33].

Symptoms:

Visual disturbance

Stroke-like symptoms

Seizures

Confusion

Reduced Consciousness

Typically, symptoms of CIE develop during or shortly after the interventional procedure or radiological imaging. The timing is closely associated with the iodine contrast administration [1, 2]. Rarely, symptoms can manifest more than 24 h after the procedure [1–3].

Sometimes the exact time of onset is unknown, especially when general anesthesia is used because the neurological exam is unreliable due to sedation/anesthetics. In such cases patients may awake with residual symptoms following acute stroke treatments during endovascular thrombectomy or may even experience worsening of their stroke symptoms [3].

12.6 Radiological Findings

The classic approach of ruling out complications and confidently making the diagnosis of CIE is by performing a non-contrast computed tomography (NCCT) of the head. The classic imaging findings can typically be observed on the ipsilateral side of the intervention, specifically in the vascular territory of the vessel into which the contrast agent was introduced during neurointerventional procedures [2, 15]. However, imaging findings can also be bilateral, especially in the absence of predilecting, localized BBB damages and in the presence of homogenous exposure of the brain to contrast media, e.g., after cardiac catheterization or intravenous contrast administration for cross-sectional imaging.

Typical signs on NCCT are sulcal effacement and swelling due to vasogenic edema (see Fig. 12.5), which can potentially lead to mass effect with midline shift or other signs of herniation. Additionally, cortical and sulcal enhancement can be observed, which is important to differentiate from subarachnoid hemorrhage. This differentiation is crucial as subarachnoid hemorrhage can also be observed after neurovascular interventions and may appear similar on imaging [34].

In difficult cases, dual-energy CT can confidently discriminate iodine from clotted blood, allowing for an accurate diagnosis. Dual-energy CT utilizes two different energy levels to distinguish between different materials based on their attenuation properties at different energy levels. This advanced imaging technique is also beneficial for avoiding overcalling edema in cases with significant amounts of contrast in the sulci, which can mimic edema. The differentiation can be achieved by creating a virtual NCCT and an iodine map from the dual-energy CT source

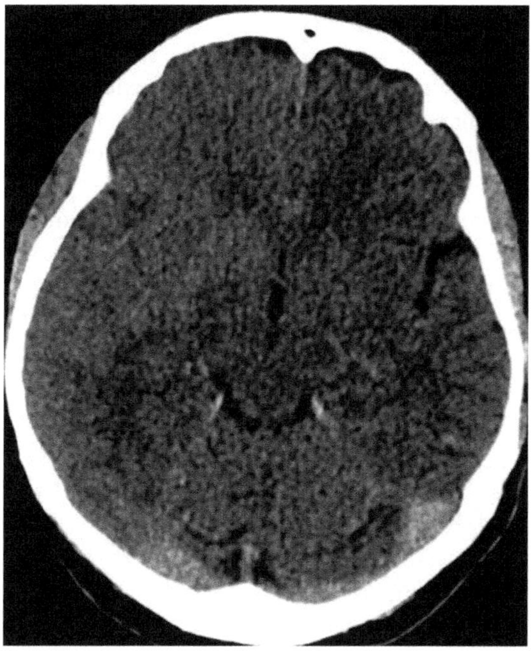

Fig. 12.5 Increased density on the right side with swelling and sulcal effacement

images, which can be compared to identify areas with contrast extravasation. Overall dual-energy CT might improve diagnostic confidence, but might not be available in all hospitals (see Fig. 12.6) [35–37].

CT perfusion imaging is rarely required for the diagnosis of CIE but can be a valuable tool in specific situations. This imaging technique makes it possible to assess the hemodynamic status of the patient's brain by determining parameters such as the cerebral blood flow (CBF), mean transit time (MTT), and cerebral blood volume (CBV) and thus to rule out a recurrent stroke or vasospasm. In some cases, CTP can also reveal signs of cerebral edema [15, 38]. However, one should keep in mind that additional contrast media is required, which could lead to symptom worsening.

Another helpful tool, if available in an emergency setting, is MRI with diffusion-weighted imaging (DWI), T2 fluid-attenuated inversion

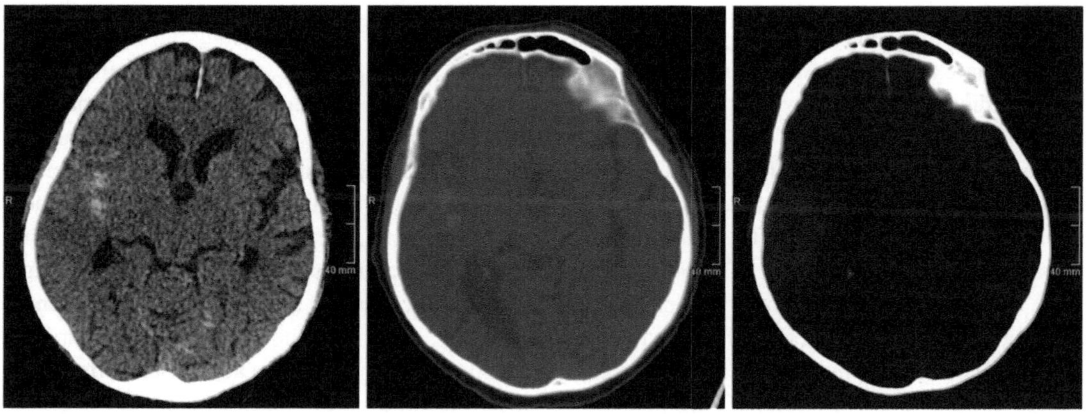

Fig. 12.6 Dual-Energy CT. From left to right: The first image shows a NCCT after an EVT procedure with infarct demarcation, and swelling and hyperdensities in the insular region. The second picture is a virtual non-contrast CT showing that the hyperdensities indeed are representing some post-procedural hemorrhage. The last imaging is showing the iodine map, revealing, contrast staining in the temporal region that was not well appreciated on the source images on the left

recovery (FLAIR), and susceptibility weighted imaging (SWI) to rule out differential diagnoses and specially identify the typical MR imaging findings of CIE, namely vasogenic edema without signs of stroke and subarachnoid hemorrhage (SAH). DWI is particularly valuable for distinguishing between cytotoxic and vasogenic edema, by showing areas of restricted diffusion, which helps differentiate CIE from acute strokes. T2 or T2/FLAIR imaging will typically show hyperintense signal in the cortical and subcortical regions corresponding to vasogenic edema. FLAIR imaging is also helpful for identification of subarachnoid hemorrhage, in which hyperintense signal in the sulci is seen. SWI is also sensitive for blood products as well as hemorrhagic transformation. MRI is especially helpful in excluding other potential causes of the patients' symptoms indirectly leading to the diagnosis of CIE [13, 39].

Although the classical imaging appearance of CIE is virtually always seen in symptomatic patients, cases of CT-negative CIE have been described [15, 40, 41].

An early proposed criterion suggestive of CIE in the context of EVT is edematous change accompanied by contrast staining extending beyond the infarct core [3, 42]. This criterion, however, does not hold up in clinical practice. Contrast extravasation/contrast staining is a relatively common CT finding after neurointerventional procedures, observed up to 30% of patients post EVT [42]. Furthermore, benign contrast staining appears regularly beyond the infarct core in 13% of stroke patients after EVT [43]. Visually, benign contrast extravasation/staining post EVT appears less dominant when compared to CIE and is generally a self-limiting, asymptomatic condition although negative outcomes after stroke have been correlated with contrast extravasation [44, 45]. In the end, diagnosis of CIE requires a combination of both radiological and clinical findings, including unequivocal clinical deterioration (i.e., an increase of ≥4 in the National Institutes of Health Stroke Scale score or a decrease ≥2 in the Glasgow Coma Scale score) or delayed improvement after EVT that could not otherwise be explained [3].

12.7 Treatment

To date, no established guidelines exist for CIE treatment. The initial approach involves the exclusion of potential differential diagnoses, like ischemic or hemorrhagic stroke or other causes of encephalopathy through imaging and clinical evaluation. The therapy for CIE is primarily supportive and depends on the patients' symptoms, with the main goal being the elimination of the contrast agent from the body, reducing inflammatory processes and edema. Most commonly used treatments are steroids and fluids [1, 2].

Treatment:

Steroids

Fluids

Mannitol

Sedatives / Antiseizure drugs

Hemodialysis

Steroids have potent anti-inflammatory properties and have been reported to protect and stabilize the BBB. This helps restore a possible BBB breakdown and prevent further leakage into the brain tissue [46]. By reducing inflammation and swelling, steroids help reduce possible intracranial pressure and structure displacements [46].

Intravenous fluids are administered to dilute the concentration of contrast media in the bloodstream, facilitating faster excretion and reducing its neurotoxic impact, particularly in patients with sufficient renal function [1]. Hemodialysis can help patients with pre-existing kidney disease to remove contrast agents from the body more effectively.

Frequently used and clinically approved is Mannitol, an osmotic diuretic, to decrease intracranial pressure. This medication is especially beneficial in cases where brain edema is prominent, and the patient is at risk of herniation. Mannitol drains fluid out of the brain and into the bloodstream, thereby reducing brain swelling and lowering intracranial pressure [1, 47].

Additional supportive medicine like sedatives in cases of agitation and confusion as well as antiseizure medications for patients with epileptic episodes can be given [1].

Overall, the treatment of CIE requires a personalized approach that depends on the patients' specific symptoms. Each case is unique, and treatment plans must be tailored to address the individual needs. Further research is needed to establish more definitive guidelines (which currently do not exist) and improve the standard of care.

12.8 Outcomes

The outcomes of CIE are generally favorable, with a high rate (~90%) of complete recovery of both clinical symptoms and imaging findings within 24–72 h [1, 2, 24]. However, longer recovery periods are often observed following neurointerventional procedures compared to cardiac catheterization [2, 48]. Patients who develop CIE after EVT for stroke tend to have less favorable functional outcomes on the modified Rankin Scale at 90 days, although the mortality rates after 90 days are similar to those seen in other contexts [3].

Even though it is rare, CIE can occasionally be very severe (see Fig. 12.7), with approximately 19% of CIE cases requiring intensive care management. There are even individual documented cases of mortality in the literature [4, 5]. The need for intensive care is not necessarily related to the type of procedure or the amount of contrast administered, highlighting the unpredictable nature of this condition [1]. These cases demonstrate the importance of prompt recognition and appropriate management of CIE to optimize patient outcomes and minimize the risk of severe complications (Fig. 12.8).

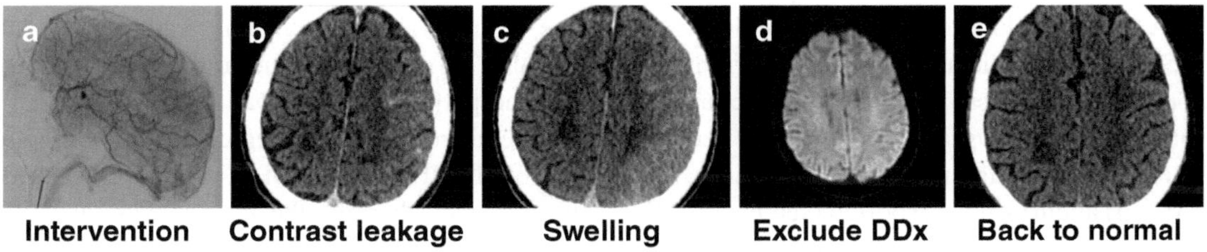

Fig. 12.7 Typical imaging sequence of a patient with CIE: After an interventional procedure (**a**) was performed, patients might develop symptoms that lead to a control non-contrast CT. The NCCT (**b**) might show some focal hyperdense foci that can be hard to distinguish from SAH but will represent contrast. Remember that not all contrast leakage after endovascular procedures will cause symptoms! The follow-up imaging (**c**) shows a significant increase in contrast staining and swelling, extending one vascular territory, which is atypical for a recurrent stroke and such brain swelling is rarely associated with SAH. Still, in unclear cases, e.g., recurrent thromboembolic infarcts including more than one territory, you should exclude other potential reasons for the clinical symptoms and imaging appearance. In this case the brain MRI (**d**) looks normal without signs of inflammation, hemorrhage, or stroke. After a short period of time, the patient should improve clinically and control NCCT (**e**) should return to normal, as was the case in this patient

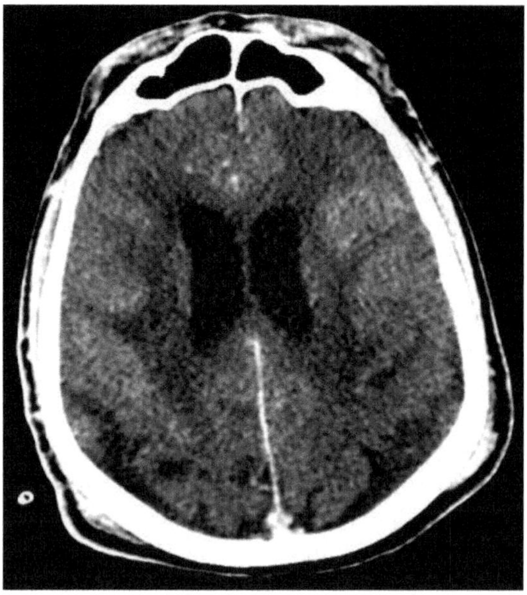

Fig. 12.8 A severe case of CIE with bilateral swelling

12.9 Case Illustrations

Case 1 CIE after aneurysm coiling.

A 51-year-old female patient underwent a NCCT scan for headache and recurrent episodes of dizziness. An additional computed tomography angiography (CTA) was acquired after a potential anterior communicating artery (ACom) aneurysm was spotted (see Fig. 12.9a). The CTA confirmed a 7 x 10 x 6 mm large ACom aneurysm (see Fig. 12.9b). After a discussion of the potential risk of aneurysm rupture, the patient consented to an endovascular treatment of the aneurysm. Besides a long history of asthma, for which she was taking medication, no comorbidities existed. The procedure (see Fig. 12.9c) went well with successful web device treatment of the aneurysm. The patient woke up from her general anesthesia with a right-sided weakness and difficulties in speaking. The NIHSS score was 4. An urgent CT scan with angiogram was performed revealing diffuse contrast staining on the left side (see Fig. 12.9d and e) but with no signs of a vessel occlusion or suspected large causative hemorrhage. Based on the clinical presentation and imaging findings, the diagnosis of CIE was made. No specific therapy was initiated, and the patient began to improve after 6 hours with a residual NIHSS score of 1. An MRI performed the next day showed some restricted diffusion in the left precentral gyrus potentially corresponding to her residual right arm weakness and paresthesia, but still no signs of hemorrhage (see Fig. 12.9f). The patient further improved and was discharged with a slight weakness of the right arm and an NIHSS score of 1.

Case 2 CIE after contrast-enhanced CT showing an acute ischemic stroke.

An 81-year-old patient presented in a peripheral hospital with a cerebrovascular ischemia in the area of the middle cerebral artery on the left side with a M1/M2 occlusion. Additionally, he had also an internal carotid artery (ICA) stenosis. The patient had a global aphasia, pure sensory hemisyndrome, and neglect to the right with an initial NIHSS score of 9. After intravenous thrombolysis therapy, the patient was taken to the nearest EVT center for endovascular recanalization of the M1/M2 occlusion. The repeat non-contrast CT showed small amounts of contrast leakage (see Fig. 12.10a), the already diagnosed high-grade ICA stenosis, and an the M1/M2 occlusion had recanalized after intravenous thrombolysis. Therefore, no intracranial intervention was performed in the absence of an intracranial target occlusion, and no carotid intervention was performed due to the increased

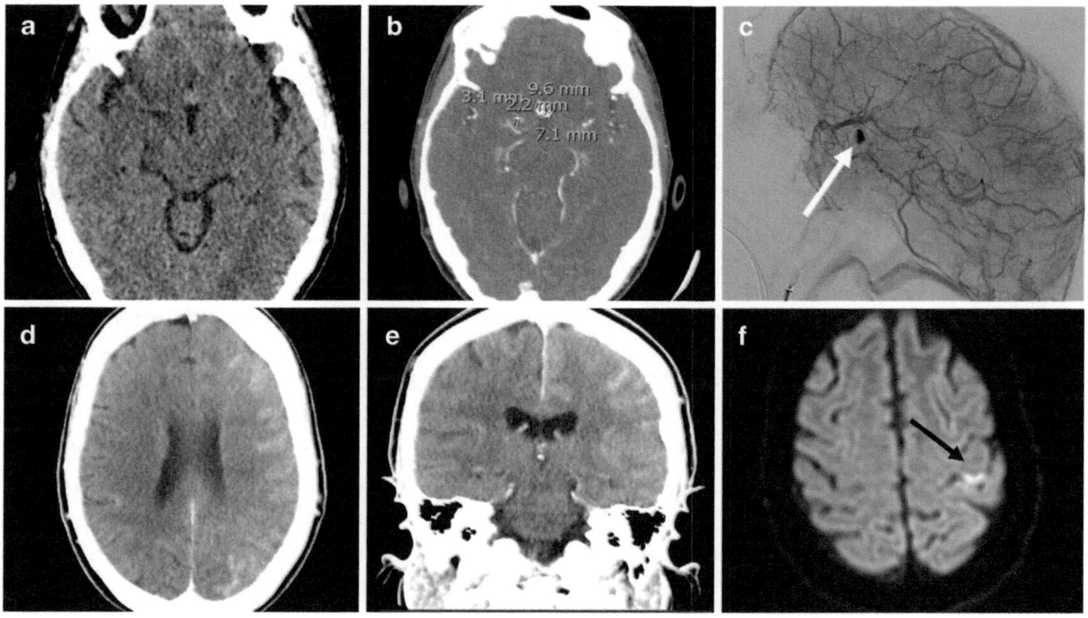

Fig. 12.9 (**a**) A NCCT with suspected ACom aneurysm. (**b**) CTA confirmed a 10 mm ACom aneurysm and additionally a small carotid-t aneurysm. (**c**) Successful web device treatment of the aneurysm (white arow). (**d**, **e**) Diffuse sulcal and cortical contrast staining and swelling without signs of infract demarcation or large causative hemorrhage. (**f**) Follow-up MRI the next day shows a small cortical infarction in the precentral gyrus on the right (black arow)

risk of cerebral reperfusion syndrome in the presence of visible contrast leakage. Over the next 6 h, the patient's symptoms progressively worsened with a transition of the initially purely sensory deficits to a combined, sensoric, and motoric hemisyndrome. The follow-up CT showed increasing edema and hyperdense material in the sulk of the left hemisphere (see Fig. 12.10b). The MRI on the next day showed small, scattered foci of diffusion restriction in the left frontal and partial lobes (see Fig. 12.10d) with some degree of edema in the FLAIR-sequence (see Fig. 12.10e), but no signs of intracranial hemorrhage. The last CT after 6 days showed complete regression of hyperdensities and edema (see Fig. 12.10f). The patient was discharged with a residual deficit of a NIHSS score of 6.

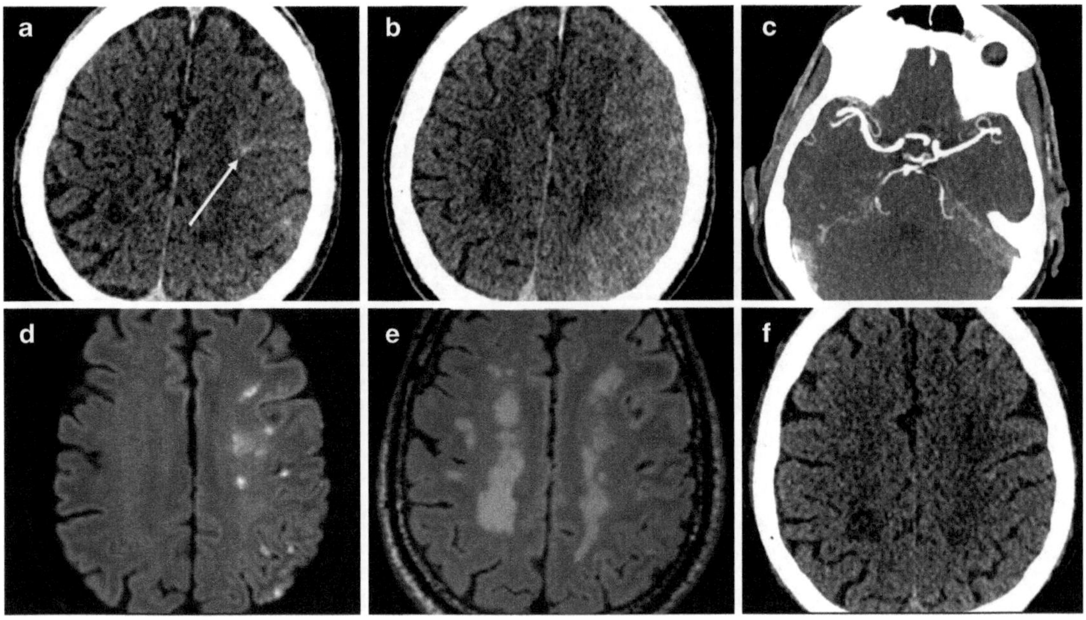

Fig. 12.10 (**a**) The follow-up NCCT, after intravenous thrombolytics, which was obtained after the patient arrived at the EVT center with minimal sulcal hyperdensities on the left hemisphere that might be mistaken for subarachnoid hemorrhage (white arrow). (**b**) A second follow-up NCCT was performed due to symptom worsening, shortly after the previous one with still some visible circulating contrast, showing a significant swelling and hyperdensities of the left hemisphere. (**c**) The CT-Angiogram showed no recurrent vessel occlusion or progressive ICA stenosis. (**d**) The MRI of the following day shows small foci of infarction on DWI in the left hemisphere. (**e**) FLAIR imaging shows white matter disease without signs of intracerebral hemorrhage and only mild swelling and hyperintensities on the right hemisphere. (**f**) The follow-up CT 5 days after the MRI--imaging shows complete regression of the swelling and hyperdensities of the left hemisphere

12.10 Summary

Contrast-induced encephalopathy is a rare, but probably underrecognized condition that requires greater awareness. Accurate diagnosis of CIE and distinguishing it from other diseases are crucial, as it is generally a benign and self-limiting condition. Further research is needed to improve our pathophysiological understanding and management of CIE, which will hopefully improve patient care.

References

1. Mariajoseph FP, Chung JX, Lai LT, et al. Clinical management of contrast-induced neurotoxicity: a systematic review. Acta Neurol Belg. 2024:20240208. https://doi.org/10.1007/s13760-024-02474-4.
2. Quintas-Neves M, Araújo JM, Xavier SA, et al. Contrast-induced neurotoxicity related to neurological endovascular procedures: a systematic review. Acta Neurol Belg. 2020;120:1419–24. 20200930. https://doi.org/10.1007/s13760-020-01508-x.
3. Chu YT, Lee KP, Chen CH, et al. Contrast-induced encephalopathy after endovascular Thrombectomy for acute ischemic stroke. Stroke. 2020;51:3756–9. 20201030. https://doi.org/10.1161/strokeaha.120.031518.
4. Zhao W, Zhang J, Song Y, et al. Irreversible fatal contrast-induced encephalopathy: a case report. BMC Neurol. 2019;19:46. 20190328. https://doi.org/10.1186/s12883-019-1279-5.
5. Nakao K, Joshi G, Hirose Y, et al. Rare cases of contrast-induced encephalopathies. Asian J Neurosurg. 2020;15:786–93. 20200828. https://doi.org/10.4103/ajns.AJNS_68_20.
6. Silverman SM, Bergman PS, Bender MB. The dynamics of transient cerebral blindness: report of nine episodes following vertebral angiography. Arch Neurol. 1961;4:333–48. https://doi.org/10.1001/archneur.1961.00450090099014.

7. Fischer-Williams M, Gottschalk PG, Browell JN. Transient cortical blindness. An unusual complication of coronary angiography. Neurology. 1970;20:353–5. https://doi.org/10.1212/wnl.20.4.353.
8. Vazquez S, Graifman G, Spirollari E, et al. Incidence and risk factors for acute transient contrast-induced neurologic deficit: a systematic review with meta-analysis. Stroke Vasc Int Neurol. 2021;2 https://doi.org/10.1161/SVIN.121.000142.
9. Zhang F, Lu Z, Wang F. Advances in the pathogenesis and prevention of contrast-induced nephropathy. Life Sci. 2020;259:118379. 20200903. https://doi.org/10.1016/j.lfs.2020.118379.
10. Rai AT, Seldon AE, Boo S, et al. A population-based incidence of acute large vessel occlusions and thrombectomy eligible patients indicates significant potential for growth of endovascular stroke therapy in the USA. J Neurointerv Surg. 2017;9:722–6. 20160715. https://doi.org/10.1136/neurintsurg-2016-012515.
11. Capasso R, Caranci F, Conforti R, et al. Contrast-induced encephalopathy after abdominal CT examination. Acta Neurol Belg. 2021;121:1325–6. 20210429. https://doi.org/10.1007/s13760-021-01690-6.
12. Maclean MA, Rogers PS, Muradov JH, et al. Contrast-induced encephalopathy and the blood-brain barrier. Can J Neurol Sci. 2024:1–10. 20240308. https://doi.org/10.1017/cjn.2024.38.
13. Liu MR, Jiang H, Li XL, Yang P. Case report and literature review on low-Osmolar, non-ionic iodine-based contrast-induced encephalopathy. Clin Interv Aging. 2020;15:2277–89. 20201204. https://doi.org/10.2147/cia.S280931.
14. Meijer FJA, Steens SCA, Tuladhar AM, et al. Contrast-induced encephalopathy-neuroimaging findings and clinical relevance. Neuroradiology. 2022;64:1265–8. 20220315. https://doi.org/10.1007/s00234-022-02930-z.
15. Zevallos CB, Dandapat S, Ansari S, et al. Clinical and imaging features of contrast-induced neurotoxicity after Neurointerventional surgery. World Neurosurg. 2020;142:e316–24. 20200704. https://doi.org/10.1016/j.wneu.2020.06.218.
16. Gonzalez-Pardo O, Ordoñez A, Roa C. Contrast-induced encephalopathy in an infant. Radiol Case Rep. 2021;16:1065–7. 20210224. https://doi.org/10.1016/j.radcr.2021.02.028.
17. Davis PW, Krisanapan P, Tangpanithandee S, et al. Contrast-induced encephalopathy in patients with chronic kidney disease and end-stage kidney disease: a systematic review and meta-analysis. Medicines (Basel). 2023;10:20230808. https://doi.org/10.3390/medicines10080046.
18. Mariajoseph FP, Lai L, Moore J, et al. Pathophysiology of contrast-induced neurotoxicity: a narrative review of possible mechanisms. Eur Neurol. 2024;87:26–35. 20231220. https://doi.org/10.1159/000535928.
19. Mariajoseph FP, Lai LT, Moore J, et al. Current knowledge and perspectives of contrast-induced neurotoxicity: a survey of Australian clinicians. J Clin Neurosci. 2023;116:8–12. 20230817. https://doi.org/10.1016/j.jocn.2023.08.014.
20. Nielsen YW, Thomsen HS. Trends in contrast media research the last 100 years. Acta Radiol. 2021;62:1515–24. 20211012. https://doi.org/10.1177/02841851211051014.
21. Currie GM. Pharmacology, part 5: CT and MRI contrast media. J Nucl Med Technol. 2019;47:189–202. https://doi.org/10.2967/jnmt.118.220012.
22. Junck L, Marshall WH. Neurotoxicity of radiological contrast agents. Ann Neurol. 1983;13:469–84. https://doi.org/10.1002/ana.410130502.
23. Andreucci M, Solomon R, Tasanarong A. Side effects of radiographic contrast media: pathogenesis, risk factors, and prevention. Biomed Res Int. 2014;2014:741018. 20140511. https://doi.org/10.1155/2014/741018.
24. Persidsky Y, Ramirez SH, Haorah J, Kanmogne GD. Blood-brain barrier: structural components and function under physiologic and pathologic conditions. J Neuroimmune Pharmacol. 2006;1:223–36. 20060706. https://doi.org/10.1007/s11481-006-9025-3.
25. Bernardo-Castro S, Sousa JA, Brás A, et al. Pathophysiology of blood-brain barrier permeability throughout the different stages of ischemic stroke and its implication on Hemorrhagic transformation and recovery. Front Neurol. 2020;11:594672. 20201209. https://doi.org/10.3389/fneur.2020.594672.
26. Ekholm SE, Reece K, Coleman JR, et al. Metrizamide–a potential in vivo inhibitor of glucose metabolism. Radiology. 1983;147:119–21. https://doi.org/10.1148/radiology.147.1.6828715.
27. Bryan RN, Centeno RS, Hershkowitz N, et al. Neurotoxicity of iohexol: a new nonionic contrast medium. Radiology. 1982;145:379–82. https://doi.org/10.1148/radiology.145.2.7134441.
28. Zevallos CB, Dai B, Dandapat S, et al. Greater intraprocedural systolic blood pressure and blood pressure variability are associated with contrast-induced neurotoxicity after neurointerventional procedures. J Neurol Sci. 2021;420:117209. 20201024. https://doi.org/10.1016/j.jns.2020.117209.
29. Goyal M, Menon BK, van Zwam WH, et al. Endovascular thrombectomy after large-vessel ischaemic stroke: a meta-analysis of individual patient data from five randomised trials. Lancet. 2016;387:1723–31. 20160218. https://doi.org/10.1016/s0140-6736(16)00163-x.
30. Tamayo A, Siepmann T. Regulation of blood flow in the cerebral posterior circulation by parasympathetic nerve Fibers: physiological background and possible clinical implications in patients with Vertebrobasilar stroke. Front Neurol. 2021;12:660373. 20211029. https://doi.org/10.3389/fneur.2021.660373.
31. Ando Y, Ono Y, Sano A, et al. Posterior reversible encephalopathy syndrome: a review of the literature. Intern Med. 2022;61:135–41. 20210717. https://doi.org/10.2169/internalmedicine.7520-21.

32. Anderson RC, Patel V, Sheikh-Bahaei N, et al. Posterior reversible encephalopathy syndrome (PRES): pathophysiology and neuro-imaging. Front Neurol. 2020;11:463. 20200616. https://doi.org/10.3389/fneur.2020.00463.
33. Li M, Liang H, Liu C, et al. Risk factors of transient cortical blindness after cerebral angiography: a Multicenter study. Front Neurol. 2019;10:1005. 20190918. https://doi.org/10.3389/fneur.2019.01005.
34. Muhammad N, Ramayya AG, Srinivasan VM. Clinical image: contrast-induced encephalopathy mimicking subarachnoid Hemorrhage. World Neurosurg. 2023;176:227–8. 20230518. https://doi.org/10.1016/j.wneu.2023.05.043.
35. Phan CM, Yoo AJ, Hirsch JA, et al. Differentiation of hemorrhage from iodinated contrast in different intracranial compartments using dual-energy head CT. AJNR Am J Neuroradiol. 2012;33:1088–94. 20120119. https://doi.org/10.3174/ajnr.A2909.
36. Postma AA, Das M, Stadler AA, Wildberger JE. Dual-energy CT: what the Neuroradiologist should know. Curr Radiol Rep. 2015;3:16. https://doi.org/10.1007/s40134-015-0097-9.
37. Pagani-Estévez GL, Nasr DM, Brinjikji W, et al. Dual-energy CT to diagnose Pseudoedema in contrast-induced encephalopathy following cerebral angiography. Neurocrit Care. 2017;27:261–4. https://doi.org/10.1007/s12028-017-0394-7.
38. Wintermark M, Flanders AE, Velthuis B, et al. Perfusion-CT assessment of infarct core and penumbra: receiver operating characteristic curve analysis in 130 patients suspected of acute hemispheric stroke. Stroke. 2006;37:979–85. 20060302. https://doi.org/10.1161/01.Str.0000209238.61459.39.
39. Wu B, Zeng L, Peng K, et al. Radiological findings of contrast-induced encephalopathy following cerebral angiography: a case report. Medicine (Baltimore). 2023;102:e33855. https://doi.org/10.1097/md.0000000000033855.
40. Babalova L, Ruzinak R, Ballova J, et al. Contrast-induced encephalopathy. Bratisl Lek Listy. 2021;122:618–20. https://doi.org/10.4149/bll_2021_098.
41. Dattani A, Au L, Tay KH, Davey P. Contrast-induced encephalopathy following coronary angiography with no radiological features: a case report and literature review. Cardiology. 2018;139:197–201. 20180202. https://doi.org/10.1159/000486636.
42. Parrilla G, García-Villalba B, Espinosa de Rueda M, et al. Hemorrhage/contrast staining areas after mechanical intra-arterial thrombectomy in acute ischemic stroke: imaging findings and clinical significance. AJNR Am J Neuroradiol. 2012;33:1791–6. 20120426. https://doi.org/10.3174/ajnr.A3044.
43. Abdalkader M, Nguyen TN, Sahoo A, et al. Contrast staining in noninfarcted tissue after endovascular treatment of acute ischemic stroke. AJNR Am J Neuroradiol. 2024. 20240502; https://doi.org/10.3174/ajnr.A8222.
44. Hoche C, Henderson A, Ifergan H, et al. Determinants and clinical relevance of iodine contrast extravasation after endovascular Thrombectomy: a dual-energy CT study. AJNR Am J Neuroradiol. 2023;45:30–6. 20231229. https://doi.org/10.3174/ajnr.A8081.
45. Xu T, Wang Y, Yuan J, et al. Contrast extravasation and outcome of endovascular therapy in acute ischaemic stroke: a systematic review and meta-analysis. BMJ Open. 2021;11:e044917. 20210707. https://doi.org/10.1136/bmjopen-2020-044917.
46. Witt KA, Sandoval KE. Steroids and the blood-brain barrier: therapeutic implications. Adv Pharmacol. 2014;71:361–90. 20140822. https://doi.org/10.1016/bs.apha.2014.06.018.
47. Kim JH, Jeong H, Choo YH, et al. Optimizing mannitol use in managing increased intracranial pressure: a comprehensive review of recent research and clinical experiences. Korean J Neurotrauma. 2023;19:162–76. 20230620. https://doi.org/10.13004/kjnt.2023.19.e25.
48. Spina R, Simon N, Markus R, et al. Contrast-induced encephalopathy following cardiac catheterization. Catheter Cardiovasc Interv. 2017;90:257–68. 20161129. https://doi.org/10.1002/ccd.26871.

Iatrogenic Cerebral Amyloid Angiopathy

13

Marialuisa Zedde, Kanishk Kaushik, Marieke J. H. Wermer, Fabrizio Piazza, and Rosario Pascarella

13.1 Introduction

Cerebral amyloid angiopathy (CAA) classically presents in the elderly with intracerebral hemorrhage (ICH) and cognitive decline, stemming from pathological changes in leptomeningeal and small cortical vessels. The impaired clearance of amyloid-beta (Aβ) protein through perivascular drainage systems is considered a central mechanism in the disease's pathogenesis [1]. Nevertheless, recent insights have emerged regarding a previously unrecognized form of CAA—iatrogenic CAA (iCAA)—which occurs in relatively young patients several decades after undergoing neurosurgical procedures in childhood. It is hypothesized that this variant is caused by prion-like transmission of Aβ from cadaveric materials used during these interventions, including cadaveric dural grafts, embolization materials, and contaminated surgical instruments [2, 3].

The transmission routes for iCAA have been proposed in several studies, with cadaveric dural grafts as a significant concern. Diagnostic criteria for iCAA were published to standardize investigations into this emerging subtype of CAA [3]. Recently, an increased rate of CAA has been associated with the exposure to blood products, in particular red cells transfusion, opening a new chapter about the potential transmissibility of CAA [4].

This chapter aims to discuss the frequency, clinical profile, neuroradiological features, and outcomes associated with iCAA.

13.2 Pathophysiology

Proteinopathies are diseases marked by misfolded proteins that can self-replicate and lead to neurodegenerative disorders, including prion diseases (e.g., Creutzfeldt-Jakob disease or CJD), Alzheimer's disease (AD), Parkinson's disease (PD), and Huntington's disease). While prion diseases are the classic example of transmissible proteinopathies, proteins associated with AD and

M. Zedde (✉)
Neurology Unit, Stroke Unit, Azienda Unità Sanitaria Locale-IRCCS di Reggio Emilia, Reggio Emilia, Italy
e-mail: zedde.marialuisa@ausl.re.it

K. Kaushik
Department of Neurology, Leiden University Medical Center, Leiden, The Netherlands

M. J. H. Wermer
Department of Neurology, Leiden University Medical Center, Leiden, The Netherlands

Department of Neurology, University Medical Centre Groningen, Groningen, The Netherlands

F. Piazza
CAA and AD Translational Research and Biomarkers Laboratory, School of Medicine and Surgery, University of Milano-Bicocca, Monza, Italy

R. Pascarella
Neuroradiology Unit, Ospedale Santa Maria della Misercordia, AULSS 5 Polesana, Rovigo, Italy

M. Zedde, R. Pascarella (eds.), *Neuroimaging of Treatment-Related Conditions in the Brain*,
https://doi.org/10.1007/978-3-032-23618-0_13

PD, such as amyloid-β, tau, and α-synuclein, also display prion-like properties, including self-replication and potential transcellular propagation [5]. In humans, protein aggregation is linked to neurodegeneration and clinical impairments [6]. In 2019, two independent studies reported cases of potential contamination from neurosurgical instruments [7, 8], widening the spectrum of transmissible proteinopathies. This discussion addresses whether proteinopathies can be transmitted between humans, the conditions for such transmission, and the necessary research to assess risks and develop safety measures. The term "prion" refers to agents causing transmissible spongiform encephalopathies, while "proteopathic seed" describes aggregated proteins with seeding properties [9].

13.2.1 Animal-to-Animal Transmission

Experimental evidence shows that the transmission of abnormally folded proteins linked to various neurodegenerative diseases can occur in animal models and cell cultures [10]. Minute amounts of proteopathic seeds, particularly amyloid-β aggregates, can induce cerebral amyloidosis in transgenic mice [11, 12], and pathological aggregates can form distant from the injection site [10]. Moreover, intravenous or intraperitoneal injection of amyloid-β seeds can lead to cerebral amyloid angiopathy in rodents [13, 14]. Cerebral microhemorrhage was also noted in wild-type mice after parabiosis with APP/human mutant PSEN1 transgenic littermates [15].

13.2.2 Animal-to-Human and Human-to-Human Transmission

The findings in animal studies have prompted the hypothesis that amyloid-β and other neurodegenerative proteins could be transmitted between humans, akin to infectious prions.

In the context of prion diseases, human-to-human amyloid transmission has been observed during mortuary feasts in Papua New Guinea [16], through medical procedures such as corneal transplants and the use of neurosurgical instruments [17], and via treatments involving human pituitary hormones from human cadavers. Notably, variant CJD has been linked to blood transfusions, with four reported cases of transmission [18, 19]. Concerns arose when the bovine agent of bovine spongiform encephalopathy crossed into humans, leading to an outbreak of variant CJD linked to contaminated meat. Between 1958 and the mid-1980s, growth hormone extracted from post-mortem pituitary glands was used for treating growth hormone deficiency [20], and human dura mater grafts were employed until the mid-1990s for various surgical procedures. Pathological amyloid deposits may be present in these tissues from donors despite the lack of neurodegenerative disease signs [21, 22]. A retrospective study of 796 individuals treated with cadaver-derived growth hormone found no increased risk of AD or PD [22], although CAA was noted in patients with iatrogenic CJD [23–26]. Histopathological analyses revealed that 34% of 92 patients treated with growth hormone had amyloid-β deposits [23–26]. Additionally, evidence indicated that human cadaveric growth hormone contained tau and amyloid-β peptides capable of inducing amyloid pathology in mice [25, 27]. In studies of 45 individuals receiving dura mater grafts, 71% exhibited pathological evidence of CAA, with a significant number showing amyloid-β deposits [21, 23, 28–33].

13.2.3 Transmission in Iatrogenic CAA

Concerns have also been raised about the transmission of amyloid-β through contaminated neurosurgical instruments, as evidenced by cases of CAA in patients who underwent procedures in early childhood [7, 8, 26]. Until 2020, 74 suspected cases of iatrogenic amyloid-β transmission have been documented (31 from c-hGH exposure, 32 through dura mater grafts, 11 from neurosurgery), primarily in younger individuals. The absence of cognitive impairment in these cases suggests a limited transmission of full Alzheimer's pathology [34].

In animal studies, CAA has been triggered by the intracerebral [34], intraperitoneal [14], and intravenous administration of amyloid-β [13, 35]. Regarding blood transfusion, prior to the implementation of leucodepletion in Europe, there were four probable cases of variant CJD transmission [36]. However, extensive studies showed no increased risk of CNS diseases among individuals with hemophilia receiving blood products [37]. A comprehensive study of over 1.4 million transfused individuals found no evidence linking blood donations from patients with neurodegenerative disorder patients to transmission in recipients [38].

While human-to-human transmission via blood transfusions has been established for prion diseases, its potential for CAA remains unexplored [21, 39]. Consequently, a recent international consortium has prioritized the investigation of possible transfusion-related transmission of CAA [34]. A recent study started from the assumption that transfusion-related transmission of CAA might be reflected in an elevated risk of spontaneous ICH among recipients who received blood from donors with spontaneous ICH [4]. To investigate this hypothesis, the authors analyzed the correlation between spontaneous ICH occurrences in blood donors and their recipients, utilizing a nationwide cohort from Sweden (759,858 patients, median age 65 [IQR, 48–73] years; 59% female) and further validating the findings with a nationwide cohort from Denmark (329,512 patients, median age 64 [IQR, 50–73] years; 58% female) with a median follow-up period of 5.8 (IQR, 1.4–12.5) and 6.1 (IQR, 1.5–11.6) years, respectively [4]. Patients who received red blood cell transfusions from donors who subsequently experienced multiple spontaneous ICHs exhibited a significantly higher risk of developing a single spontaneous ICH compared to those receiving blood from donors without spontaneous ICH. This was evident in both the Swedish cohort (unadjusted incidence rate [IR], 3.16 vs. 1.12 per 1000 person-years; adjusted hazard ratio [HR], 2.73; 95% CI, 1.72–4.35; $P < 0.001$) and the Danish cohort (unadjusted IR, 2.82 vs. 1.09 per 1000 person-years; adjusted HR, 2.32; 95% CI, 1.04–5.19; $P = 0.04$). In contrast, no significant differences were observed for patients receiving transfusions from donors who had experienced a single spontaneous ICH in the Swedish cohort (unadjusted IR, 1.35 vs. 1.12 per 1000 person-years; adjusted HR, 1.06; 95% CI, 0.84–1.36; $P = 0.62$) or the Danish cohort (unadjusted IR, 1.36 vs. 1.09 per 1000 person-years; adjusted HR, 1.06; 95% CI, 0.70–1.60; $P = 0.73$) [4]. These findings may point to a transfusion--transmissible agent linked to certain types of spontaneous ICH; however, they could be influenced by selection bias and residual confounding. Further research is essential to determining whether transfusion transmission of CAA could elucidate this association. Two further small cohorts of patients with CAA potentially acquired through transfusion have been reported [40, 41]. The implication of the biological plausibility of CAA transmission through transfusion has been explored, concluding that future studies with well-characterized definitions and temporal ascertainment of exposure and outcomes are needed to ascertain whether CAA is transfusion--transmissible [42]. Currently, there's insufficient evidence to warrant any public health implications.

The concept of prion-like transmission of Aβ has gained substantial traction in understanding iCAA. Evidence from animal models suggests that exogenous Aβ seeds can lead to vascular deposition of Aβ, potentially through mechanisms involving the glymphatic and hematogenic systems [27, 28]. However, the precise pathways of Aβ propagation remain unclear. Although some studies have indicated spatial colocalization of CAA markers with surgical sites, there is no definitive correlation established in most cases [3]. The implications of these findings are significant, particularly given the historical use of cadaveric materials in various surgical interventions. The potential population at risk for developing iCAA may be substantial, highlighting the necessity for awareness among clinicians regarding this condition, especially in older patients who may not typically be evaluated for iCAA [43, 44].

13.3 Diagnostic Criteria

Iatrogenic CAA usually manifests at an earlier age than sporadic CAA, often presenting in individuals under the age of 50 with a history of prior medical interventions, particularly those during childhood. The latency between exposure and clinical symptoms may span several decades [45]. The proposed diagnostic criteria come from an analysis of 23 previously reported cases and include five issues [3]:

1. Age at onset
2. History of potential exposure
3. Clinical and neuroradiological features consistent with a diagnosis of CAA
4. Evidence of amyloid-beta (Aβ) accumulation in the CNS
5. Exclusion of genetic causes of Aβ CNS disease.

According to these criteria, symptom onset <55 years is strongly suggestive, but diagnosis cannot be excluded based on age alone, and should be considered in people aged >55 years or above, if they meet the other criteria. The surgical exposure means exposure to cadaveric human CNS tissues (i.e., brain, meninges, pituitary-derived hormones), being strongly suggestive, or neurosurgical procedure involving the brain, spinal cord, and posterior eye. However, in the last case diagnosis can be considered if history of alternative potential exposure and all other criteria are met. The clinical features consistent with CAA are intracerebral hemorrhage or convexity subarachnoid hemorrhage (single or multiple), transient focal neurological episodes ("amyloid spells"), focal seizures (with or without secondary generalization), and cognitive impairment not attributable to another cause (including acute stroke). To consider the diagnosis, at least one among these manifestations should occur, either at presentation or during disease course. Neuroradiological features are bot CT- and MRI-based and include the following:

- CT: lobar intracerebral hemorrhage and/or convexity subarachnoid hemorrhage.
- MRI (T2*-GRE, SWI): cerebral microbleeds with predominantly lobar distribution, distant from sites of parenchymal intracerebral hemorrhage and/or cortical superficial siderosis (focal or disseminated).

Evidence of amyloid-beta accumulations can be provided through positive amyloid-PET scan (not specific for vascular Aβ deposition) and CSF (reductions of Aβ − 42, Aβ − 40). Otherwise, a brain biopsy demonstrating vascular Aβ deposition, in the absence of significant inflammation is needed [46]. A positive amyloid-PET scan in isolation might not necessarily be specific for Aβ accumulation, depending on the tracer used [39]; correlation with either CSF Aβ measures, brain biopsy findings, and/or genetic testing for non-Aβ CAAs is advised.

Finally, the differential diagnosis should consider genetic causes: APP duplications (including Trisomy 21), mutations of APP, PSEN1, PSEN2, and, in cases where CNS Aβ deposition has not been confirmed by other means, mutations resulting in non-Aβ CAA (CST3, TTR, GSN, PRNP, ITM2B).

Figures 13.1, 13.2, 13.3, and 13.4 illustrate the non-contrast computed tomography (NCCT) pattern of iCAA, including inflammation (Figs. 13.3

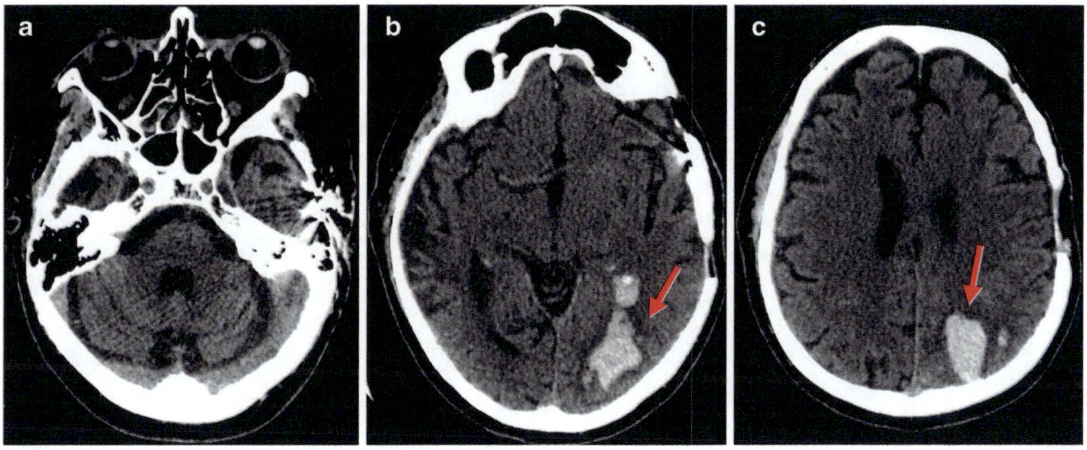

Fig. 13.1 Non-contrast computed tomography (NCCT) in axial plane in caudo-cranial direction from panel a to panel c in a 67-year-old patient with a past TBI requiring surgery with dural graft when he was 24 years old. A left occipito-parietal lobar ICH is evident, as hyperdense lesion with island sign (red arrows)

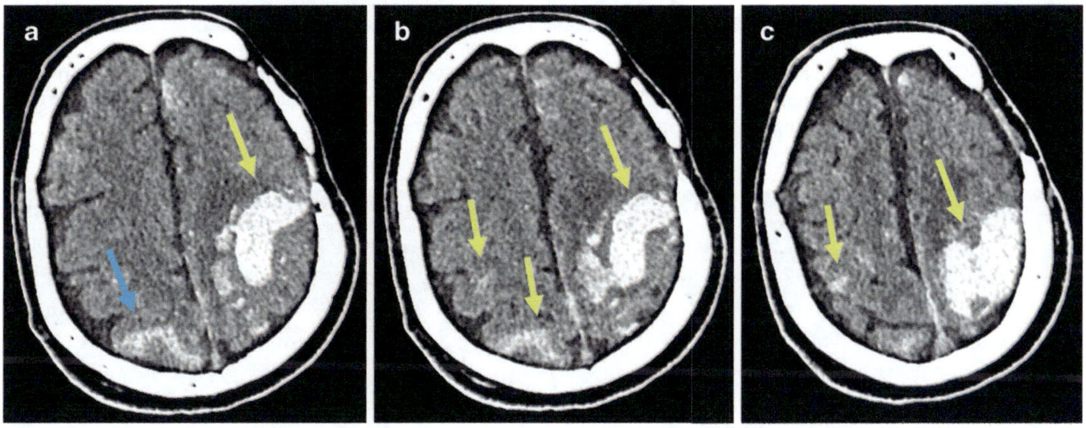

Fig. 13.2 NCCT (panels **a–c**) after 3 months in the same patient as in Fig. 13.1 showing a new ICH in left frontal posterior lobe with cortical extension (yellow arrow) and subarachnoid hemorrhage in the right posterior frontal and parietal sulci (blue arrow)

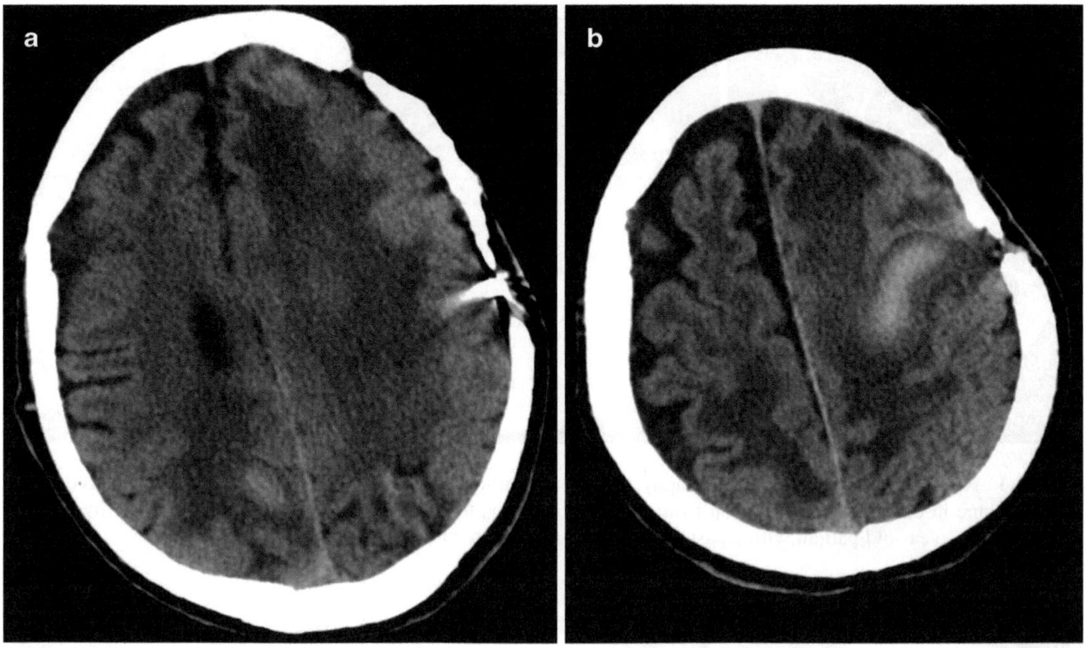

Fig. 13.3 NCCT in the same patient as in Figs. 13.1 and 13.2, at 30 days from the recurrent ICH (Fig. 13.2), showing a partial clearance of bleeding and the appearance of an extensive white matter hypointensity up to the cortico--subcortical junction in the left hemisphere and in the right parietal lobe

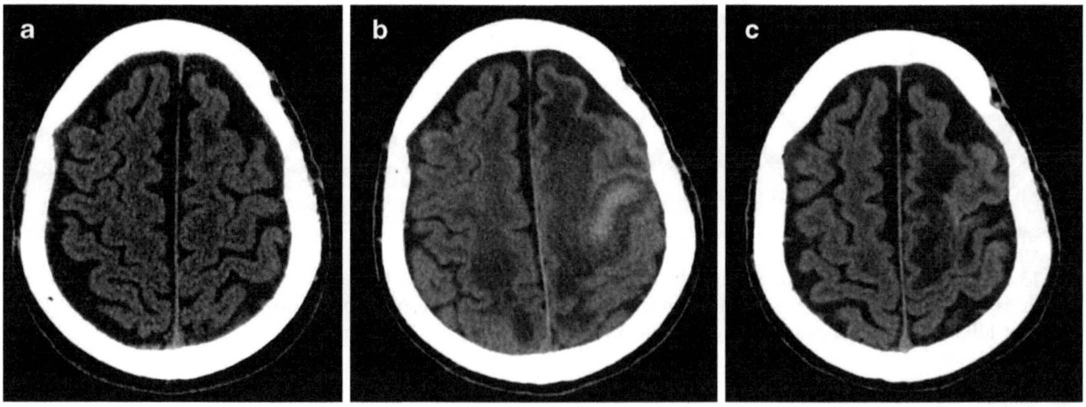

Fig. 13.4 Sequential NCCT changes in the same patient as in Figs. 13.1, 13.2, and 13.3 from the first ICH (panel **a**), through the recurrent one (panel **b**) up to the bleeding clearance and probable inflammatory sign in the left hemisphere (panel **c**)

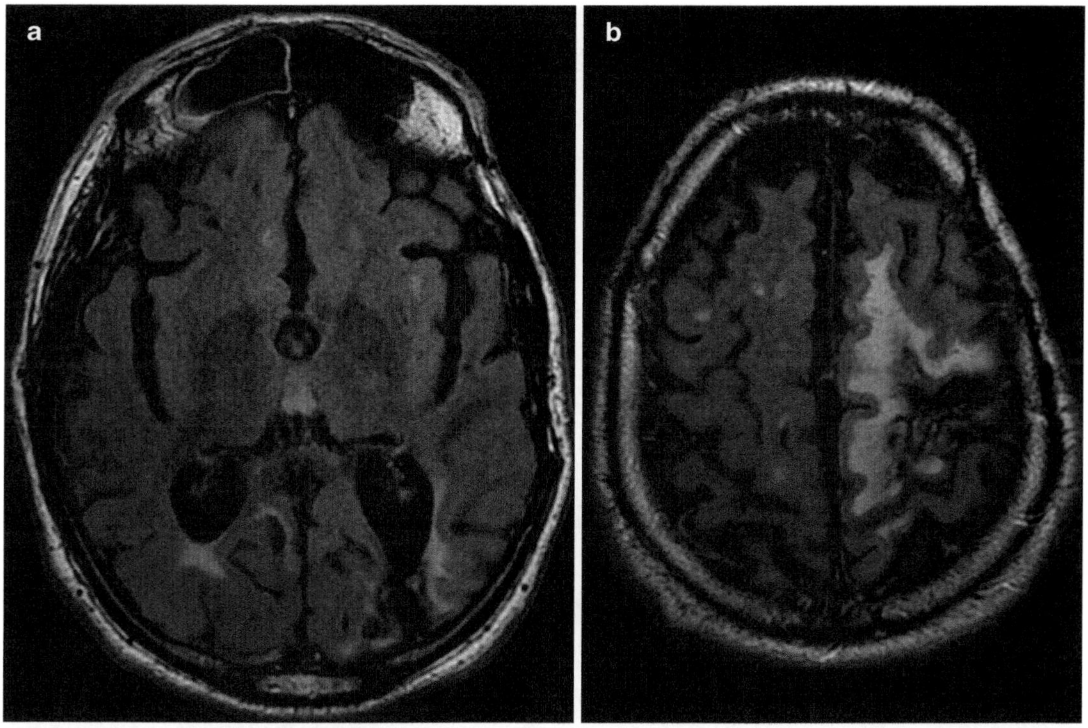

Fig. 13.5 Brain MRI 6 months after the first ICH (Fig. 13.1), showing axial fluid attenuated inversion recovery (FLAIR) sequence with ICH consequences (left occipital lobe in panel **a** and left frontal lobe in panel **b**) and wide white matter hypointensity in the left frontal lobe

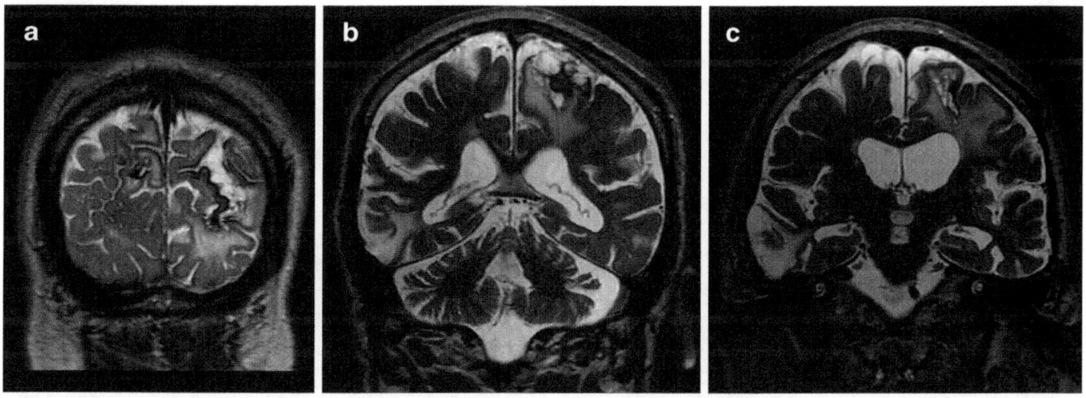

Fig. 13.6 Brain MRI in coronal plane (T2W sequence) in a posterior-anterior direction (from panel **a** to **c**), showing the hypointense lining of the cerebral cortex in the left and right occipital-parietal lobes (panel **a**–**c**), the hyperintense white matter lesions in the left frontal lobe (panel **b**, **c**), and a diffuse widening of the pericerebral CSF spaces

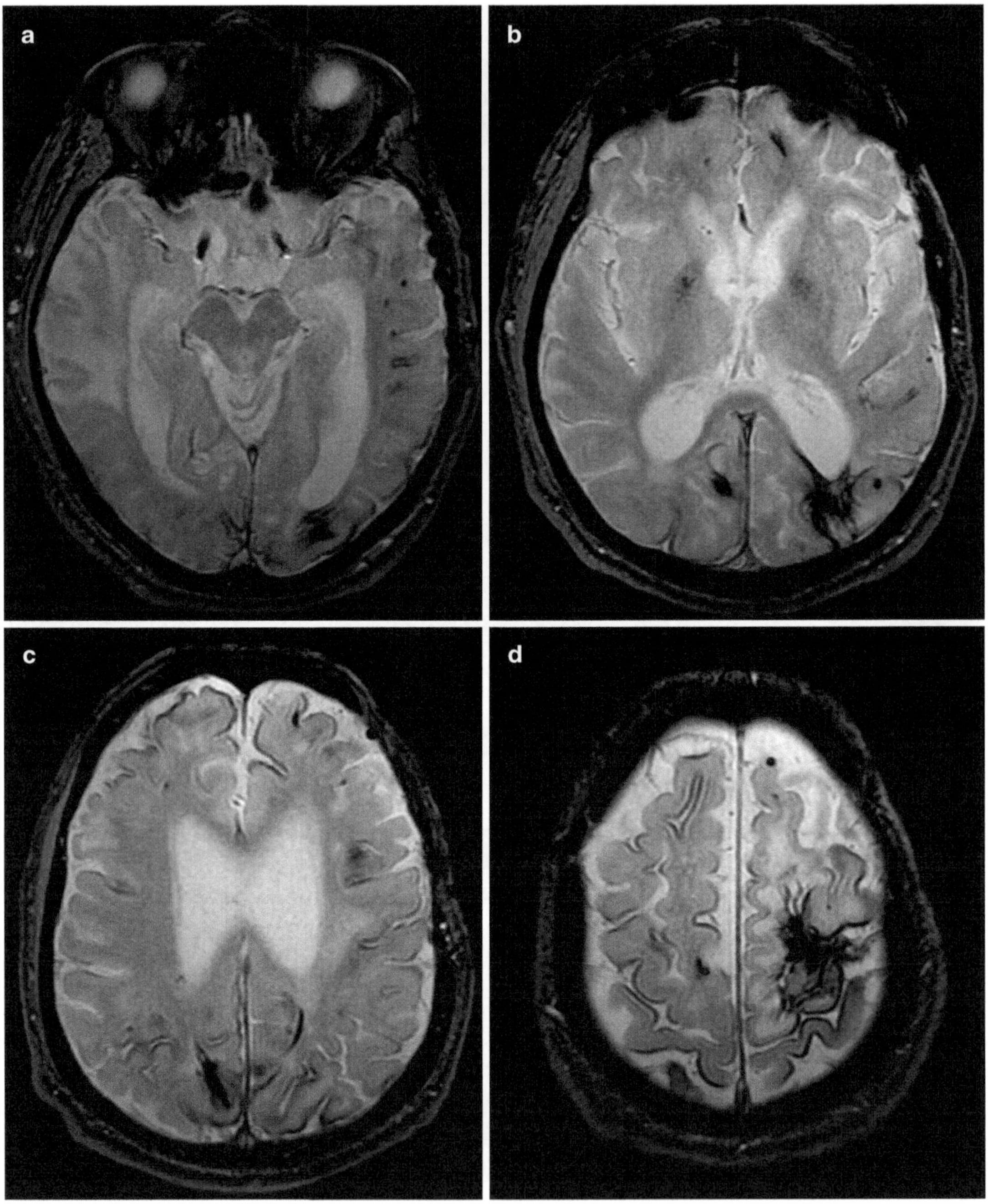

Fig. 13.7 Brain MRI (axial T2* sequence) in caudal-cranial direction, showing diffuse and almost ubiquitous cSS as hypointense cortical lining with only a few isolated CMBs in axial ascending slices from **a** to **d**

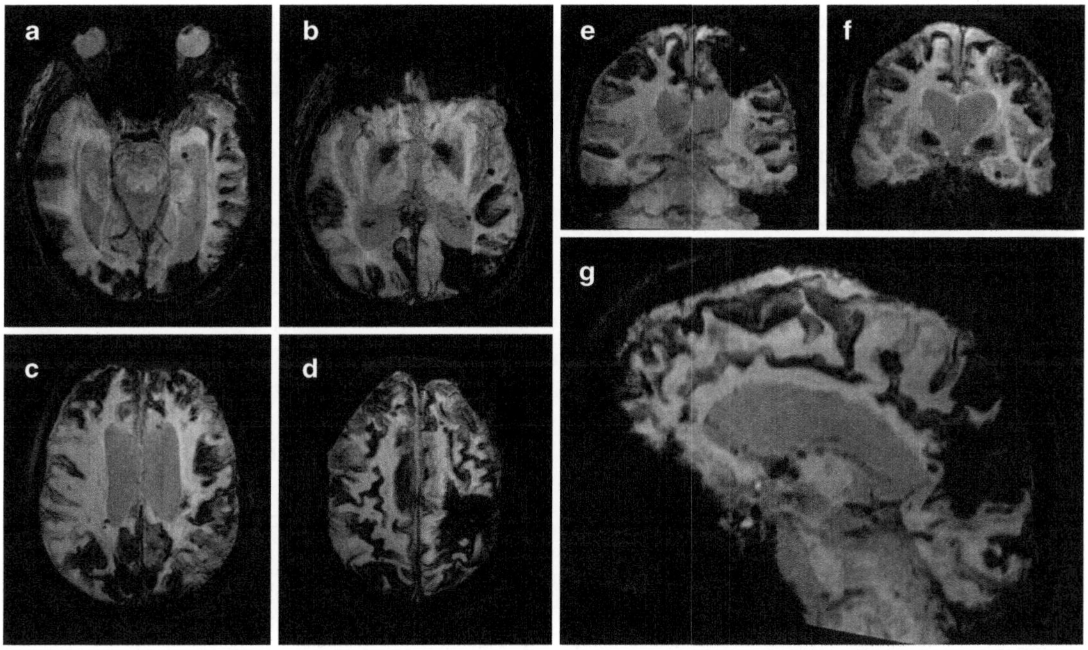

Fig. 13.8 Brain MRI (susceptibility-weighted imaging—SWI—reconstructed with minimum intensity projections/multiplanar protocol) in axial planes (panels **a–d**), coronal planes (panels **e**, **f**), and in sagittal plane (panel **g**), showing diffuse and almost ubiquitous cSS as hypointense cortical lining with only a few isolated CMBs. The different sensitivity of the two sequences (T2* and SWI) for blood degradation products is well evident, with better visualization in SWI-MRI

and 13.4). Figures 13.5, 13.6, 13.7, and 13.8 illustrate the brain MRI pattern of iCAA.

13.4 Clinical Presentation

In a comprehensive study, 49 patients with suspected iCAA were classified according to the proposed diagnostic criteria [2]. Of these, 43% were classified as probable iCAA and 57% as possible iCAA. The findings showed that lobar ICH was the most frequent presentation (57%), followed by transient focal neurological episodes (12%) and seizures (8%). Notably, the recurrence rate of ICH was lower in newly identified patients compared to previously documented cases from the literature, suggesting potential variations in disease course, although publication bias is present. The clinical profiles of patients with iCAA in this case series reveal important similarities and differences when compared to sporadic CAA. While both conditions exhibit a potential male predominance, iCAA cases are typically younger at presentation, and there is a notable lack of specific associations with the ApoE ε2 and ε4 alleles, which are often seen in sporadic CAA [3]. Furthermore, the presence of rapidly progressive cognitive symptoms, recurrent ICH and seizures, which are less common in sporadic CAA, emphasizes the need for clinicians to consider the possibility of iCAA in younger patients presenting with these features. The main factor conditioning the age at diagnosis (and the age of symptoms' onset) is the incubation period. When patients present at a young age, they will then necessarily have had the procedure during childhood, but when patients present at older age, the procedure is not necessarily during childhood, considering the latency a constant [47].

In a neuroradiological systematic review with restrictive inclusion criteria, data are similar [48]. Only patients with probable iCAA were included, cases involving patients with concurrent CJD and CAA were excluded, and patients were excluded if the surgical site was not clearly described or if there were multiple potential routes of amyloid introduction (for example, cases that involved both spinal surgery and ventriculoperitoneal shunting or bilateral supratentorial surgeries). A total of 24 patients from 19 reports met the inclusion criteria. The age at exposure varied significantly, ranging from the neonatal period to 23 years, with a median age of 20 months (interquartile range 8.25–60 months). The latency period between the surgical intervention and the occurrence of ICH ranged from 25 to 49 years. In half of the cases ($n = 12$), there was confirmation of the use of lyophilized dura; in 6 cases, the use was explicitly denied, while in the remaining 6, the status of lyophilized dura usage remained unverified. Among these patients, 19 underwent supratentorial surgeries, while 5 had infratentorial or spinal procedures. Notably, many neurosurgical interventions ($n = 11$) were performed following some form of trauma. The latency between the initial exposure and the first ICH ranged from 25 to 49 years, with a notable peak in the third to fourth decade following exposure.

In a comprehensive study [45] involving 51 patients (68.6% male), the median age at presentation was 48 years, with a notable 51% classified as having probable iCAA and 49% as possible iCAA. The median age at the time of exposure to relevant medical procedures was 9 years (IQR 2–21 years). The most common exposure events included cranial neurosurgery (70.6%), spinal neurosurgery (21.6%), and vascular embolization procedures (7.8%). Among these patients, 27.5% had confirmed usage of lyophilized cadaveric dura [45].

It should be noted that this study [45] pooled individual patient data from the aforementioned cohorts, reporting clinical symptoms at presentation ranging from ICH (45.1%) to transient focal neurological episodes (TFNEs) (35.3%), seizures (7.8%), and cognitive decline (5.9%). The latency from exposure to symptom onset averaged 38 years (IQR 34–41 years), highlighting the long-term implications of these procedures [45].

A final issue is that cognitive changes are currently poorly investigated and reported in iCAA in comparison with CAA and AD patients. This point could be the focus of a longitudinal study together with clinical and neuroimaging follow-up.

13.5 Neuroimaging Features

Neuroimaging plays a crucial role in the diagnosis and monitoring of iCAA. The role of neuroradiological markers comes directly from the definition of iCAA as an uncommon variant of CAA characterized by the introduction of amyloid fibrils into the human CNS via external seeding from sources such as human cadaveric dura mater grafts, other cadaveric materials, and contaminated neurosurgical instruments [26]. In fact, although the clinical presentation and age of onset may differ slightly from those of spontaneous CAA, the imaging markers are largely analogous [2]. In a recently published cohort, baseline MRI revealed that 94.1% of patients had cerebral microbleeds (CMBs), with a median count of 18 (IQR 6–45) [45]. Notably, 19.6% of patients presented with deep CMBs, which are typically not found in sporadic CAA, indicating a unique characteristic of iCAA. Additionally, cortical superficial siderosis (cSS) was observed in 68.6% of patients, often with a disseminated pattern [45]. During follow-up, which had a median duration of 3.7 years, there were 43 symptomatic recurrent ICHs, translating to a rate of 16.7 per 100 patient-years. A substantial number of asymptomatic ICHs were also detected, indicating a high burden of cerebral hemorrhages in this patient population [45].

In the above-reported multicenter cohort [45], longitudinal analysis revealed significant progression of hemorrhagic markers over time. The median number of CMBs increased from 16 at baseline to 55 at the last follow-up, with a marked increase in the proportion of patients exhibiting ≥50 lobar CMBs (from 21.6% to 51.1%). Additionally, inflammatory changes, characterized by cortical edema and parenchymal hyperintensities, were noted in 27.4% of patients, suggesting a potential inflammatory component to the disease's progression [45].

In cases of iCAA, it is hypothesized that the introduced amyloid triggers a prion-like propagation throughout the brain tissue. Recent attempts have been made to map this propagation using diffusion MRI techniques in CJD, another type of prion disease [49]. Diffusion-weighted MRI has proven to be an effective modality for detecting lesions and tracking their progression in CJD. In the context of iCAA, ICH have been consistently reported; however, the early indicators of amyloid-related damage that precede these hemorrhages, as well as their temporal relationship, remain poorly understood. Consequently, in vivo assessment of iCAA-related damage, particularly in at-risk patients, is highly sought after. This issue has been recently addressed by a systematic review and neuroradiological meta-analysis [48] aiming to assess the hypothesis that there is a correlation between the surgical site and both hemorrhagic and non-hemorrhagic imaging markers of iCAA, as suggested by some previous case reports [50, 51]. This correlation could serve as an indicator of damage propagation from the initial site of surgery to surrounding brain regions. In contrast, a previous study [47] did not find such a correlation for hemorrhagic markers, but it did not investigate the temporal pattern and the number of iCAA patients with available MRI scans was limited. Of these, three occurred in the thalamus, while the remainder were located in lobar regions. Notably, 69% ($p = 0.0498$, Fisher's exact test) of the initial ICHs occurred ipsilateral to the surgical site, whereas 59% of all ICHs ($n = 63$, $p = 0.126$, Fisher's exact test) were also found ipsilaterally, considering only patients with supratentorial surgeries. Importantly, no cerebellar or spinal hemorrhages were reported, even among those with infratentorial or spinal surgeries. CMBs were identified in 21 patients. In 7/18 (39%) patients who underwent supratentorial surgery, CMBs appeared ipsilateral to the surgical site. The latency between surgery and the appearance of CMBs was slightly shorter (33.1 ± 3.3 years vs. 38.5 ± 6.8 years, $p = 0.069$) for those with ipsilateral CMBs. In six patients, CMBs were noted prior to or without the occurrence of ICH. Additionally, infratentorial CMBs were reported in three patients. Cortical superficial siderosis (cSS) was observed in nine patients, showing no lateralization toward the surgical site. Infratentorial cSS was reported in two cases. Subarachnoid hemorrhage (SAH) occurred in only two patients. White matter lesions were noted in ten patients, with no side differences observed (0%). Ischemic lesions, either diffusion-weighted imaging (DWI) lesions or chronic ischemic lesions, were identified in three patients, again showing no lateralization. Both enlarged perivascular spaces (EPVS) and contrast enhancement with swelling were reported in only two patients, with no side differences noted. Among the eight patients who presented before the onset of symptoms and/or occurrence of ICH, CMBs were present in one patient, while SAH preceded ICH in two cases. Ischemic lesions were identified in two patients, all located ipsilateral to the surgical site.

In this cohort [48], the side of the initial ICH correlated with the side of the initial surgery. Notably, 5/8 (62%) patients exhibited both hemorrhagic and non-hemorrhagic signs before the onset of symptoms or ICH. This contrasts with findings by Kaushik et al. [2], who did not find a spatial correlation between surgery sites and hemorrhagic manifestations in a Dutch cohort of eight patients with iCAA. In prion diseases, such as CJD, the spread of prions is theorized to occur in two phases: an initial phase of misfolded protein accumulation, followed by a second phase marked by cell damage and clinical symptoms [52, 53]. The occurrence of CMB may serve as an indicator of initial brain damage. The first ICH could signify more severe damage near the surgical site, with subsequent ICHs occurring elsewhere in the brain. This pattern might clarify the presence of thalamic hemorrhages and lacunar ischemia, typically seen in hypertensive arteriopathy rather than amyloid-related conditions [54–56], especially given the absence of reported arterial hypertension in these cases. Interestingly, no cerebellar hemorrhages were noted, despite the cerebellum being a common site for ICH in CAA [57, 58], leaving the reason for this observation unclear. Some imaging markers were seldom reported, raising questions about their actual presence or significance in relation to amyloid pathology, as seen with enlarged perivascular spaces (EPVS), which were only recently included in the Boston criteria 2.0 [55]. The observed presence and potential colocalization of CMB with the surgical site may suggest a marker for disease progression in iCAA. Another interesting consideration is that the described hypothesis contrasts with the current pathophysiological framework of CAA, stating that the pre-hemorrhagic stage, characterized by WMH and EPVS, always comes first and before the hemorrhagic stages in sporadic and Dutch-type hereditary CAA [59].

In a recently published cohort of patients with iCAA [45], 23 patients underwent unilateral supratentorial brain surgery and distinct focal patterns of hemorrhagic markers associated with CAA were observed both at baseline and follow-up. At baseline, patients showed a higher median number of CMBs in the ipsilateral hemisphere compared to the contralateral side (10 vs. 5) and a trend toward more cSS and ICH on the ipsilateral side. At the final follow-up, similar patterns persisted for ipsilateral CMBs and cSS, although the number of ipsilateral ICHs remained unchanged. At baseline, 60.9% of patients exhibited ipsilateral dominance of CMBs, while only 21.7% showed contralateral dominance. For cSS, 52.9% patients had ipsilateral dominance. Among patients with ICH, 72.2% showed ipsilateral dominance. Follow-up MRI indicated even stronger evidence of ipsilateral dominance for CMBs (65.2% vs. 8.7%), cSS (73.7% vs. 5.3%), and recurrent ICH (55.0% vs. 15.0%), as for sporadic CAA [60]. However, no focal patterns of non-hemorrhagic markers were detected at either time point. In contrast, patients who had infratentorial or spinal surgery did not exhibit any lateralization patterns, with a similar distribution of CMBs on both sides [45].

Summarizing the issues from different studies, iCAA seems to be characterized by a marked progression in hemorrhagic markers of CAA (CMBs, cSS, ICH) over a median MRI follow-up time of 3 years. This suggests an active hemorrhage-prone phase of CAA, following a prolonged latent period post presumed exposure (inoculation). Alongside a substantial number of symptomatic ICH cases, many patients also exhibited asymptomatic smaller (often intragyral) ICHs. In addition, hemorrhagic lesions were frequently found in deep brain regions, which are typically not included in the diagnostic criteria for "sporadic" CAA and may be supportive of a copathology in these last patients more than in younger iCAA patients. These hemorrhagic CAA markers show a lateralized progression in a subset of patients, which may hold pathophysiological relevance. Additionally, asymptomatic findings indicative of transient inflammation were common, potentially implicating inflammation in the pathophysiology of iCAA, as well as in CAA [61–64]. Throughout the follow-up period, nearly half of the patients experienced at least one symptomatic (recurrent) ICH, and the median number of CMBs increased by more than threefold. An interesting point is that over 40% of patients had deep CMBs, and therefore it would not have been possible to diagnose them as CAA based on the Boston criteria 2.0 [55]. Amyloid-β deposition in CAA is generally thought to occur almost exclusively in the leptomeningeal and cortical arteries and arterioles [65]; however, neuropathological studies show that in severe stages, CAA can also affect deep structures, particularly the deep gray nuclei (which include the thalamus and basal ganglia) [66].

Additionally, a recent case series found MRI findings suggestive of inflammation in patients with iCAA [45]. While such changes are sometimes observed in CAA-related inflammation or as amyloid-related imaging abnormalities (ARIA) in immunotherapy trials for AD, the proportion of patients with inflammatory signs on MRI in iCAA (nearly one in three) is higher than reported rates in patients with sporadic CAA [46, 59, 67]. Moreover, the exact prevalence of

CAA-related inflammation in patients with sporadic CAA may be largely underestimated [46].

Several fields of research are open in iCAA and most of them are shared with CAA. In particular, an attractive issue may be to assess Blood Oxygenation Level Dependent (BOLD) MRI changes in iCAA to see how it relates to sporadic CAA in terms of lateralization [68].

13.6 CSF and PET

In the proposed diagnostic criteria of iCAA, both CSF analysis and PET with amyloid tracers are proposed in order to assess the amyloid deposition in vivo in these patients, although a minority of reported cases provide this information. One of the reasons for this is that in several countries PET and CSF analysis are not commonly used for supporting CAA diagnosis outside research, not being formally part of the current diagnostic criteria. Sporadic CAA is frequently associated with changes in CSF levels of amyloid-beta 40 and 42 and total tau and phosphorylated tau proteins. It is not surprising that in iCAA, the same pattern has been found, independently from the association with AD [69]. These changes in CAA are more pronounced when some neuroradiological markers are present. One study [69] investigated the association between cSS and CSF levels of β-amyloid in 101 patients diagnosed with probable (79%) or possible (21%) CAA (61% with cSS) and mild cognitive impairment. Patients with cSS had significantly lower levels of β-amyloid 42 compared to those without cSS (odds ratio [OR] 0.2; $p = 0.0052$). No significant differences were found in levels of β-amyloid 40, total tau, or phosphorylated tau between cSS and non-cSS patients. There was no significant correlation between the number of CMB and CSF biomarkers. A recent study on a small sample of iCAA patients did not find significant differences in CSF profile among young iCAA patients and old CAA patients, suggesting common pattern of CSF findings in both diseases [70].

PET with amyloid tracers has been proposed as an ancillary diagnostic technique in patients with CAA, trying to differentiate the spatial pattern of tracer distribution between CAA and AD. In a recently published scoping review [70], PET imaging indicates significantly higher global amyloid deposition in CAA patients compared to healthy controls and those with deep ICH. A distinctive occipital-predominant pattern of amyloid deposition is observed in CAA, helping differentiate it, particularly in young patients, from AD, which typically shows more diffuse amyloid distribution. Finally, amyloid PET has shown promise in supporting the diagnosis of CAA, particularly in cases of ICH, where it can predict recurrence with high sensitivity and specificity. Despite its utility, current amyloid-PET tracers lack specificity for vascular amyloid, complicating the differentiation from other conditions. Until now, a single study on a small cohort of patients with iCAA has been published [71].

13.7 Discussion and Differential Diagnosis

The diagnostic criteria for iCAA are obviously related with the CAA diagnostic criteria and their update (Boston criteria 2.0) [56], with some differences that deserve to be mentioned: (1) iCAA criteria include deep CMBs and macrobleeds although Boston criteria exclude them; (2) the current criteria for iCAA do not require pathological confirmation; (3) the age limit of the Boston criteria (actually 50 years) does not apply to iCAA, the exposure to the iatrogenic trigger being possible during childhood with an age at diagnosis <50 years, as for CAA-ri criteria [46], including patients >40 years.

The clinical and radiological presentation of iCAA showcases distinctive features that differentiate it from sporadic CAA [58]. The presence of deep CMBs, the tendency for ipsilateral spread of hemorrhagic markers, and the high rates of both symptomatic and asymptomatic ICHs underscore the need for heightened awareness and appropriate diagnostic strategies in managing patients with a history of relevant medical procedures. Further investigation into the underlying mechanisms of iCAA could yield important insights into its pathophysiology and implications for treatment.

The utilization of cadaveric human materials is highly regulated in many countries due to the associated risk of iatrogenic CJD. However, determining the exact number of individuals exposed to such materials is complicated by inconsistencies in centralized record-keeping. Transmission of prions can occur through contaminated neurosurgical instruments and blood transfusions, with documented cases of iatrogenic CJD linked to both exposure routes [34]. Moreover, accurately verifying neurosurgical procedures through historical records poses significant challenges as documentation is often found missing. Research involving transgenic mice has demonstrated that Aβ can be transmitted via steel wires, and while plasma sterilization can prevent this transmission, boiling is ineffective [28]. The role of transfusion is less extensively investigated than in CJD, but there is some recent evidence supporting a role in CAA occurrence [54]. In fact, experimental evidence suggests that Aβ transmission may occur through this route [27]. Comprehensive epidemiological studies are essential to thoroughly assessing the risk of Aβ transmission through contaminated instruments, which will guide future protocols for sterilization methods aimed at preventing such transmission. Further investigation into these transmission pathways is warranted.

Previous iterations of the MRI-based Boston criteria for CAA required the absence of alternative diagnoses [46]; for patients with sporadic CAA, the most common alternative is arteriolosclerosis, which is characterized by hemorrhages in deep structures. The most recent version of the Boston criteria explicitly excludes patients with deep hemorrhagic features from receiving a CAA diagnosis, but deep CMBs were found in patients with Dutch-type hereditary CAA, an inherited form of amyloid-β CAA [72]. The coexistence of arteriolosclerosis is less likely to explain deep hemorrhagic changes in iCAA, given the younger age of these patients and their relative absence of vascular risk factors such as hypertension. Therefore, it seems most probable that these deep hemorrhagic changes, reported in previously published cases of iCAA [65], are related to CAA, indicating either a high degree of CAA severity or a unique neuroimaging feature of iatrogenic disease (e.g., due to regional vulnerability to amyloid-β prions). Post-mortem reports have demonstrated amyloid-β deposition in the basal ganglia and thalamus in iatrogenic cases, supporting this perspective [26].

While iCAA shares many features with sporadic and hereditary CAA, it may not be identical to these disease forms; one recognized difference is the age of onset with a male predominance, raising a question about a potential hormonal protective effect for women. The rapid progression of hemorrhagic markers and the large number of both symptomatic and smaller intragyral ICHs suggest an active hemorrhage-prone vasculopathy in iCAA. Similar well-recognized clinical and radiological differences are observed between acquired (iatrogenic and variant) and sporadic forms of CJD [73].

In most patients where exposure to amyloid-β was unilateral and supratentorial, a lateralized spread of hemorrhagic lesions, with ICH, CMB, and cSS was predominantly found in the ipsilateral hemisphere [45, 48]. The lateralization of these hemorrhages suggests a locally active pathophysiological process at later disease stages. Prions exhibit "two-stage kinetics," characterized by distinct periods of first propagation (an exponential increase in prion titer) and subsequent toxicity (where cell death occurs) [74]; if amyloid-β behaves similarly, a model for which there is some supporting experimental data [75], then the observed vasculopathy and subsequent hemorrhages would occur during the later toxicity stage. The reasons for selective vulnerability to toxicity near the presumed inoculation site in those who underwent supratentorial brain surgery remain unknown, but lateralization of amyloid-β pathology after intracerebral inoculation has been observed in animal models of amyloid-β transmission [75, 76]. This is particularly perplexing, as there is evidence of vascular toxicity at sites far removed from the presumed inoculation site in patients with iCAA following spinal surgery, supporting the notion of widespread propagation of amyloid-β following

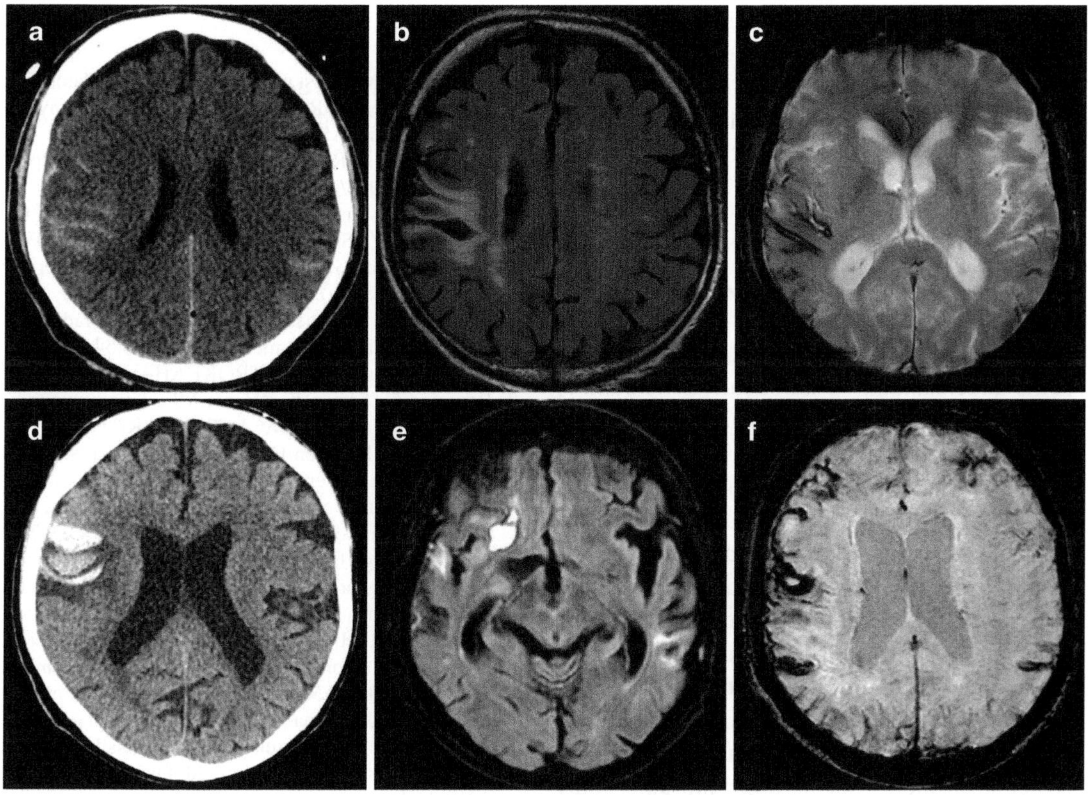

Fig. 13.9 An example of TBI-triggered CAA. Panel **a**: NCCT at the time of head injury, showing diffuse subarachnoid hemorrhage (sulcal hyperdense signal in the right and left frontal cortex). Panel **b**: brain MRI (axial FLAIR) showing the consequences of TBI. Panel **c**: brain MRI (T2*) showing the cSS, mainly in the sulci previously involved by the subarachnoid hemorrhage. Panel **d**: NCCT at the first spontaneous ICH occurrence. Panel **e**: recurrent ICH in the right fronto-orbital region found at the control MRI (axial FLAIR). Panel **f**: brain MRI (SWI) with increased extension of cSS

exposure. Further exploration of these hypotheses in experimental models will be relevant to understanding both iatrogenic and other forms of CAA.

Alternative explanations have been suggested for the emergence of early-onset CAA in patients, particularly concerning the impact of traumatic brain injury (TBI). Research indicates that Aβ rapidly accumulates in the acute phase following TBI, potentially due to disruption of the blood-brain barrier, and this accumulation typically resolves over a matter of days [77, 78]. However, disentangling the influence of TBI can be complex, as the injuries sustained by individuals in reported cases may have necessitated neurosurgical interventions, whether or not cadaveric materials were utilized. The timeline between brain injury and the clinical presentation of symptomatic CAA aligns with the latency expected for iatrogenic Aβ transmission. It is noteworthy that the reports do not clarify whether neurosurgical procedures were performed, leaving ambiguity about the historical context of these cases. Additionally, not all patients with early-onset CAA exhibited a prior history of TBI (Fig. 13.9). This includes individuals who were exposed to cadaveric dura mater through embolization procedures or those who received cadaveric human growth hormone during childhood [3, 79]. These cadaveric materials are well-documented as potential vectors for prion protein transmission, particularly in the context of CJD [28, 34]. Considering these factors alongside the substantial experimental evidence suggesting Aβ transmission, the putative mechanism underlying early-onset CAA in TBI cases is likely related to iatrogenic protein transmission. A recent review summarizes the evidence underlying amyloid deposition and CAA in TBI patients, highlighting this neglected situation and proposing a case, which is very similar to iCAA in spatial and time pattern and natural history, in an adult patient [80].

13.8 Conclusions

As the understanding of iatrogenic CAA continues to evolve, it is critical for clinicians to remain vigilant for its manifestations, particularly in young patients with a history of neurosurgery. Standardizing diagnostic criteria and promoting systematic inquiries into surgical histories will aid in the identification of this underrecognized subtype of CAA. Standardizing diagnostic criteria and promoting systematic inquiries into surgical histories will aid in the identification of this underrecognized subtype of CAA. Utilizing an array of epidemiological techniques, such as case-control studies, standardized mortality rates and triangulative estimation methods, could yield valuable insights into the relative risk of developing iCAA in exposed patients. Given that the use of lyophilized dura was largely discontinued in the mid-1990s, such research could yield valuable insights into the relative risk of developing iCAA in exposed patients. It should me mentioned that ethical issues are a main concern in this field.

In addition, future research must focus on elucidating the mechanisms of Aβ transmission, exploring long-term outcomes for patients with iCAA, and establishing national and international registries to enhance data collection and analysis. Through these efforts, the medical community can better address the public health implications of iCAA and improve patient outcomes for patients with CAA in general. In fact, iCAA and hereditary CAA are the unique cases that can help advance care for patients with CAA in general, allowing to study and understand particular disease mechanisms (e.g., propagation and development).

References

1. Greenberg SM, Bacskai BJ, Hernandez-Guillamon M, Pruzin J, Sperling R, van Veluw SJ. Cerebral amyloid angiopathy and Alzheimer disease – one peptide, two pathways. Nat Rev Neurol. 2020;16:30–42. https://doi.org/10.1038/s41582-019-0281-2.
2. Kaushik K, van Etten ES, Siegerink B, Kappelle LJ, Lemstra AW, Schreuder FHBM, Klijn CJM, Peul WC, Terwindt GM, van Walderveen MAA, Wermer MJH. Iatrogenic cerebral amyloid angiopathy post neurosurgery: frequency, clinical profile, radiological features, and outcome. Stroke. 2023;54:1214–23. https://doi.org/10.1161/STROKEAHA.122.041690.
3. Banerjee G, Samra K, Adams ME, Jaunmuktane Z, Parry-Jones AR, Grieve J, Toma AK, Farmer SF, Sylvester R, Houlden H, Mead S, Brandner S, Schott JM, Collinge J, Werring DJ. Iatrogenic cerebral amyloid angiopathy: an emerging clinical phenomenon. J Neurol Neurosurg Psychiatry. 2022;93:693–700. https://doi.org/10.1136/jnnp-2022-328792.
4. Zhao J, Rostgaard K, Lauwers E, Dahlén T, Ostrowski SR, Erikstrup C, Pedersen OB, de Strooper B, Lemmens R, Hjalgrim H, Edgren G. Intracerebral hemorrhage among blood donors and their transfusion recipients. JAMA. 2023;330(10):941–50. https://doi.org/10.1001/jama.2023.14445.
5. Jaunmuktane Z, Brandner S. Transmissible human proteopathies: an expanding field. Diagn Histopathol. 2019;25:16–22.
6. Duyckaerts C, Clavaguera F, Potier MC. The prionlike propagation hypothesis in Alzheimer's and Parkinson's disease. Curr Opin Neurol. 2019;32:266–71.
7. Hamaguchi T, Komatsu J, Sakai K, et al. Cerebral hemorrhagic stroke associated with cerebral amyloid angiopathy in young adults about 3 decades after neurosurgeries in their infancy. J Neurol Sci. 2019;399:3–5.
8. Giaccone G, Maderna E, Marucci G, et al. Iatrogenic early onset cerebral amyloid angiopathy 30 years after cerebral trauma with neurosurgery: vascular amyloid deposits are made up of both Aβ40 and Aβ42. Acta Neuropathol Commun. 2019;7:70.
9. Jucker M, Walker LC. Propagation and spread of pathogenic protein assemblies in neurodegenerative diseases. Nat Neurosci. 2018;21:1341–9.
10. Vaquer Alicea J, Diamond MI. Propagation of protein aggregation in neurodegenerative diseases. Annu Rev Biochem. 2019;88:785–810.
11. Eisele YS, Bolmont T, Heikenwalder M, et al. Induction of cerebral βamyloidosis: intracerebral versus systemic Abeta inoculation. Proc Natl Acad Sci USA. 2009;106:12926–31.
12. Meyer Luehmann M, Coomaraswamy J, Bolmont T, et al. Exogenous induction of cerebral betaamyloidogenesis is governed by agent and host. Science. 2006;313:1781–4.

13. Burwinkel M, Lutzenberger M, Heppner FL, SchulzSchaeffer W, Baier M. Intravenous injection of beta amyloid seeds promotes cerebral amyloid angiopathy (CAA). Acta Neuropathol Commun. 2018;6:23.
14. Eisele YS, Obermüller U, Heilbronner G, et al. Peripherally applied Abeta-containing inoculates induce cerebral beta amyloidosis. Science. 2010;330:980–2.
15. Bu XL, Xiang Y, Jin WS, et al. Blood-derived amyloid-β protein induces Alzheimer's disease pathologies. Mol Psychiatry. 2018;23:1948–56.
16. Collinge J, Whitfield J, McKintosh E, et al. Kuru in the 21st century—an acquired human prion disease with very long incubation periods. Lancet. 2006;367:2068–74.
17. Heckmann JG, Lang CJ, Petruch F, et al. Transmission of Creutzfeldt-Jakob disease via a corneal transplant. J Neurol Neurosurg Psychiatry. 1997;63:388–90.
18. Ironside JW, Ritchie DL, Head MW. Prion diseases. Handb Clin Neurol. 2017;145:393–403.
19. Urwin PJM, Mackenzie JM, Llewelyn CA, Will RG, Hewitt PE. Creutzfeldt-Jakob disease and blood transfusion: updated results of the UK transfusion medicine epidemiology review study. Vox Sang. 2016;110:310–6.
20. Ranke MB, Wit JM. Growth hormone—past, present and future. Nat Rev Endocrinol. 2018;14:285–300.
21. Kovacs GG, Lutz MI, Ricken G, et al. Dura mater is a potential source of Aβ seeds. Acta Neuropathol. 2016;131:911–23.
22. Irwin DJ, Abrams JY, Schonberger LB, et al. Evaluation of potential infectivity of Alzheimer and Parkinson disease proteins in recipients of cadaver-derived human growth hormone. JAMA Neurol. 2013;70:462–8.
23. Cali I, Cohen ML, Haik S, et al. Iatrogenic Creutzfeldt-Jakob disease with amyloid-β pathology: an international study. Acta Neuropathol Commun. 2018;6:5.
24. Ritchie DL, Adlard P, Peden AH, et al. Amyloid β accumulation in the CNS in human growth hormone recipients in the UK. Acta Neuropathol. 2017;134:221–40.
25. Duyckaerts C, Sazdovitch V, Ando K, et al. Neuropathology of iatrogenic Creutzfeldt-Jakob disease and immunoassay of French cadaver-sourced growth hormone batches suggest possible transmission of tauopathy and long incubation periods for the transmission of Abeta pathology. Acta Neuropathol. 2018;135:201–12.
26. Jaunmuktane Z, Mead S, Ellis M, et al. Evidence for human transmission of amyloid-β pathology and cerebral amyloid angiopathy. Nature. 2015;525:247–50.
27. Purro SA, Farrow MA, Linehan J, et al. Transmission of amyloid-β protein pathology from cadaveric pituitary growth hormone. Nature. 2018;564:415–9.
28. Hamaguchi T, Taniguchi Y, Sakai K, et al. Significant association of cadaveric dura mater grafting with subpial Aβ deposition and meningeal amyloid angiopathy. Acta Neuropathol. 2016;132:313–5.
29. Iwasaki Y, Imamura K, Iwai K, et al. Autopsied case of non-plaque type dura mater graft-associated Creutzfeldt-Jakob disease presenting with extensive amyloid-β deposition. Neuropathology. 2018;38:549–56.
30. Frontzek K, Lutz MI, Aguzzi A, Kovacs GG, Budka H. Amyloid-β pathology and cerebral amyloid angiopathy are frequent in iatrogenic Creutzfeldt-Jakob disease after dural grafting. Swiss Med Wkly. 2016;146:w14287.
31. Hervé D, Porché M, Cabrejo L, et al. Fatal Aβ cerebral amyloid angiopathy 4 decades after a dural graft at the age of 2 years. Acta Neuropathol. 2018;135:801–3.
32. Banerjee G, Adams ME, Jaunmuktane Z, et al. Early onset cerebral amyloid angiopathy following childhood exposure to cadaveric dura. Ann Neurol. 2019;85:284–90.
33. Raposo N, Planton M, Siegfried A, et al. Amyloid-β transmission through cardiac surgery using cadaveric dura mater patch. J Neurol Neurosurg Psychiatry. 2020;91:440–1.
34. Lauwers E, Lalli G, Brandner S, et al. Potential human transmission of amyloid β pathology: surveillance and risks. Lancet Neurol. 2020;19(10):872–8. https://doi.org/10.1016/S1474-4422(20)30238-6.
35. Meyer-Luehmann M, Coomaraswamy J, Bolmont T, et al. Exogenous induction of cerebral beta-amyloidogenesis is governed by agent and host. Science. 2006;313(5794):1781–4. https://doi.org/10.1126/science.1131864.
36. Morales R, Duran-Aniotz C, Bravo-Alegria J, et al. Infusion of blood from mice displaying cerebral amyloidosis accelerates amyloid pathology in animal models of Alzheimer's disease. Acta Neuropathol Commun. 2020;8(1):213. https://doi.org/10.1186/s40478-020-01087-1.
37. Holmqvist J, Wikman A, Pedersen OBV, et al. No evidence of transfusion transmitted sporadic Creutzfeldt-Jakob disease: results from a binational cohort study. Transfusion. 2020;60:694–7.
38. Darby SC, Kan SW, Spooner RJ, et al. Mortality rates, life expectancy, and causes of death in people with hemophilia A or B in the United Kingdom who were not infected with HIV. Blood. 2007;110:815–25.
39. Edgren G, Hjalgrim H, Rostgaard K, et al. Transmission of neurodegenerative disorders through blood transfusion: a cohort study. Ann Intern Med. 2016;165:316–24.
40. Kaushik K, Wermer MJH, van Etten ES. Cerebral amyloid angiopathy decades after red blood cell transfusions: a report of two cases from a prospective cohort. Eur J Neurol. 2024;31:e16277. https://doi.org/10.1111/ene.16277.
41. DiFrancesco JC, Tabaee Damavandi P, Pretnar-Oblak J, Frol S, de la Riva Juez P, Albajar Gomez I, Jensen-Kondering U. Iatrogenic cerebral amyloid angiopathy after red blood cell transfusion? Eur J Neurol. 2024;31(8):e16366. https://doi.org/10.1111/ene.16366.

42. Muir RT, Callum JL, Yu AYX, Kapral MK, Swartz RH, Black SE, MacIntosh BJ, Fergusson DA, Kleinman S, Demchuk AD, Stys PK, Smith EE, Hill MD. Beta-amyloid related neurodegenerative and neurovascular diseases: potential implications for transfusion medicine. Transfus Med Rev. 2024;38(4):150858. https://doi.org/10.1016/j.tmrv.2024.150858.
43. Brown P, Brandel JP, Sato T, et al. Iatrogenic Creutzfeldt-Jakob disease, final assessment. Emerg Infect Dis. 2012;18(6):901–7. https://doi.org/10.3201/eid1806.120116.
44. Fandler-Höfler S, Kaushik K, Storti B, et al. Clinical-radiological presentation and natural history of iatrogenic cerebral amyloid angiopathy. J Neurol Neurosurg Psychiatry. 2025;0:1–10. https://doi.org/10.1136/jnnp-2024-335164.
45. Auriel E, Charidimou A, Gurol ME, et al. Validation of clinicoradiological criteria for the diagnosis of cerebral amyloid angiopathy-related inflammation. JAMA Neurol. 2016;73:197–202.
46. Panteleienko L, Mallon D, Oliver R, Toosy A, Hoshino Y, Murakami A, Kaushik K, Wermer MJH, Hara H, Yakushiji Y, Banerjee G, Werring DJ. Iatrogenic cerebral amyloid angiopathy in older adults. Eur J Neurol. 2024;31(6):e16278. https://doi.org/10.1111/ene.16278.
47. Jensen-Kondering U. Spatial colocalization of imaging markers in iatrogenic cerebral amyloid angiopathy with the site of surgery: a metaanalysis. J Neurol Sci. 2024;458:122931. https://doi.org/10.1016/j.jns.2024.122931.
48. Pascuzzo R, Oxtoby NP, Young AL, et al. Prion propagation estimated from brain diffusion MRI is subtype dependent in sporadic Creutzfeldt–Jakob disease. Acta Neuropathol. 2020;140:169–81. https://doi.org/10.1007/s00401-020-02168-0.
49. Jensen-Kondering U, Heß K, Flüh C, et al. A rare case of iatrogenic prion-like pathogenesis of cerebral amyloid angiopathy. Dtsch Arztebl Int. 2024;121:68–9. https://doi.org/10.3238/arztebl.m2023.0215.
50. Romero AL, Loscertales CM, Moreno EM. Unilateral cerebral amyloid angiopathy after neurointervention. Neurologia (Engl Ed). 2022;37:310–2. https://doi.org/10.1016/j.nrleng.2021.05.009.
51. Baker HF, Ridley RM, Duchen LW, et al. Experimental induction of β-amyloid plaques and cerebral angiopathy in primates. Ann N Y Acad Sci. 1993;695:228–31. https://doi.org/10.1111/j.1749-6632.1993.tb23057.x.
52. Collinge J. Mammalian prions and their wider relevance in neurodegenerative diseases. Nature. 2016;539:217–26. https://doi.org/10.1038/nature20415.
53. Smith EE, Nandigam KRN, Chen Y-W, et al. MRI markers of small vessel disease in lobar and deep hemispheric intracerebral hemorrhage. Stroke. 2010;41:1933–8. https://doi.org/10.1161/STROKEAHA.110.579078.
54. Duering M, Biessels GJ, Brodtmann A, Chen C, Cordonnier C, de Leeuw FE, Debette S, Frayne R, Jouvent E, Rost NS, Ter Telgte A, Al-Shahi Salman R, Backes WH, Bae HJ, Brown R, Chabriat H, De Luca A, deCarli C, Dewenter A, Doubal FN, Ewers M, Field TS, Ganesh A, Greenberg S, Helmer KG, Hilal S, Jochems ACC, Jokinen H, Kuijf H, Lam BYK, Lebenberg J, MacIntosh BJ, Maillard P, Mok VCT, Pantoni L, Rudilosso S, Satizabal CL, Schirmer MD, Schmidt R, Smith C, Staals J, Thrippleton MJ, van Veluw SJ, Vemuri P, Wang Y, Werring D, Zedde M, Akinyemi RO, Del Brutto OH, Markus HS, Zhu YC, Smith EE, Dichgans M, Wardlaw JM. Neuroimaging standards for research into small vessel disease-advances since 2013. Lancet Neurol. 2023;22(7):602–18. https://doi.org/10.1016/S1474-4422(23)00131-X.
55. Charidimou A, Boulouis G, Frosch MP, et al. The Boston criteria version 2.0 for cerebral amyloid angiopathy: a multicentre, retrospective, MRI–neuropathology diagnostic accuracy study. Lancet Neurol. 2022;21:714–25. https://doi.org/10.1016/S1474-4422(22)00208-3.
56. Pasi M, Marini S, Morotti A, et al. Cerebellar hematoma location. Stroke. 2018;49:207–10. https://doi.org/10.1161/STROKEAHA.117.019286.
57. Gavriliuc P, Molad J, Yaghmour N, et al. Cerebellar hemorrhages in patients with cerebral amyloid angiopathy. J Neurol Sci. 2019;405:116418. https://doi.org/10.1016/j.jns.2019.08.003.
58. Ohashi SN, DeLong JH, Kozberg MG, Mazur-Hart DJ, van Veluw SJ, Alkayed NJ, Sansing LH. Role of inflammatory processes in hemorrhagic stroke. Stroke. 2023;54:605–19. https://doi.org/10.1161/STROKEAHA.122.037155.
59. Koemans EA, Chhatwal JP, van Veluw SJ, van Etten ES, van Osch MJP, van Walderveen MAA, Sohrabi HR, Kozberg MG, Shirzadi Z, Terwindt GM, van Buchem MA, Smith EE, Werring DJ, Martins RN, Wermer MJH, Greenberg SM. Progression of cerebral amyloid angiopathy: a pathophysiological framework. Lancet Neurol. 2023;22(7):632–42. https://doi.org/10.1016/S1474-4422(23)00114-X.
60. Goeldlin MB, Fandler-Höfler S, Pezzini A, Manikantan A, Rauch J, Hald SM, Kristensen ML, Obergottsberger L, Sembill JA, Haupenthal D, Larsen KT, Avramiotis NS, Polymeris AA, Periole C, Thiankhaw K, Rangus I, Puy L, Pasi M, Morotti A, Silvestrelli G, Giacalone G, Paciaroni M, Zedde M, Giorli E, Tassi R, Delgado-Romeu M, Fischer U, Volbers B, Hakim A, Z'Graggen WJ, Nolte CH, Werring DJ, Raposo N, Engelter ST, Kristoffersen ES, Kuramatsu J, Gattringer T, Gaist D, Seiffge DJ. EURECA collaborators. Location and timing of recurrent, nontraumatic intracerebral hemorrhage. JAMA Neurol. 2025;82(4):355–63. https://doi.org/10.1001/jamaneurol.2025.0026.
61. Greenberg SM, Bax F, van Veluw SJ. Amyloid-related imaging abnormalities: manifestations, metrics and mechanisms. Nat Rev Neurol. 2025; https://doi.org/10.1038/s41582-024-01053-8.
62. Kozberg MG, Yi I, Freeze WM, Auger CA, Scherlek AA, Greenberg SM, van Veluw SJ. Blood-brain barrier leakage and perivascular inflammation in cerebral

amyloid angiopathy. Brain Commun. 2022;4:fcac245. https://doi.org/10.1093/braincomms/fcac245.
63. Piazza F, Caminiti SP, Zedde M, Presotto L, DiFrancesco JC, Pascarella R, Giossi A, Sessa M, Poli L, Basso G, Perani D. Association of microglial activation with spontaneous ARIA-E and CSF levels of anti-Aβ autoantibodies. Neurology. 2022;99(12):e1265–77. https://doi.org/10.1212/WNL.0000000000200892.
64. Biffi A, Greenberg SM. Cerebral amyloid angiopathy: a systematic review. J Clin Neurol. 2011;7:1–9.
65. Thal DR, Ghebremedhin E, Orantes M, et al. Vascular pathology in Alzheimer disease: correlation of cerebral amyloid angiopathy and arteriosclerosis/lipohyalinosis with cognitive decline. J Neuropathol Exp Neurol. 2003;62:1287–301.
66. Cogswell PM, Andrews TJ, Barakos JA, Barkhof F, Bash S, Benayoun MD, Chiang GC, Franceschi AM, Jack CR, Pillai JJ, et al. Alzheimer's disease anti-amyloid immunotherapies: imaging recommendations and practice considerations for ARIA monitoring. AJNR Am J Neuroradiol. 2024;46:24–32. https://doi.org/10.3174/ajnr.A8469.
67. Sperling R, Salloway S, Brooks DJ, Tampieri D, Barakos J, Fox NC, Raskind M, Sabbagh M, Honig LS, Porsteinsson AP, et al. Amyloid-related imaging abnormalities in patients with Alzheimer's disease treated with bapineuzumab: a retrospective analysis. Lancet Neurol. 2012;11:241–9. https://doi.org/10.1016/S1474-4422(12)70015-7.
68. Catak C, Zedde M, Malik R, Janowitz D, Soric V, Seegerer A, Krebs A, Düring M, Opherk C, Linn J, et al. Decreased CSF levels of ß-amyloid in patients with cortical superficial Siderosis. Front Neurol. 2019;10:439. https://doi.org/10.3389/fneur.2019.00439.
69. Pollaci G, Potenza A, Gorla G, Carrozzini T, Marinoni G, De Toma C, Canavero I, Rifino N, Boncoraglio GB, Difrancesco JC, Damavandi PT, Stanziano M, Erbetta A, Caroppo P, Di Fede G, Catania M, Zulueta A, Parati EA, Bersano A, Gatti L, Storti B. CSF and plasma biomarkers in patients with iatrogenic cerebral amyloid angiopathy. Neurology. 2024;103(8):e209828. https://doi.org/10.1212/WNL.0000000000209828.
70. Zedde M, Piazza F, Pascarella R. Positron emission tomography in cerebral amyloid angiopathy: a scoping review. Appl Sci. 2025;15:3973. https://doi.org/10.3390/app15073973.
71. Michiels L, Van Weehaeghe D, Vandenberghe R, Demeestere J, Van Laere K, Lemmens R. The role of amyloid PET in diagnosing possible transmissible cerebral amyloid angiopathy in young adults with a history of neurosurgery: a case series. Cerebrovasc Dis. 2021;50(3):356–60. https://doi.org/10.1159/000514139.
72. van Rooden S, van der Grond J, van den Boom R, et al. Descriptive analysis of the Boston criteria applied to a Dutch-type cerebral amyloid angiopathy population. Stroke. 2009;40:3022–7.
73. Collinge J. Molecular neurology of prion disease. J Neurol Neurosurg Psychiatry. 2005;76:906–19.
74. Sandberg MK, Al-Doujaily H, Sharps B, et al. Prion propagation and toxicity in vivo occur in two distinct mechanistic phases. Nat New Biol. 2011;470:540–2.
75. Rother C, Uhlmann RE, Müller SA, et al. Experimental evidence for temporal uncoupling of brain Abeta deposition and neurodegenerative sequelae. Nat Commun. 2022;13:7333.
76. Kane MD, Lipinski WJ, Callahan MJ, et al. Evidence for seeding of beta-amyloid by intracerebral infusion of Alzheimer brain extracts in beta-amyloid precursor protein-transgenic mice. J Neurosci. 2000;20:3606–11.
77. Roberts GW, Gentleman SM, Lynch A, et al. Beta amyloid protein deposition in the brain after severe head injury: implications for the pathogenesis of Alzheimer's disease. J Neurol Neurosurg Psychiatry. 1994;57:419–25. https://doi.org/10.1136/jnnp.57.4.419.
78. Roberts GW, Gentleman SM, Lynch A, et al. Beta A4 amyloid protein deposition in brain after head trauma. Lancet. 1991;338:1422–3. https://doi.org/10.1016/0140-6736(91)92724-G.
79. Ritchie DL, Adlard P, Peden AH, et al. Amyloid-β accumulation in the CNS in human growth hormone recipients in the UK. Acta Neuropathol. 2017;134:221–40. https://doi.org/10.1007/s00401-017-1703-0.
80. Zedde M, Piazza F, Pascarella R. Traumatic brain injury and chronic traumatic encephalopathy: not only trigger for neurodegeneration but also for cerebral amyloid angiopathy? Biomedicine. 2025;13:881. https://doi.org/10.3390/biomedicines13040881.

GPSR Compliance

The European Union's (EU) General Product Safety Regulation (GPSR) is a set of rules that requires consumer products to be safe and our obligations to ensure this.

If you have any concerns about our products, you can contact us on ProductSafety@springernature.com

In case Publisher is established outside the EU, the EU authorized representative is:

Springer Nature Customer Service Center GmbH
Europaplatz 3
69115 Heidelberg, Germany

Batch number: 10731385

Printed by Printforce, the Netherlands